MANUAL FOR PULMONARY AND CRITICAL CARE MEDICINE

T0195125

MANUAL FOR PULMONARY AND CRITICAL CARE MEDICINE

JUDD W. LANDSBERG MD
Professor of Medicine,
University of California San Diego School of Medicine,
Section Chief for Pulmonary and Critical Care Medicine,
Medical Director for Respiratory Therapy,
VA San Diego Healthcare System.

ELSEVIER

ELSEVIER

1600 John F. Kennedy Blvd.
Ste 1800
Philadelphia, PA 19103-2899

MANUAL FOR PULMONARY AND CRITICAL CARE MEDICINE   ISBN: 978-0-323-39952-4

Content Strategist: Robin R Carter
Content Development Specialist: Joan Ryan
Project Manager: Srividhya Vidhyashankar
Design Direction: Ryan Cook

Working together to grow libraries in developing countries

www.elsevier.com • www.bookaid.org

Printed in India

Last digit is the print number: 9 8 7

PREFACE

This book represents teaching materials and illustrative cases that have been compiled and refined over more than a decade, focused on basic topics that are taught poorly, fraught with misunderstanding, and for which no clear management algorithms exist. I wish I had this book when I started my training, and I am glad that I have it now to teach my trainees. My hope is that this book will help you every day in your clinical practice and your teaching.

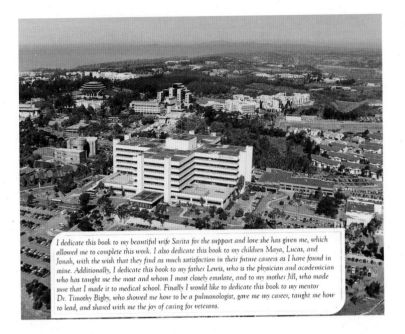

I dedicate this book to my beautiful wife Sarita for the support and love she has given me, which allowed me to complete this work. I also dedicate this book to my children Maya, Lucas, and Jonah, with the wish that they find as much satisfaction in their future careers as I have found in mine. Additionally, I dedicate this book to my father Lewis, who is the physician and academician who has taught me the most and whom I most closely emulate, and to my mother Jill, who made sure that I made it to medical school. Finally I would like to dedicate this book to my mentor Dr. Timothy Bigby, who showed me how to be a pulmonologist, gave me my career, taught me how to lead, and shared with me the joy of caring for veterans.

ACKNOWLEDGMENTS

I want to individually acknowledge and thank **Dr. Philippe Montgrain**, my colleague and specialized content editor, who read every word of this book, on his own time, to ensure that I said what I meant and meant what I said. I also want to thank **Dr. Laura Crotty Alexander** and **Dr. Jess Mandel** for providing me the opportunities that ultimately resulted in this finished book. Finally I would like to thank the veterans who have taught me about service, longevity, and family and pulmonary disease, and who have allowed me to use our experiences together to teach others.

Special thanks go to the teaching attendings who have shaped my thoughts and practice of medicine:

Vincent Andriole, MD
William Auger, MD
Thomas Balcezak, MD
Frank Bia, MD, MPH
Margaret (Peggy) Bia, MD
Timothy Bigby, MD
Antonino Catanzaro, MD
Geoffrey Chupp, MD
David Coleman, MD
Douglas Conrad, MD
Leo Cooney, MD
Thomas Duffy, MD
Jack Elias, MD
Franklin Epstein, MD
Daniel Federman, MD
Peter Fedullo, MD
Joshua Fierer, MD
John Forrest, MD
Mark Fuster, MD
James Harrell, MD
Eric Holmboe, MD
Fred Kantor, MD

Kim Kerr, MD
Samuel Kushlan, MD
Philip LoBue, MD
Jose Loredo, MD, MS, MPH
Richard Matthay, MD
Timothy Morris, MD
Vincent Quagliarello, MD
Asghar Rastegar, MD
Andrew Ries, MD, MPH
William Ring, MD
Lewis Rubin, MD
Frederick Sachs, MD
Kenneth Serio, MD
Mark Siegel, MD
Patricio Silva, MD
Robert Smith, MD
Roger Spragg, MD
Lynn Tanoue, MD
Angela Wang, MD
Aaron Waxman, MD, PhD
Jason Yuan, MD, PhD
Gordon Yung, MD

CONTENTS

APPROACH TO OXYGENATION, HYPOXEMIA, AND HYPOXEMIC RESPIRATORY FAILURE

CHAPTER 1

COMMON MISCONCEPTIONS AND MISTAKES

- Hypoxemia is a significant cause of dyspnea
- A cutaneous O_2 sat $\geq 92\%$ predicts adequate oxygenation and is the appropriate target for O_2 orders
- 100% O_2 suppresses respiratory drive in CO_2 retainers
- O_2 supplementation for patients with COPD is given to improve exercise tolerance
- Confusing failure of oxygen delivery to tissues, hypoxia (the job of the circulatory system) with hypoxemia, and failure to maintain an adequate Pao_2 (the job of the respiratory system)

OXYGENATION

- **Normal oxygenation** (at sea level) predicts:
  - A partial pressure of oxygen (Pao_2) of 75–100 mm Hg with 21% Fio_2 (room air) and a Pao_2 of **~660 mm Hg** with **100% Fio_2**
- **Impaired oxygenation** exists on a spectrum from mild (abnormal A-a gradient) to severe (shunt):
  - $Pao_2 < 200$ mm Hg on Fio_2 of 100% = "shunt physiology"
  - **Without "shunt physiology"** an $Fio_2 > 40\%$ ($\sim > 6$ L/min via nasal cannula (NC)) should give a **$Pao_2 > 60$ mm Hg**, despite pathology causing an abnormally increased A-a gradient
- Patients demonstrating shunt physiology are at high risk for hypoxemic respiratory failure, necessitating a search for the underlying cause, as well as close observation and aggressive support (e.g. chest imaging, 100% FiO_2)
- What defines adequate oxygenation Pao_2, O_2 sat, or *it depends?* Correct answer, Pao_2:
  - Tissue oxygenation is a function of the circulatory system (primarily cardiac output (CO) and hemoglobin (Hb))
    - Systemic hypox**ia**, the result of failed oxygen delivery to tissue (e.g. distributive shock), leads to systemic lactic acidosis
      - Increasing Pao_2 does **not** meaningfully increase oxygen delivery to tissues or decrease lactate
  - The job of the respiratory system is to maintain a Pao_2 **>60 mm Hg**
    - When Pao_2 drops acutely to **<60 mm Hg** (hypox**emia**), organ specific symptomatic hypox**ia** may occur
      - Especially in the **brain, heart,** and **kidney** (high metabolic demand)
  - When treating hypoxemia hypox**emia** target, a **$Pao_2 > 60$ mm Hg**
- **Hypoxemic respiratory failure** is practically **defined as a $Pao_2 < 60$ mm Hg**
- An **acute drop in $Pao_2 < 60$ mm Hg** (but >54 mm Hg), ie, "mild hypoxemia," **may cause** a range of symptoms:
  - **Tachypnea** (hypoxic hyperventilation reflex)

- Designed to increase alveolar O_2 by decreasing alveolar CO_2, thereby increasing work of breathing
- Tachycardia
  - The right ventricle (RV) attempts to maintain CO in the face of rising pulmonary artery pressure (PAP) (hypoxic vasoconstriction) and decreased stroke volume (SV) by increasing heart rate (HR)
- **Mental status changes** (agitation, confusion, and decreased sensorium)
- **Increased left ventricular end-diastolic pressure (LVEDP)** (a.k.a. heart failure) from diastolic dysfunction
  - Hypoxia stiffens the left ventricle (LV) and tachycardia shortens diastole, both impairing ventricular filling
- **Decreased glomerular filtration rate (GFR)** from increased LVEDP (cardio-renal physiology) or hypoxic renal injury

- Additionally, **asymptomatic** patients with an acute drop in PaO_2 (<60 mm Hg) are at increased risk for sudden profound/life-threatening desaturations (steep portion of the hemoglobin–oxygen [Hb–O_2] dissociation curve)

- When patients in hypoxemic respiratory failure achieve a PaO_2 > 60 mm Hg (without hyperventilation) **no** further increase in respiratory support aimed at improving oxygenation is required
  - Efforts then focus on resolution of the underlying cause of hypoxemia
  - A low O_2 saturation, occurring with a PaO_2 > 60 mm Hg, indicates acidosis (causing Hb desaturation), **not** hypoxemic respiratory failure
    - Efforts then focus on resolving the acidosis (eg, renal replacement therapy)

- Symptomatic hypoxemia can be effectively ruled out by demonstrating a PaO_2 > 60 mm Hg
  - And, to a lesser extent, screened for by a cutaneous O_2 saturation (with a good wave form) >94%

- Pulse oximeter readings >92% (but <95%) may mask a PaO_2 < 60 mm Hg because of alkalosis or error (Figs. 1.1 and 1.2)

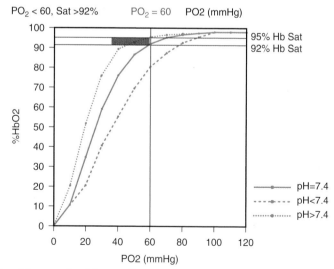

Fig. 1.1 Hemoglobin–oxygen dissociation curve. Shown is the Bohr effect (eg, shift in Hb saturation based on pH) where, for any given PaO_2 value, alkalosis promotes increased saturation and acidosis decreases it. The shaded area in red shows individuals whose cutaneous pulse oximetry readings will be >92% but whose PaO_2 values will be <60 mm Hg (because of alkalemia). Pulse oximetry readings of >94% ensure a PaO_2 > 60 mm Hg over a wide range of pH values, making it a more appropriate target for pulse oximetry orders (aimed at screening for hypoxemia, ie, a PaO_2 < 60 mm Hg)

- Patient admitted for heart failure with a preserved ejection fraction (HFpEF)
- Intubated for increased work of breathing and hypoxemia
- Admit CXR with increased interstitial markings, small effusions
- Despite a ~ 4L negative fluid balance over the first 24 hours the PT suffers ↓ oxygenation
- CXR on HD # 1 shows worsening pulmonary edema:
  - ↑Perihilar ground glass and interstitial edema with worsening effusions (L > R)
- EKG, troponins and a STAT cardiac echo were unchanged from admission
- Blood pressure overnight 150–160/80–85, HR: 60–90 sinus rhythm

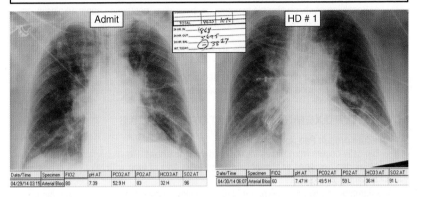

Date/Time	Specimen	FIO2	pH AT	PCO2 AT	PO2 AT	HCO3 AT	SO2 AT
04/29/14 03:15	Arterial Bloo	80	7.39	52.9 H	83	32 H	96

Date/Time	Specimen	FIO2	pH AT	PCO2 AT	PO2 AT	HCO3 AT	SO2 AT
04/30/14 06:07	Arterial Bloo	60	7.47 H	49.5 H	59 L	36 H	91 L

- Inspection of the flow sheet shows the ↓ in FiO_2 to 60% at 4:30 am lead to hypoxemia
- Not recognized until a routine ABG was obtained at 6:00 am
- The hypoxemia was missed because of:
  - Pulse oximeter 3 point error despite a good wave form
    - Cutaneous O_2 sat 94%, calculated O_2 sat 91%
  - Alkalosis shifting the Hb–O_2 dissociation curve

SPO₂	99	98	98	96	95	93	94	100	100%
MODE; VC/PC	AC	AC	AC	AC	AC	AC	AC	AC	AC
Fio2 / PEEP	70 8	70 8	70 8	70 8	70 8	60	60 8	70 8	100 /8
RATE SET / OBSRV	14/14	14/16	14/17	14/14	14/14	14/14	14/14	14/14	14/14
TV SET / OBSRV	550	590	540	580	559	631	560	572	562
INSP PRESS SET / Pip	31	34	31	31	31	33	32	41	35
PH	7.45				7.60		7.47		7.42
PO2/PCO2	90 /49.3						60 /49.9		100 /56.2
PEO2									

Date/Time	Specimen	FIO2	pH AT	PCO2 AT	PO2 AT	HCO3 AT	SO2 AT
04/30/14 06:07	Arterial Bloo	60	7.47 H	49.5 H	59 L	36 H	91 L

- The hypoxemia caused worsening pulmonary edema by provoking diastolic dysfunction
  - Hypoxemia → subendocardial hypoxia → causing LV stiffing → impaired filling
- Leading to ↑ LVEDP and pulmonary edema despite a negative fluid balance
- Note, increased peak inspiratory pressures occurring during the same time frame indicative of pulmonary edema and worsening pulmonary mechanics

Fig. 1.2 Encapsulated case. Worsening pulmonary edema, despite aggressive diuresis because of diastolic dysfunction provoked by hypoxemia during oxygen weaning, targeting a cutaneous O_2 saturation of 92%. Because of error and alkalosis, the patient had PaO_2 values <60 mm Hg, leading to subendocardial hypoxia, left-ventricular (LV) stiffening, impaired filling, and increased left-ventricular end-diastolic pressure (LVEDP) physiology despite a 4 L negative fluid balance.

Teaching point: pulse oximetry readings should be used to screen for hypoxemia (PaO_2 values <60 mm Hg), and thus one should target cutaneous O_2 saturations >94%.

- Hb is designed to bind O_2 tightly (increase O_2 sat) in the alkalotic lungs and unload O_2 (decrease O_2 sat) in acidotic muscle
  - **Alkalemia elevates Hb sat** (steepening the Hb–O_2 dissociation curve, increasing the risk of rapid desaturation)
  - **Acidemia decreases Hb sat** (flattening the Hb–O_2 dissociation curve buffering against rapid desaturation)
- **Alkalosis** occurs commonly in:
  - Hypoxemia (hypoxic hyperventilation reflex)
  - Resolving acute on chronic hypercapnic failure (eg, posthypercapnic alkalosis), as ventilation improves and the previously compensatory metabolic alkalosis becomes the primary disorder
  - Aggressive diuresis (contraction alkalosis)
- **Error** occurs commonly:
  - Secondary to a poor signal (e.g. inadequate wave form)
  - Even with a good waveform, pulse oximetry devices have a ±3 point error range

ACUTE HYPOXEMIC RESPIRATORY FAILURE

- An acute drop in $Pao_2 < 60$ mm Hg
  - Typically occurs from the spectrum of **low VQ to shunt** (Fig. 1.3)
    - Sudden decrease or absent ventilation to an area of lung with relatively preserved perfusion
  - Confusion; tachycardia common; dyspnea (mild or absent) and work of breathing normal or mildly increased, unless the Pao_2 drop is severe (i.e. < 55 mm Hg)
- VQ mismatch (ie, low VQ) will respond to 100% Fio_2 (shunt will not)
  - With normal lungs 100% Fio_2 should lead to a $Pao_2 \approx 660$ mm Hg
  - A $Pao_2 < 200$ mm Hg on 100% Fio_2 implies shunt (physiologic more common than anatomic)
  - The **cause** of **shunt physiology** should be either:
    - Radiographically apparent (eg, diffuse alveolar filling, lung collapse [Fig. 1.4], or bilateral lower lobe atelectasis in the mechanically ventilated obese patient [Fig. 1.5]) or
    - Obvious on physical examination (eg, diffuse wheeze, or no airflow)
  - If the cause of shunt physiology is not obvious consider anatomic shunt (intracardiac or intrapulmonary)

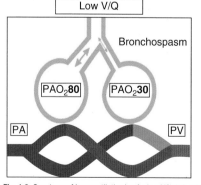 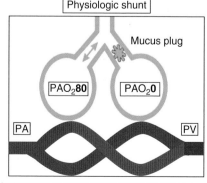

Fig. 1.3 Spectrum of low ventilation/perfusion (VQ) (a.k.a. VQ mismatch) to physiologic shunt. Schematic depicting two lung units (left and right). The left lung unit demonstrates normal aeration ($Pao_2 = 80$ mm Hg), and the right lung unit shows decreased aeration (bronchospasm) leading to low VQ or no ventilation (mucus plug) leading to physiologic shunt. Low VQ and physiologic shunt allow deoxygenated blood to mix with oxygenated blood, the major mechanism of hypoxemia.

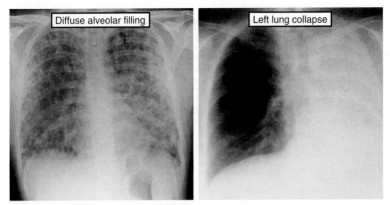

Fig. 1.4 Two frontal views of the chest showing the dramatically abnormal imaging typically associated with shunt physiology and hypoxemic respiratory failure (eg, a $PaO_2 < 60$ mm Hg despite FiO_2 of 100%). Left shows alveolar edema (either cardiogenic or noncardiogenic), and right shows complete lung collapse from endobronchial obstruction. Note the volume loss associated with the opacified hemithorax.

- A-a gradient screens for more subtle derangements in oxygenation, removing the confounding variable of CO_2 displacement in alveoli (as is seen in hypoventilation syndromes)

CHRONIC HYPOXEMIC RESPIRATORY FAILURE (PHYSIOLOGY AND UNDERLYING DISEASE)

- Mild chronic hypoxemic respiratory failure where PaO_2 falls gradually over time (typical PaO_2 values in the 55-59 range)
  - Caused by heterogeneous lung destruction, most commonly seen in chronic obstructive pulmonary disease (COPD)
    - Hypoxemia occurs from VQ mismatch (pink puffers) or hypoventilation (blue bloaters)
  - Causes mild symptoms of cognitive impairment (not exercise limitation), and increases the risk of heart failure
    - In COPD Exercise is limited by ventilation
  - Treat to prevent heart failure, arrhythmia, and risk of sudden death (not to improve exercise tolerance)
- Chronic severe hypoxemic respiratory failure, $PaO_2 < 55$ mm Hg
  - Commonly seen in pulmonary fibrosis
    - Fibrotic thickening of the pulmonary interstitium leads to diffusion limitation
  - Less commonly caused by small vessel pulmonary vascular disease (eg, idiopathic pulmonary arterial hypertension [IPAH])
    - Loss of vascular cross-sectional area from obliteration of small to medium pulmonary arterioles
  - In both cases, exercise limitation and dyspnea may be caused by profound hypoxemia (Fig. 1.6)

CLINICAL APPROACH TO ACUTE HYPOXEMIC RESPIRATORY FAILURE

- Goal of O_2 support is a $PaO_2 > 60$ mm Hg **without** hyperventilation
  - Target an O_2 sat >94% or get an ABG to ensure $PaO_2 > 60$ mm Hg
  - Impending hypoxemic respiratory failure (ie, hypoxemia despite supplemental O_2 at ≥ 6 L/min) should be given 100% FiO_2
    - O_2 can be titrated down when a $PaO_2 > 60$ mm Hg is demonstrated, do not worry about O_2 causing CO_2 retention in patients with impending hypoxemic respiratory failure

```
Pulm Crit Resident H&P
CC: Hypoxic respiratory failure s/p sacral tumor resection
HPI:
53M with h/o CAD s/p 3v CABG (2012), HFrEF (EF 49%), OSA on CPAP, and morbid obesity,
here s/p sacral tumor resection , still intubated and noted to be hypoxic on 100% FiO2.
On admission to the ICU, his ABG was 7.33 / 44 / 71 / 26 (on 100% FiO2 and 5 PEEP).
```

1) Initial PaO_2 393 mm Hg (100% FiO_2, PEEP of 5 cm H_2O)
2) PaO_2 drops to < 90 mm Hg during the surgery
3) Hypoxemia and shunt physiology persist on postoperative day # 1
4) Postoperative CXR shows only LLL atelectasis (**NOT** clearly explaining shunt physiology)

| Wt (lbs): | 302.5 |
| BMI | 38.92 |

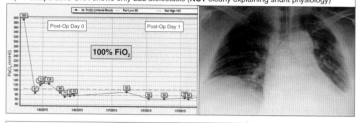

5) CT angiography negative for PE, reveals bilateral lower lobe atelectasis instead (subtle on CXR)

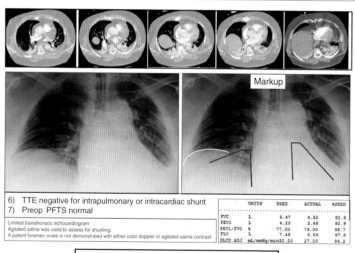

Markup

6) TTE negative for intrapulmonary or intracardiac shunt
7) Preop PFTS normal

Limited transthoracic echocardiogram
Agitated saline was used to assess for shunting.
A patent foramen ovale is not demonstrated with either color doppler or agitated saline contrast.

	UNITS	PRED	ACTUAL	%PRED
FVC	L	5.47	4.52	82.6
FEV1	L	4.20	3.48	82.9
FEV1/FVC	%	77.00	76.00	98.7
TLC	L	7.48	6.53	87.3
DLCO ADJ	mL/mmHg/min	32.20	27.10	84.2

Pre-discharge CXR and ABG (POD # 14) shows
resolution of lower lobe atelectasis and shunt physiology

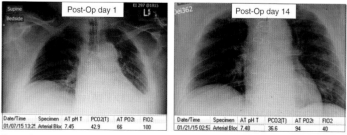

Date/Time	Specimen	AT pH T	PCO2(T)	AT PO2	FIO2
01/07/15 13:2	Arterial Bloc	7.45	42.9	66	100

Date/Time	Specimen	AT pH T	PCO2(T)	AT PO2	FIO2
01/21/15 02:5	Arterial Bloc	7.48	36.6	94	40

Fig. 1.5 Encapsulated case. Intraoperative and postoperative shunt physiology occurring in a morbidly obese individual undergoing general anesthesia and mechanical ventilation for an uncomplicated nonthoracic procedure. The patient had no underlying lung disease, evidence of anatomic shunt, or obvious radiographic explanation (by portable chest x-ray) for his profound hypoxemia, despite an FiO_2 of 100%. A computed tomography scan showed near complete bilateral lower

See the opposite page

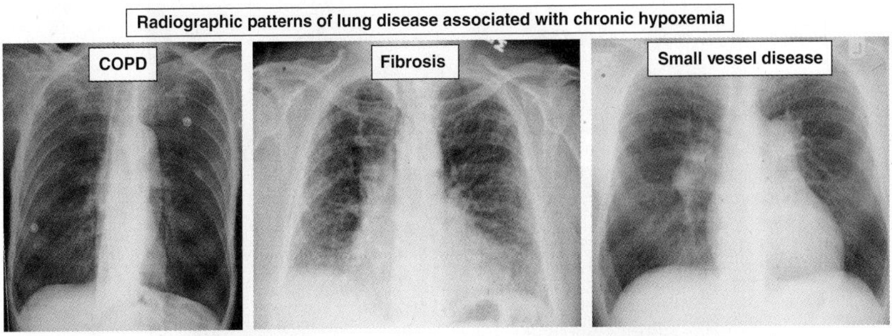

Radiographic patterns of lung disease associated with chronic hypoxemia

| COPD | Fibrosis | Small vessel disease |

Fig. 1.6 Common radiographic patterns for patients with chronic hypoxemic respiratory failure. In chronic obstructive pulmonary disease (COPD) and idiopathic pulmonary arterial hypertension (a.k.a. small vessel disease) the hypoxemia is caused by a loss of pulmonary arterial vascular cross sectional area. In pulmonary fibrosis, the hypoxemia is caused by diffusion limitation, secondary to a thickened pulmonary capillary interstitium.

- Deliver O_2 via high-flow system or reservoir device
  - Achieve ~100% FiO_2 by preventing entrainment of surrounding room air (when minute ventilation is high)
- A $PaO_2 < 60$ mm Hg on a 100% FiO_2 is life-threatening and mandates mechanical ventilation
  - Noninvasive (eg, Bi-level positive airway pressure [BiPAP]) or invasive (endotracheal intubation)
- Mechanical ventilation is used to increase mean airway pressure and recruit atelectatic lung (not primarily to ventilate)

CO_2 RETENTION AND HIGH FiO_2

- Patients with severe parenchymal disease and chronic CO_2 retention (ie, blue bloaters) *occasionally* increase their PcO_2 (~6 mm Hg) when given a high FiO_2
  - **Not** primarily by suppression of respiratory **drive**
    - Will not lead to progressive central hypercapnic respiratory failure
  - But rather by release of hypoxic vasoconstriction and subsequent steal phenomenon
    - Leading to an increase in dead space fraction
  - Ventilated units are suddenly underperfused as blood is "stolen" to poorly ventilated units (effectively increasing dead space) (Fig. 1.7)
- Average PcO_2 increase is ~6 mm Hg and is of little clinical significance (unlike hypoxemic respiratory arrest, which occurs when oxygen is withheld)
  - Anecdotally, **very rarely** a high FiO_2 and PaO_2 *may* suppress respiratory drive (**but this is *not* proven**) and should not dictate routine management

Fig. 1.5, cont'd lobe atelectasis (subtle on chest x-ray). His hypoxemia improved with spontaneous breathing, and his shunt physiology ultimately resolved with extubation and resolution of his lower lobe atelectasis.

Teaching point: obese patients are vulnerable to shunt physiology from lower lobe atelectasis occurring when they receive general anesthesia and mechanical ventilation, likely from the collapsing forces of their abdominal and thoracic adipose tissue, no longer opposed by abdominal musculature (because of sedation). High positive end-expiratory pressure (PEEP) (possibly guided by esophageal manometry) and awake spontaneous breathing trials can often improve lower lobe aeration and oxygenation. It is likely that the shunt physiology in this case (and ones like it) is made worse by overdistention of lung apices (more complaint lung units). This overdistension decreases apical blood flow. The combination leads to extremely low ventilation/perfusion (VQ) physiology, where the lung apices receive most of the ventilation and the bases receive all of the blood flow.

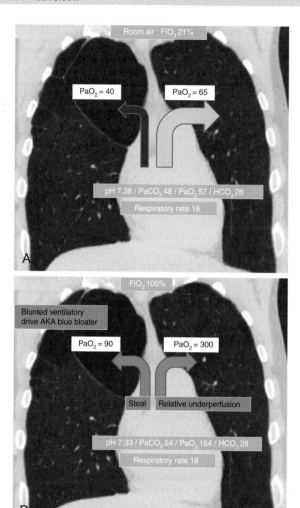

Fig. 1.7 Graphic depiction of the likely mechanism explaining acute CO$_2$ retention occurring in response to an increased Fio$_2$ in a patient with chronic obstructive pulmonary disease (COPD) and chronic CO$_2$ retention. (A)The heterogeneous ventilation and perfusion relationships between a diseased lung and a relatively normal lung in a patient with COPD while breathing room air. The profound hypoxemia in the bullae leads to a low Pao$_2$ in the pulmonary artery supplying the area. This causes hypoxic vasoconstriction, which attempts to improve ventilation/perfusion (VQ) matching in the lung by decreasing perfusion to the area of decreased ventilation and oxygenation (graphically depicted by the smaller darker blue arrow). (B) The same individual while breathing 100% Fio$_2$. Note, the oxygen level in the poorly ventilated bullae rises enough to increase the Pao$_2$ such that hypoxic vasoconstriction is released. This inappropriately "steals" blood from the normal lung to the diseased lung, effectively increasing dead space, as the increased blood flow to the right apex is **not** accompanied by increased ventilation. Because of this, the individual must either increase their minute ventilation (and work of breathing) or allow their Pco$_2$ to rise (and their pH to fall). Individuals with chronic CO$_2$ retention, **by definition**, have a blunted ventilatory drive, such that the increased dead space causes an increase in Pco$_2$ and concomitant fall in pH, leading to an acute, uncompensated, respiratory acidosis that is nearly uniformly asymptomatic and of no clinical significance.

COMMON CAUSES AND INITIAL TREATMENT OF ACUTE HYPOXEMIC RESPIRATORY FAILURE

- Pneumonia (PNA)
  - VQ mismatch from alveolar filling, mucus plugging, and atelectasis
  - Rx with O_2, antibiotics, and pulmonary toilet (chest physiotherapy)
  - If supplemental O_2 fails, BiPAP may be difficult with copious secretions; often have to intubate

- Cardiogenic pulmonary edema
  - VQ mismatch from alveolar and interstitial edema, and effusions with compressive atelectasis
  - Common cause of shunt physiology
  - Rx with O_2, IV loop diuretics at adequate dose (eg, $\geq$ 80 IV Lasix, 2 IV Bumex)
  - BiPAP works great (rarely have to intubate)

- Noncardiogenic pulmonary edema (a.k.a. acute respiratory distress syndrome [ARDS])
  - VQ mismatch from diffuse alveolar filling (not believed to be secondary to HF)
  - Common cause of shunt physiology
  - Can be primary pulmonary inflammation vs. systemic infection or inflammation
  - Treat underlying cause, support and time, consider steroids, and avoid HF
  - Typically requires intubation (slow to resolve)
  - Common DDx (bronchoscopy useful):
    - Eosinophilic pulmonary inflammation (spectrum of acute to chronic eosinophilic PNA)
      - Bronchoscopy with significant bronchoalveolar lavage (BAL) eosinophilia (> then 25%, often 40–80%)
      - Responds well to steroids
    - Diffuse alveolar hemorrhage
      - Bronchoscopy with progressively bloody lavage
      - Search for underlying disease (eg, anti-glomerular basement membrane disease)
      - Treat provocative factors (eg, thrombocytopenia, PNA)
      - Consider steroids
    - Acute interstitial pneumonitis
      - Bronchoscopy shows a BAL with neutrophil predominance
      - Consider trial of high-dose steroids

- Bronchospasm
  - VQ mismatch from poorly ventilated lung
  - Rx with O_2, steroids, and β-agonists
  - Rarely requires intervention beyond supplemental O_2 **for hypoxemia**

- Large volume gastric aspiration
  - VQ mismatch from alveolar filling (initially pneumonitis)
  - Treat with O_2, often requires intubation, consider Abx; limited role for acute bronchoscopy
    - Urgent BAL does not mitigate the instantaneous injury of aspirated digestive contents
      - Should be reserved for segmental collapse and large particle removal

- Pulmonary embolism
  - VQ mismatch from atelectasis secondary to inflammatory mediator release (not increased dead space)
  - Rarely requires intervention beyond supplemental O_2 for hypoxemia

- Hypoventilation
  - Hypoxemia from CO_2 accumulation and displacement of O_2 from the alveoli
  - Seen commonly with blunted ventilatory drive (eg, obesity or narcotic effect)
  - Hypoxemia is easily reversed with supplemental oxygen

COMMON QUESTIONS GENERATED BY THIS TEACHING

1. **How should I write my oxygen orders?**
   Titrate oxygen to sat >94%, or Pao_2 > 60 mm Hg

2. **Do I have to get an ABG?**
   If you are unable to obtain an O_2 sat >94% on $\geq$6 L O_2 then obtain an ABG to ensure your Pao_2 is >60 mm Hg

3. **When should I use a 100% FiO_2 empirically, before a blood gas is obtained?**
   In any patient whose cutaneous Patients with an O_2 sat <94% on $\geq$6 L O_2

4. **I once had a patient who stopped breathing when I gave them 100% oxygen – question implied by tone…**
   The most common scenario where this misinterpretation occurs is the following: An obese patent (with baseline blunted ventilatory drive) has a procedure requiring conscious sedation. During recovery he is noted by nursing to be "sleeping comfortably … sleeping comfortably … sudden O_2 desaturation, patient unarousable, placed on 100% FM", ABG shows pH 7.27/Pco_2 57/Pao_2 360, and oxygen is blamed for the arrest. In actuality the patient was hypoventilating while sleeping, unarousable from CO_2 narcosis, which is finally detected as a desaturation (CO_2 displacing O_2 in the alveoli). The hypoxemia is easily reversed, but the patient completes his hypercapnic arrest – unrelated to the oxygen administration.

5. **Shouldn't I target O_2 sats 88–92% in my hospitalized patients with severe COPD?**
   No. Oxygen does not significantly inhibit respiratory drive. More importantly, in the setting of acute illness, hypoxemia (PaO_2 <60 mm Hg) will complicate and worsen any disease presentation. In contrast, a lower than normal O_2 sat (88–92%) is tolerated in outpatients with severe chronic lung disease, pragmatically because it is not feasible to deliver oxygen at more than 6 L/min in the home setting. Therefore, when hospitalized, patients with chronic lung disease should have the same oxygenation goal as everybody else.

VENTILATION AND HYPERCAPNIC RESPIRATORY FAILURE

CHAPTER 2

COMMON MISCONCEPTIONS AND MISTAKES

- 100% O_2 sat is reassuring with regard to impending respiratory failure in a tachypneic, dyspneic patient

- Hypercapnic respiratory failure is ruled out by $Pco_2 < 45$ mm Hg

- Chronic CO_2 retention in chronic obstructive pulmonary disease (COPD) is caused by the **severity** of the obstructive defect

- Ventilation is driven by Pco_2 alone

- Thinking about (and reporting) pH as either normal or abnormal when in actuality it is always acidemic, pH <7.40, or alkalemic pH ≥7.40

- Diagnosing (or worse, treating) a primary anxiety disorder in a tachypneic patient **without** an arterial blood gas (ABG) measurement

NORMAL VENTILATION

- The role of ventilation is to remove dissolved CO_2 (the ultimate metabolic waste product of all metabolism) from the blood
    - Dissolved CO_2 acidifies blood, threatening to decrease pH (a big problem)
        - pH is one of the mostly tightly regulated parameters in humans
            - The "cost–benefit" ratio of evolution has selected for enzymes that function extremely efficiently (benefit) but do so over a tiny range of pH (cost)

- The minute-to-minute regulation of blood pH is controlled by, the medullary respiratory center, in the brainstem
    - Under normal physiologic conditions, the respiratory center aggressively targets $Pco_2 \approx 40$ mm Hg (normal range 35–45 mm Hg), yielding a pH of ≈7.4 (normal range 7.35–7.45)
    - To maintain tight control over CO_2 and pH, minute ventilation (MV), defined as tidal volume x respiratory rate, varies widely throughout the day (between 5 and 10 L/min) based on metabolic activity (mainly body temperature and the degree of skeletal muscle activity)
        - As temperature increases (ie, fever), or more muscle groups are activated (ie, physical activity), more glucose is metabolized to CO_2, which threatens to increase Pco_2 above 40 mm Hg
        - This triggers the respiratory center to increase MV
            - This is achieved by effortlessly increasing tidal volume and rate (ie, not noticed by the individual)

- When pH is in the normal range, **normal**, MV varies, targeting $Pco_2 \approx 40$ mm Hg

- When pH is abnormal, MV varies targeting the normal pH range

COMPENSATORY VENTILATORY RESPONSES TO ACIDEMIA AND ALKALEMIA (A.K.A. ABG INTERPRETATION)

- **Protecting** a normal **pH** is **more important** physiologically **than protecting a normal** Pco_2 (ie, **pH trumps** Pco_2) with regard to control of ventilation
- **Metabolic acidosis increases ventilation**, decreasing Pco_2, increasing pH toward, but never >7.35
- **Metabolic alkalosis inhibits ventilation**, increasing Pco_2, decreasing pH toward, but never <7.45
- When a metabolic process occurs that either lowers pH (eg, lactic acidosis) or raises pH (eg, contraction alkalosis) MV either increases (acidosis) or decreases (alkalosis) in an attempt to compensate, without overcompensating
  - No overcompensation means the pH defines the primary disorder
    - If the pH is ≥7.40 the primary disorder is the one producing the alkalemia
    - If the pH is <7.40 the primary disorder is the one producing the acidemia
  - Pco_2 determines whether or not respiratory compensation is appropriate
  - Appropriate compensation suggests a single acid–base disorder
  - Inappropriate compensation implies a mixed acid–base disorder
- Checking for appropriate respiratory compensation **without** math, equations, or the "nomogram"
  - Ensuring that respiratory compensation is appropriate for the degree of metabolic acidosis is crucial, since inappropriate compensation may signal impending respiratory failure
    - The last two digits of the pH **are** the predicted Pco_2 (spectacularly convenient), observe:
      - Appropriate compensation for metabolic acidosis with a pH of 7.32 is $Pco_2 \approx 32$ mm Hg (± 1–2 mm Hg)
      - Appropriate compensation for metabolic acidosis with a pH of 7.27 is $Pco_2 \approx 27$ mm Hg (± 1–2 mm Hg)
        - Note that this rule begins to fall apart when pH is <7.20 because the maximum ventilation a normal person can achieve is $Pco_2 \approx 20$–25 mm Hg (even though some young individuals with diabetic ketoacidosis [DKA] can do much better, ie, $Pco_2 < 10$ mm Hg)
      - The appropriate respiratory compensation for a pH of 7.16 should be "maximum ventilation," which should generate a Pco_2 in the low 20s mm Hg (not necessarily 16 mm Hg as the rule implies)
    - Example: metabolic acidosis with a serum HCO_3 of 18 mEq/L will give a pH of 7.35 and a Pco_2 of 35 mm Hg
      - Because the pH is <7.40 we know the primary disorder is an acidosis; Because the $Pco_2 < 40$ mm Hg we know that the acidosis is metabolic
      - Since a pH of 7.35 should drive the Pco_2 down to 35 mm Hg, compensation is appropriate, which means there is a single acid–base disorder present
      - Overcompensation **(which does not occur)** would suggest that an HCO_3 of 18 mEq/L could give you a pH of 7.41 and a Pco_2 of 30 mm Hg
        - Instead, this ABG represents a primary respiratory alkalosis, obvious by the fact that the pH is >7.40 (alkalosis) and the Pco_2 is <35 mm Hg (low)
  - Ensuring that respiratory compensation is appropriate for the degree of metabolic alkalosis is also crucial, since inappropriate compensation may signal superimposed hypercapnic respiratory failure
    - The last two digits of the pH **are** still the predicted Pco_2 (with more variability [± 5 mm Hg])

- Often more helpful is the fact that a metabolic alkalosis with compensatory respiratory hypoventialtion will never yield a pH < 7.45 (overcompensation dos not occur):
  - A pH <7.45 in a patient with metabolic alkalosis **always** implies a superimposed respiratory acidosis (lowering the pH to the normal range)
- Example: A metabolic alkalosis with a serum HCO_3 of 38 mEq/L will give a pH of 7.49 and cause compensatory hypoventilation (ie, decreased MV) giving a PCO_2 of ≈49 mm Hg
  - Because the pH is >7.40, a primary alkalosis has occurred; Because the $PCO_2 > 40$ mm Hg we know the alkalosis is metabolic
  - Since a pH of 7.49 should cause the PCO_2 to rise to 49 mm Hg, compensation is appropriate, which means there is a single acid–base disorder present
  - Overcompensation **(which does not occur)** would suggest that an HCO_3 of 38 mEq/L could give a pH of 7.42 and a PCO_2 of 55 mm Hg
    - Instead, this ABG represents primary metabolic alkalosis (pH >7.40) with a superimposed respiratory acidosis
      - Because a metabolic alkalosis should give a pH >7.45, the PCO_2 must be higher than expected which implies additional hypoventilation = , or hypercapnic respiratory failure (often central, from CO_2 narcosis)

- Relevant mixed acid–base disorders (a.k.a. **never** missing a "hidden" acidosis):
  - The most important thing **not to miss** in a mixed acid–base disorder is a "**hidden**" **acidosis**, either:
    - Metabolic acidosis:
      - A PCO_2 <35 mm Hg occurring with a normal pH reveals a hidden metabolic acidosis
      - As occurs when there is a superimposed respiratory alkalosis (eg, pH 7.38, PCO_2 29 mm Hg)
      - No equations or math required to spot the metabolic acidosis
      - pH is <7.40, so the primary disorder is an acidosis; $PCO_2 < 40$ mm Hg, so it is **not** a respiratory acidosis (lactate was elevated)
        - Furthermore a $PCO_2 > 35$ mm Hg should yield a pH > 7.45
    - Respiratory acidosis:
      - A $PCO_2 > 45$ mm Hg occurring with a normal pH reveals a hidden acute respiratory acidosis
      - As occurs when there is a superimposed metabolic alkalosis (eg, pH 7.42, PCO_2 55 mm Hg)
      - No equations or math required to spot the respiratory acidosis
      - pH is >7.40, so the primary disorder is an alkalosis; $PCO_2 > 40$ mm Hg, so there **is** an additional respiratory acidosis
        - The question is, "Is the respiratory acidosis an appropriate compensation for the metabolic alkalosis, or does it represent superimposed hypoventilation?"
        - The answer is, "A compensatory respiratory acidosis **never** gives a pH <7.45; therefore hypoventilation is present" (the patient was lethargic and required intubation for hypercapnic failure)
  - "Failing to compensate" for a metabolic acidosis = implies hypercapnic failure, often occurring with a normal (or occasionally low) PCO_2 (important not to miss)
    - For a patient without chronic CO_2 retention "failing to compensate" = is detected by a PCO_2 that is higher than anticipated:
      - Example: DKA patient has an ABG showing a pH of 7.19 and a PCO_2 of 33 mm Hg
        - Even though the **PCO_2 is low** (with regard to the normal range), it represents **significant hypoventilation** (expected $PCO_2 < 25$ mm Hg)
        - If this patient demonstrates increased work of breathing (WOB), intubation should be considered for impending hypercapnic respiratory failure

- If the patient does not demonstrate increased WOB it implies the patient has blunted ventilation (ie, a central component to their hypoventilation), as seen in narcotic use, obesity, and CO_2-retaining COPD patients
  - This is a more stable situation than the individual with the same ABG who demonstrates an increased WOB, because it is less likely to progress to respiratory failure
- Individuals with chronic CO_2 retention tend to not fully compensate for their metabolic acidemia
  - The decision to support them should be made on clinical grounds or when their pH is <7.35

- Evaluation of tachypnea and increased WOB
  - Patients with an intact respiratory drive suffering impending respiratory failure experience extreme anxiety
    - The anxiety is **not** the primary problem; the respiratory failure is
    - Treating the anxiety of respiratory failure with "anxiolytics" precipitates respiratory arrest
      - This should **only** be done in patients in whom comfort is the primary goal
  - It is **not** possible to determine whether an anxious tachypneic patient is in respiratory failure or suffering a panic attack **without** an ABG
    - Alkalemia = anxiety
    - Acedemia = threatened or actual respiratory failure

- Obtain an arterial blood gas to check pH, P_{CO_2}, and PaO_2 (Fig. 2.1)
  - Even if the pH is in the "normal range" decide if it is acidemic (ie, pH <7.40) or alkalemic (ie, pH ≥7.40)
  - Then decide if the P_{CO_2} is high (ie, >45 mm Hg) or low (ie, <35 mm Hg)
    - Patients with visibly increased WOB and tachypnea rarely have a normal P_{CO_2}
  - Acidemic patients with a high P_{CO_2} have acute hypercapnic respiratory failure
  - Acidemic patients with a low P_{CO_2} are attempting to, or adequately compensating for their acidosis ($\pm$ additional hyperventilation component)
  - Alkalemic patients with a high P_{CO_2} (and tachypnea) have chronic hypercapnic respiratory failure with superimposed acute respiratory alkalosis (driven by either hypoxemia or anxiety/pain)
  - Alkalemic patients with a low P_{CO_2} have acute respiratory alkalosis (driven by either hypoxemia or anxiety/pain)

ACUTE HYPERCAPNIC RESPIRATORY FAILURE

- **Acute hypercapnic** respiratory **failure** (ie, inadequate CO_2 removal) is the **most common cause** of **respiratory arrest** because ventilation takes work (unlike oxygenation)
  - Increased MV demands (as in acidosis), or normal MV demands with increased airway resistance (as in an asthma exacerbation), or decreased compliance (as in pulmonary edema) ultimately lead to diaphragmatic fatigue and acute hypercapnia

- Acute hypercapnic failure can be defined as a **pH <7.35** and **P_{CO_2} > 45 mm Hg**

- **Acute on chronic hypercapnic failure** (individuals with baseline CO_2 retention) can be defined as a **pH <7.35** and **P_{CO_2} elevated above baseline**

- Physiologic effects of acute hypercapnia:
  - CO_2 narcosis:
    - A sudden rise in P_{CO_2} ~ 5–15 mm Hg above baseline causes somnolence progressing to obtundation
    - Gradually P_{CO_2} may rise to the limit of human tolerance 90–120 mm Hg, before CO_2 narcosis occurs

EVALUATION OF TACHYPNEA

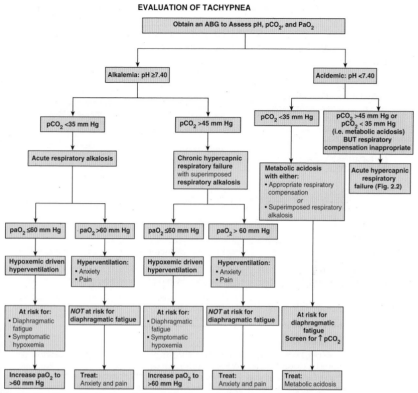

Fig. 2.1 Flow diagram showing the evaluation and management of tachypnea, which hinges on pH and P_{CO_2} assessment. Individuals with an increased respiratory rate are hyperventilating; compensating for metabolic acidosis, which they may not be able to continue indefinitely (ie, at risk for diaphragmatic fatigue); or in hypercapnic respiratory failure. Individuals who are hyperventilating do not need, and should not be given, positive pressure ventilatory support. Instead they should have their Pa_{O_2} checked to rule out hypoxemia-mediated hyperventilation (treated with oxygen). Nonhypoxemic hyperventilating patients should not be given support because this may worsen their respiratory alkalosis. A significant alkalosis (ie, pH >7.60) can be life-threatening, shifting K+ into cells and causing arrhythmia. They also do not need support because individuals with a primary hyperventilation syndrome (defined as a pH >7.4, P_{CO_2} < 35 mm Hg, and Pa_{O_2} > 60 mm Hg), as seen with pain and anxiety, will **not** suffer diaphragmatic fatigue (instead they will pause respirations and/or slow their breathing). Individuals who are appropriately compensating for metabolic acidosis should be screened for failure (ie, rising P_{CO_2}) rather than routinely supported. Nonfatigued, spontaneously breathing individuals will be able to produce a much higher minute ventilation than they would with a non-invasive positive pressure ventilation (NIPPV) mask or an ET tube and a mechanical ventilator. Tachypneic patients with acute hypercapnic respiratory failure require ventilatory support.

- Acidosis (important thresholds):
  - With a pH <7.35, individuals are at risk for dramatic dyspnea and increased WOB
    - Otherwise there is a central component to respiratory failure (blunted ventilatory drive)
  - With a **pH <7.25**, individuals are at risk for **hypotension, tachyarrhythmia** (atrial more common than ventricular)
  - With a pH <7.15, individuals are at risk for pulseless electrical activity (PEA) arrest
- Evaluation and initial management of acute hypercapnic respiratory failure (Fig. 2.2)
  - Individuals with **acute hypercapnic failure** suffering **diaphragmatic fatigue** (increased WOB with a pH <7.35 and P_{CO_2} > 45 mm Hg) or CO_2 narcosis require **ventilatory support**:
    - Patients with an intact mental status deserve a trial of NIPPV
    - Obtunded patients require emergent intubation and mechanical ventilation

EVALUATION AND INITIAL MANAGEMENT OF ACUTE HYPERCAPNIC RESPIRATORY FAILURE

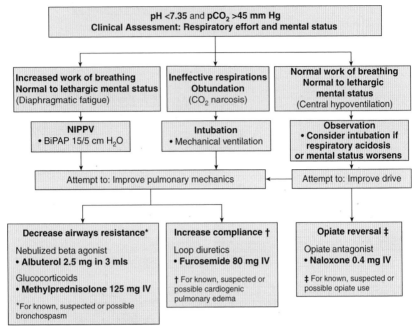

Fig. 2.2 Flow diagram showing the evaluation and management of acute hypercapnic respiratory failure, which hinges on the clinical evaluation of the patient. There are only three ways a human can experience a pH <7.35 and P_{CO_2} > 45 mm Hg: (1) with extreme dyspnea and increased work of breathing (WOB), (2) obtunded with ineffective respiration, or (3) completely comfortable and asymptomatic. Acute hypercapnic respiratory failure is often precipitated by a sudden change in pulmonary mechanics such that an attempt to improve mechanics should be made simultaneously with an attempt to support the patient's ventilation. Patients in respiratory distress with a history of obstructive lung disease or obvious wheezing should be given nebulized β-agonists. New onset wheezing in an inpatient should be presumed to represent cardiogenic (submucosal) edema until proven otherwise. Because **all** patients in respiratory distress are prone to superimposed diastolic dysfunction (via tachycardia and hypoxemia), hemodynamically stable (or hypertensive) patients with impending respiratory failure from diaphragmatic fatigue should be given a trial of empiric diuresis. This is safe and often provides dramatic improvement/resolution for the acute respiratory failure (even in individuals without a known history of heart failure [HF]). Individuals with central hypoventilation as the cause for their acute hypercapnic respiratory failure are more stable than individuals suffering from diaphragmatic fatigue, and are less likely to benefit from non-invasive positive pressure ventilation (NIPPV) (because their drive is the issue). Individuals with a blunted ventilatory drive (as seen in obesity or narcotic use) tend to further hypoventilate in the face of worsening pulmonary mechanics, rather than complain of dyspnea and increase their WOB. Therefore, improving pulmonary mechanics by increasing compliance (ie, diuresis) or decreasing airway resistance (ie, bronchodilators) often leads to improved ventilation.

- Individuals with central hypoventilation (ie, no increased WOB, no dyspnea) and an intact mental status may be closely observed
  - Ventilatory assistance does little (or nothing) to increase ventilation in those whose respiratory drive is decreased
    - Acute central hypoventilation, not secondary to sedative administration (ie, obesity related), is often triggered by worsening pulmonary mechanics (ie, decreased compliance from cardiogenic pulmonary edema)
      - Improving mechanics (ie, increasing compliance back to normal with diuresis) improves ventilation
  - Patients with central hypoventilation and obtundation require intubation and mechanical ventilation

OVERVIEW COMMON CAUSES OF ACUTE OF HYPERCAPNIC RESPIRATORY FAILURE RESULTING IN DIAPHRAGMATIC FATIGUE

- Exacerbation of obstructive lung disease (COPD and asthma)
  - Increased airways resistance from infection and inflammation, lead to an increased WOB
  - Inability to maintain the increased WOB leads to diaphragmatic fatigue
    - Pco_2 climbs and pH falls (to <7.35)
  - Support with NIPPV
  - Treat bronchospasm with nebulized short-acting β-agonist
  - Treat inflammation with IV glucocorticoids

- Exacerbation of left heart failure (LHF)
  - Seen commonly with HFpEF secondary to volume overload and diastolic dysfunction
  - Causes decreased compliance (interstitial edema and pleural effusion), leading to an increased WOB
  - Inability to maintain the increased WOB leads to diaphragmatic fatigue
    - Pco_2 climbs and pH falls (to <7.35)
  - Support with NIPPV
  - Treat with high-dose IV loop diuretic

- Overwhelming metabolic acidosis (lactate, ketones, organic acids, and ingestions)
  - Causes increased MV demand in an attempt to decrease Pco_2 to compensate for the metabolic acidosis
  - Leads to increased WOB
  - Inability to maintain the increased WOB leads to diaphragmatic fatigue
    - Pco_2 climbs and pH falls (to <7.35)
  - Patients are typically **extremely dyspneic** with an obvious **increased ventilatory effort** (a.k.a. Kussmaul respirations)
  - Individuals who are **appropriately compensating** for their metabolic acidosis should **not** have their ventilation routinely assisted
    - Individuals without lung disease can achieve a much higher MV (ie, 30–40 L/min) than is possible with support devices (ie, 20–25 L/min)
  - Intubation comes with a **significant risk of PEA arrest** from symptomatic acidosis
    - An acidotic individual who is breathing 30–40 L/min is vulnerable to a life-threatening drop in pH when ventilation is interrupted during rapid sequence intubation
      - This should be avoided by:
        - Preintubation HCO_3 administration
        - Rapid intubation
        - Initial ventilator settings aimed at maximizing MV (while avoiding volutrauma)
  - Occurs in either anion **gap (**lactate, ketones) or **mixed gap/nongap acidosis** (organic acids)
    - Anion gap acidosis:
      - Lactic acidosis (treatment of underlying cause and respiratory support):
        - Treat shock (if present) and support ventilation with NIPPV if tolerated by mental status
        - In the absence of shock, look for bowel or limb ischemia
          - In the absence of shock and regional ischemia, consider type B lactic acidosis and d/c potential offending medications (eg, metformin)
        - Support hypercapnic failure (failure to appropriately compensate) initially with NIPPV (especially if acidosis likely to resolve quickly, ie, BP improved)
      - Ketoacidosis (DKA or alcoholic ketoacidosis [AKA])
        - Treat DKA with IV insulin
        - Treat AKA with IV dextrose
        - Rarely have to assist ventilation (unless concomitant lung disease exists)

- Uncleared organic acids (ie, renal failure)
  - Consider HCO_3 and renal replacement therapy
  - Respiratory failure in this situation is typically from volume overload (not acidosis)
- Nongap acidosis
  - Commonly seen in renal failure or diarrhea (HCO_3 deficit)
  - Consider HCO_3 supplementation and renal replacement therapy
    - Patients without lung disease rarely need respiratory support
    - Patients with underlying lung disease may need NIPPV

ACUTE HYPERCARBIC RESPIRATORY FAILURE FROM CENTRAL HYPOVENTILATION

- Suppressed respiratory drive leads to hypoventilation, leading to hypercapnia

- Individuals with blunted respiratory drive (ie, obesity, narcotic use) may hypoventilate in response to worsening pulmonary mechanics (see Chapter 8)

- Patients with central hypoventilation:
  - Do not complain of dyspnea
  - Have a normal respiratory effort and WOB despite acidemia and an elevated P_{CO_2}
  - Have a lethargic-to-obtunded mental status

- Hypercapnia is often detected as oxygen desaturation in the "sleeping" inpatient
  - Occurs when hypoventilation leads to excessive CO_2 accumulation in the alveoli, thereby displacing O_2

- HFpEF and pulmonary edema commonly complicate hypoventilation
  - Hypoxemia and tachycardia impair left ventricle (LV) filling, leading to left ventricular end-diastolic pressure (LVEDP) elevations

- Differential diagnosis of central hypoventilation syndromes
  - Oversedation
    - Narcotics (ie, opiate receptor agonists)
      - Treat with naloxone
    - GABAergic drugs (benzodiazepines, muscle relaxants)
      - Support patient during drug metabolism and excretion
    - Atypical antipsychotics and gabapentin (often in the setting of renal failure and toxic accumulation)
      - Support patient during drug metabolism and excretion
  - Encephalopathy
    - Hepatic encephalopathy
      - Treat with lactulose
    - Postictal state (transient)
      - Rarely requires support beyond oxygen (unless status epilepticus occurs)
  - CNS catastrophe (eg, brainstem or meningitis)
    - Head CT, consider LP

ACUTE ON CHRONIC HYPERCAPNIC RESPIRATORY FAILURE AND MIXED ACUTE HYPERCAPNIC FAILURE

- Acute on chronic hypercapnic respiratory failure
  - Patients with chronic hypercapnic respiratory failure are extremely vulnerable to superimposed acute hypercapnic respiratory failure because they have no reserve (already have a baseline increase in their WOB or P_{CO_2})
    - Example:
      - An individual with COPD who develops a renal tubular acidosis (RTA), may experience respiratory failure from the increased MV demand

- An individual without lung disease, renal failure may only complain of fatigue and a decreased exercise tolerance when faced with a RTA

- Mixed acute hypercapnic failure
  - Any combination of impaired pulmonary mechanics, metabolic acidosis, and blunted respiratory drive may (and commonly do) occur
  - Example:
    - An individual with LHF and pulmonary edema (decreased compliance) experiences bowel ischemia (lactic acidosis)
      - Leading to an increased acid load
    - The same patient is then given narcotics for abdominal pain, which blunt respiratory drive
      - Leading to hypoventilation (blunted drive) in the setting of impaired mechanics and increased acid load

CHRONIC HYPERCAPNIC RESPIRATORY FAILURE AND VENTILATORY DRIVE

- Chronic hypercapnic respiratory failure is defined as a pH of 7.35–7.39 with a $Pco_2 > 45$ mm Hg
  - The pH range reflects compensation, without overcompensation

- Chronic hypercapnic respiratory failure **only** occurs in individuals with a **blunted ventilatory drive**

- Parenchymal lung disease (most commonly COPD) challenges humans with the problem of inefficient lungs (ie, breathing requires more work):
  - Inefficient lungs force a choice (based on ventilatory drive)
    - Either increase resting MV and thus WOB (lots of metabolic energy) in an effort to maintain a normal Pco_2 and pH (normal ventilatory drive)

OR

  - Allow Pco_2 to rise and pH to fall (gradually hypoventilating), thereby allowing for renal compensation
    - Starting a cycle of hypoventilation, followed by renal compensation, followed by further hypoventilation (blunted ventilatory drive)

- "Pink puffers" vs "blue bloaters" (Fig. 2.3)
  - Individuals with a normal ventilatory drive have classically been referred to as "pink puffers"
    - Pink (ie, not cyanotic) because they avoid CO_2 retention and subsequent displacement of O_2 from the alveoli (a common cause of hypoxemia in COPD)
    - Cachectic from the metabolic cost of breathing >10 L/min at baseline
    - Chronically dyspneic; unable to augment their MV when faced with exercise and increased CO_2 generation
  - Individuals with a **blunted ventilatory drive** have classically been referred to as "blue bloaters"
    - **Blue bloaters** maintain a normal MV (inadequately low given the inefficiency of the diseased lungs), allowing Pco_2 to rise and pH to fall slightly (until renal compensation occurs in days), establishing a cycle of gradual CO_2 retention, leaving them:
      - Blue (ie, cyanotic/hypoxemic) because the retained CO_2 displaces O_2 in the alveoli
      - Bloated (ie, edematous) because of volume overload from HFpEF, secondary to diastolic dysfunction, provoked by hypoxemia and tachycardia (more commonly than isolated right-sided heart failure, ie, cor pulmonale)
      - Less dyspneic and more comfortable than pink puffers but with a higher mortality, given concomitant heart failure

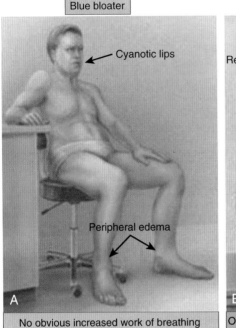

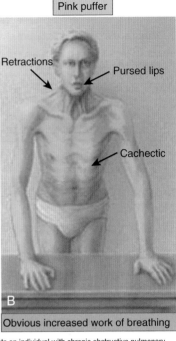

Fig. 2.3 (A) A drawing of the prototypical "blue bloater." This represents an individual with chronic obstructive pulmonary disease whose inefficient lungs, combined with a baseline blunted ventilatory drive, have caused him to hypoventilate (instead of increasing his work of breathing [WOB]). Although he enjoys the benefits (ie, minimal dyspnea, no increased WOB), he also suffers the consequences, namely hypoxemia (without an A-a gradient) from alveolar CO_2 accumulation (and subsequent O_2 displacement), and heart failure with volume overload and peripheral edema. Traditionally heart failure was attributed to isolated right ventricle (RV) failure (ie, cor pulmonale), but in reality these patients more commonly suffer from left-sided heart failure (HFpEF) as a result of diastolic dysfunction. This is often easily proven by the presence of pleural effusions. Cor pulmonale occurs when over 50% of the vasculature has been destroyed as a part of the parenchymal loss seen with chronic obstructive pulmonary disease (COPD) (evidenced by a diffusing capacity of the lung for carbon dioxide (DLCO) <50%). Said differently, Cor pulmonale should not be confidently diagnosed in an individual with a predicted DLCO >50%. Either way, decompensated isolated right-sided heart failure and biventricular failure both deserve diuresis to euvolemia. (B) The prototypical "pink puffer." This represents an individual with the same severity of chronic obstructive pulmonary disease as the "blue bloater," leading to the same degree of lung inefficiency, BUT combined with a normal ventilatory drive, which forces the individual to increase their WOB in an attempt to prevent pH fall and P_{CO_2} rise. This leaves him or her chronically dyspneic with a baseline increased WOB, which causes cachexia from the energy expenditure of breathing.

- Patients with chronic CO_2 retention and end-stage renal disease (ESRD) (or renal tubular acidosis [RTA]) will have a baseline ABG that erroneously suggests acute hypercapnic respiratory failure
  - Actually, the hypoventilation and CO_2 retention occur gradually over time
    - In RTA, this occurs because the kidney lacks the ability to reclaim HCO_3, and thus it cannot compensate for the acidosis caused by the hypoventilation
    - In ESRD, nephrologists (hesitant to cause worsening hypoventilation) do not completely compensate chronically hypercapnic individuals; instead they choose to leave them mildly acidotic

COMMON QUESTIONS GENERATED BY THIS TEACHING

1. **Why is 100% oxygen saturation not reassuring in a patient who has increased WOB?**
   Increased WOB is worrisome for hypercapnic failure (oxygenation is irrelevant)

2. **Why does hyperventilation driven by acidosis or hypoxemia lead to diaphragmatic fatigue, but hyperventilation driven by pain or anxiety does not?**

   When an individual's respiratory rate is increased by the respiratory center pacemaker, responding to normal physiologic stimuli or to a supratentorial stimulus (eg, pain and/or anxiety), it will not lead to diaphragmatic fatigue. If the respiratory rate is driven by an abnormal physiologic stimulus like a pH <7.35 or $Pao_2 < 60$ mm Hg, diaphragmatic fatigue may ensue.

3. **Does severe COPD cause CO_2 retention?**

   No. Severe COPD causes lung inefficiency. This means that more breathing effort is required to remove the same amount of CO_2. Individuals with a normal ventilatory response will increase their resting WOB (not allowing CO_2 to rise). COPD patients with chronic CO_2 retention have a blunted ventilatory drive (by definition) such that they do not increase their WOB but instead allow for hypercapnia to ensue (effectively "quitting on ventilation").

CHAPTER 3

PULMONARY FUNCTION TESTING

COMMON MISCONCEPTIONS AND MISTAKES

- Believing that a significant bronchodilator response on PFTs equals a diagnosis of asthma
- Obtaining pulmonary function testing (PFT) during an acute illness involving cardiopulmonary disease
- Not commenting on, or working up, a DLCO decrease out of proportion to the degree of obstruction (often indicative of additional disease)
- Believing that the DLCO is an assay for pulmonary capillary interstitial thickening (only)

PULMONARY FUNCTION TESTING

- The primary role for PFTs is to determine if abnormal lung function is present, and if so, is it significant enough to explain an individuals exercise limitation
- There are three major types of pulmonary pathophysiologic malfunction that are screened for by PFT: **obstructive** physiology, **restrictive** physiology, and **pulmonary vascular disease:**
  - Spirometry screens for **obstructive** physiology
    - Obstructive disease limits exercise by causing a prolonged exhalation, which limits the individual's ability to increase his or her minute volume (MV)
    - An inability to increase MV limits exercise as symptomatic lactic acidosis ensues instead of appropriate respiratory compensation
  - Lung volumes screen for **restrictive** physiology
    - Restrictive disease associated with parenchymal lung disease (DPLD) limits exercise by increasing the work of breathing (small, stiff lungs are more work to inflate) and by profound exercise-induced oxygen desaturation (as diffusion is severely limited by interstitial fibrosis or alveolar filling)
  - A DLCO measurement screens for **pulmonary vascular disease and interstitial lung disease**
    - Pulmonary vascular disease limits exercise by increasing dead space (vascular obstruction creates physiologic dead space) and by right ventricular (RV) afterload, which limits RV cardiac output (CO) and thus left ventricular (LV) CO
- PFTs are also used to determine the severity of lung disease, where the:
  - Obstructive defect is based on the FEV1 % predicted
  - Restrictive Defect, is based on the TLC % predicted
- PFTs are also essential in the assessment of lung resection tolerability for individuals with early-stage lung cancer (see lung cancer chapter)
- Serial PFT measurements may be used to screen for:
  - Pulmonary drug toxicity (eg, amiodarone, biologics)
  - Progression of DPLD
    - Total lung capacity (TLC), forced vital capacity (FVC) and DLCO are relatively sensitive measures of disease progression
  - Progression of neuromuscular disease

- Serial PFT measurements in individuals with asthma are useful to:
  - Demonstrate disease control (ie, normal PFTs)
  - Screen for the transition from reversible to fixed obstruction (eg, loss of a previously demonstrated bronchodilator response)
    - Which may prompt escalating therapy (eg, biologics)
- Serial PFT measurements are much less useful in the management of chronic obstructive pulmonary disease (COPD)
  - Relegated to ensuring that worsening exercise limitation is attributable to declining lung function and not a new problem (eg, angina)

SPIROMETRY

- Spirometry involves measuring airflow and lung volume while the subject forcefully exhales from TLC to residual volume, otherwise known as a forced vital capacity maneuver (Fig. 3.1).
- During forced expiration from TLC, **normal** airflow is almost immediately limited in the medium-sized airways by dynamic airway compression and collapse (Fig. 3.2)
- Dynamic airway collapse is:
  - Provoked by positive intrathoracic pressure generated during forced exhalation, which exerts a compressive force on intrathoracic structures (including medium-sized airways)
  - Resisted by the radial traction provided to the walls of the medium-sized airways by surrounding alveolar tissue (elastic recoil)
  - Responsible for the **normal** airway resistance encountered during forced expiration leading to the sloping nature of the exhalation limb of a normal flow volume loop
  - Effort independent, being a phenomenon of the elastic recoil properties of the lung at any given lung volume
    - As the lung deflates, its elastic recoil force decreases such that at a certain lung volume, positive intrathoracic pressure normally provokes dynamic collapse limiting airflow (normally at a low lung volume near complete exhalation)
    - Obstructive lung physiology occurs when dynamic collapse occurs early, limiting airflow at a relatively high lung volume
- In patients with COPD/emphysema, loss of alveolar tissue leads to decreased radial traction, increasing the tendency of the medium-sized airways to collapse pathologically early during exhalation (at relatively high lung volumes), leading to a scooped exhalation limb of the **obstructed** flow volume loop

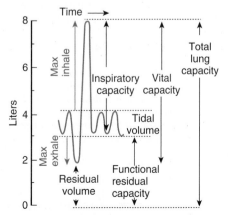

Fig. 3.1 Classic spirometry tracing showing volume over time during normal tidal breathing, followed by maximum exhalation and inhalation, with the key volumes and capacities (sums of volumes) labeled.

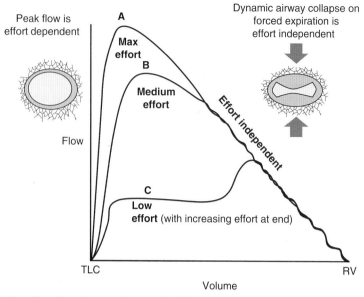

Fig. 3.2 Three different flow volume loops (showing exhalation limb only) from the same subject, with varying degrees of effort, illustrating how the peak flow rate is effort dependent. Schematic drawing of the medium-sized airway in cross section, embedded in a lattice of normal alveolar tissue, depicting the airway open at the onset of forced expiration (ie, approaching peak flow). Almost immediately, as lung volume drops from total lung capacity (TLC), the flow rate begins to decline, as positive intrathoracic pressure causes dynamic airway collapse (represented schematically by the medium-sized airway, collapsing, despite being embedded in a lattice of normal alveolar tissue). This decline in flow rate for a given lung volume is a function of the mechanical properties of the lung (ie, elastic recoil airway resistance) and is thus effort independent. Note how all three loops ultimately converge.

- In patients with asthma, the medium-sized airway lumen is narrowed by airway tone and inflammation, leading to a similar premature (for a given lung volume) pathologic dynamic collapse
- Importantly, the inspiratory limb of the flow volume loop appears as a uniform arc (in normal and emphysematous individuals alike), as the negative thoracic pressure of inspiration exerts an opening force on intrathoracic structures (including medium-sized airways), minimizing airway resistance (Fig. 3.3)
- With normal pulmonary mechanics, most of the air is exhaled from the lung in the first second
  - Said another way, the ratio of the forced expiratory volume in 1 second (FEV_1) to the total forced volume exhaled, or forced vital capacity (FVC), should be high
    - The FEV_1/FVC should be >70% (ratio of volumes, **not** percent)
- In obstructive lung disease, dynamic airway collapse occurs pathologically early during exhalation, reducing airflow prematurely and increasing exhalation time
  - Said another way, the ratio of the FEV_1 to the FVC (ie, total forced volume exhaled) should be low
    - The ratio of FEV_1 to the FVC will be <70%
- This ratio of airflow for a given lung volume is a function of pulmonary mechanics (ie, airway resistance and elastic recoil) and is thus effort independent, making the FEV_1/FVC ratio superior to peak flow measurements in the determination of obstructive lung disease
  - Although the peak airflow rate will be reduced in obstructive lung disease, it is an effort-dependent measure, making it less reliable (see Fig. 3.2)

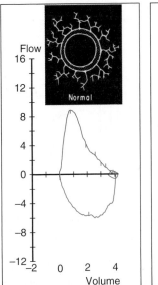 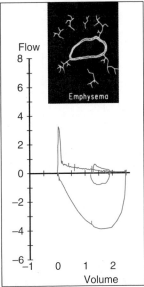

Fig. 3.3 Normal flow volume loop on the left, with a schematic insert depicting a medium-sized airway, embedded in normal alveolar tissue, providing radial traction resisting airway collapse until the end of exhalation when lung volume is low. The flow volume loop on the right demonstrates a severe obstructive defect, with a schematic insert depicting a medium-sized airway prone to premature collapse at the beginning of exhalation when lung volume is still high, secondary to decreased radial traction.

- A proportionate reduction in FVC and FEV1 with a preserved ratio (ie, FEV1/FVC> 70%) suggests a restrictive defect vs poor effort
  - TLC measurement required to confirm the diagnosis of a restrictive physiology
- If lung volumes are not attainable, spirometry may strongly suggest a restrictive defect secondary to pulmonary fibrosis when the FVC is <80% predicted and the FEV_1/FVC ratio is pathologically high (ie, >115% predicted), implying increased elastic recoil, as occurs when areas of fibrosis stent open the medium sized airways, resisting normal dynamic airway collapse

FLOW VOLUME LOOP

- The flow volume loop provides a visual representation of airflow during inhalation and exhalation
- Although the inspiratory limb of the flow volume loop appears similar (as an arc) in most normal individuals, the shape of the expiratory slope demonstrates more variability as a function of individual effort and pulmonary mechanics (Fig. 3.4)
- Inspection of the flow volume loop is **necessary** to screen for obstruction of the large airways, as can occur in the setting of upper airway tumors, tracheal tumors, mediastinal masses (via external compression), subglottic stenosis, vocal cord paralysis/impingement, and tracheomalacia
- **Variable extrathoracic obstruction**
  - Commonly caused by squamous cell cancers involving the larynx, subglottic stenosis, and vocal cord paralysis (as occurs as a complication of intubation or tracheostomy)
  - Variable obstruction of the upper extrathoracic portion of the airway leads to a flow limitation on inhalation **only**
    - This causes the normal arc of the inspiratory limb to be cut like an upside down plateau

NORMAL FLOW VOLUME LOOPS

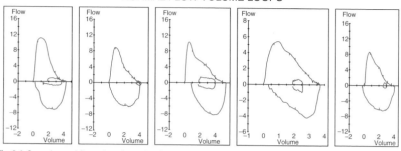

Fig. 3.4 Several normal flow volume loops showing the wide range of shapes based on effort and individual lung mechanics.

- Because the flow limitation is **only present during inhalation** (when negative intrathoracic pressure exerts a collapsing force on the extrathoracic airway), it is called **variable extrathoracic** obstruction (Fig. 3.5A)
  - During exhalation, positive intrathoracic pressure exerts an opening force on the extrathoracic airway such that expiratory flow is not affected
- It is common for subjects to volitionally limit airflow (at their mouths) during the slow inspiratory vital capacity (VC) maneuver that generates the inspiratory limb of the flow volume loop
  - Because of this, a flow limitation should be evident on multiple trials to raise concern for upper airway obstruction
  - Additionally, some individuals experience a paradoxical vocal cord closure during the inspiratory maneuver (producing audible stridor), which they can often be "coached" out of by the PFT technician
- **Variable intrathoracic obstruction**
  - Commonly caused by squamous cell tumors of the trachea, tracheomalacia, and external compression from mediastinal tumors/adenopathy
  - Variable obstruction of the intrathoracic portion of trachea leads to a flow limitation during exhalation **only**
    - This causes the normal sloped exhalation limb to be cut, as peak flow plateaus until lung volume is low enough that dynamic airway collapse supervenes and limits the remainder of the expiratory flow
    - Because the flow limitation is **only present during forced exhalation** (when positive intrathoracic pressure exerts a collapsing force on the intrathoracic airway), it is called **variable intrathoracic** obstruction (Fig. 3.5B)
    - During inhalation, negative intrathoracic pressure exerts an opening force on the intrathoracic airway such that inspiratory flow is not affected
- **Fixed intrathoracic or extrathoracic obstruction**
  - Commonly caused by squamous cell tumors of the trachea and the larynx (extending down into the thorax), or by a fixed narrowing anywhere in the main airway, commonly from tumor or scarring
  - Fixed obstruction of either the intrathoracic and extrathoracic airway leads to flow limitation during inhalation and exhalation
    - This causes the flow volume loop to appear ovoid as both inspiratory and expiratory limbs demonstrate plateauing of airflow
    - Because the airway obstruction does not vary normally with inspiration or expiration, it is called fixed intrathoracic-extrathoracic obstruction (Fig. 3.5C)
- Though not used for diagnosis, the flow volume loops of obstructive disease, restrictive disease, and mixed obstructive restrictive disease have a characteristic appearance (Fig. 3.6)

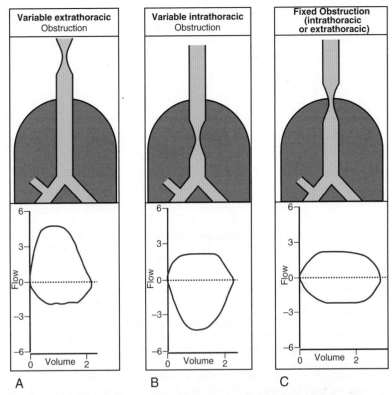

Fig. 3.5 Schematic representation paired with idealized flow volume loops illustrating the flow limitation patterns of large airway obstruction. **(A)** Variable extrathoracic obstruction. Schematic representation of extrathoracic airway narrowing, with an anticipated flow volume loop below showing pathologic inspiratory flow limitation. **(B)** Variable intrathoracic airway obstruction. Schematic representation of intrathoracic airway narrowing, with an anticipated flow volume loop below showing pathologic expiratory flow limitation. **(C)** Fixed intrathoracic or extrathoracic obstruction. Schematic representation of a fixed airway narrowing spanning the intrathoracic and extrathoracic airway, with an anticipated flow volume loop below, showing pathologic inspiratory and expiratory flow limitation.

LUNG VOLUMES

- Measuring lung volume dynamically, by spirometry (ie, FVC), has one major limitation
  - If the patient has obstructive disease with air trapping, his or her RV will be increased
    - As the RV increases, it reduces the available space for ventilation (despite TLC increase, because there is limited space in the thorax), decreasing the VC
    - This is known as pseudorestriction
- Pseudorestriction (secondary to obstructive lung disease) can only be distinguished from obstructive disease with concomitant restriction (aka mixed obstructive-restrictive disease), by measuring the TLC
  - TLC = the vital capacity (easy to measure via spirometry) + the residual volume (requires body plethysmography or the helium dilution technique)
- Measuring TLC by helium dilution and body plethysmography
  - The helium dilution technique takes advantage of the fact that helium is not absorbed by the blood:
    - The subject breathes helium from a reservoir with a known amount of helium, effectively diluting the helium from the reservoir
      - Amount of helium in the reservoir = concentration of helium (C_1) × volume of gas (V_1)

OBSTRUCTED, RESTRICTED AND MIXED OBSTRUCTED –
RESTRICTED FLOW VOLUME LOOPS

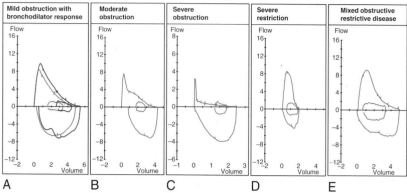

Fig. 3.6 Flow volume loops illustrating classic disease patterns. **(A)** Mild obstructive disease, with a positive bronchodilator response (red loop). Notice the improvement in the scooped appearance of the expiratory limb after bronchodilator administration. **(B)** Moderate obstruction. **(C)** Severe obstruction. Note the y-axis scale difference. **(D)** Severe restriction. Note the A shape to the flow volume loop, created by the pathologically fast flows during exhalation as the increased elastic recoil of fibrosis resists dynamic airway collapse despite forced exhalation. **(E)** Mixed obstructive restrictive disease appearing as a combination of a restricted loop and an obstructed loop.

- After several breaths the helium equilibrates between the reservoir and the lung, leading to a new, reduced concentration of helium in the reservoir (C_2)
- The change in concentration allows a calculation of TLC (V_2)
  - $V_2 = V_1(C_1 - C_2)/C_2$
- The major limitation to the helium dilution technique is that only ventilated lung is measured such that patients with air trapping and bullous lung disease will have their **lung volumes underestimated**
  - This can erroneously lead to pseudorestriction being misinterpreted as true mixed obstructive restrictive disease
- Body plethysmography enables measurement of RV or functional residual capacity (FRC), from which TLC is calculated by adding the VC or inspiratory capacity (maximum inhalation from a normal exhale during tidal breathing), respectively
  - Because body plethysmography assesses the total volume inside the thorax (ventilated and unventilated areas alike), it more accurately measures TLC in patients with poorly ventilated areas of the lung (eg, those with air trapping and bullous disease)
  - Body plethysmography technique:
    - The subject is seated in a sealed chamber (in which pressure is measured closely) and then instructed to exhale normally to FRC or RV
    - Next the subject is instructed to make repetitive inspiratory efforts against a sealed tube (effectively panting **without** moving any air)
      - As the diaphragm contracts, pressure decreases inside the thorax and the volume of air in the FRC and/or RV increases
    - Pressure in the box increases proportionately, allowing FRC or RV to be calculated
      - FRC can then be added to the inspiratory capacity (maximum inhale maneuver) to give TLC, where TLC = FRC + IC
      - RV can be added to the VC to give TLC, where TLC = RV + VC
    - Although measuring RV directly is more intuitive, it is difficult for older individuals to exhale maximally before "panting" against a closed circuit, occasionally causing syncope

DIFFUSION CAPACITY

- The diffusion capacity of the lung depends on the pulmonary capillary surface area available for gas exchange
- Thus the DLCO can be thought of as an assay for pulmonary vascular health
  - A low DLCO indicates one of the following: pulmonary interstitial thickening (diffuse parenchymal lung disease [DPLD]); a loss of vasculature, as seen in COPD; or pulmonary vascular disease (ie, chronic thromboembolic pulmonary hypertension [CTEPH] or idiopathic pulmonary arterial hypertension [IPAH])
- It is measured in the PFT laboratory by having subjects hold their breaths at TLC for 10 seconds after breathing a dilute mixture of a known amount of carbon monoxide (CO)
  - During the breath hold, the CO diffuses into the blood (assessing the diffusion capacity of the lung)
- The amount of CO exhaled after the 10-second breath hold is measured and subtracted from the initial amount, giving the quantity of CO diffused in a 10-second period
  - Without a diffusion limitation, 20–30 mL of CO will diffuse into the blood per minute
- Some patients either inhale two slowly (>2.5 seconds), are unable to hold their breaths for 10 seconds, or are unable to reach ≥85% of there previous VC measurement, any of which will lead to a falsely **reduced** DLCO measurement (and should be reported by the technician)
- Most laboratories add helium (He) to the CO gas mixture to obtain an additional TLC measurement via helium dilution (measuring only ventilated units)
  - In **normal individuals,** the TLC obtained from He dilution will be similar to the TLC obtained by body plethysmography
    - Because normal individuals do not have a significant volume of unventilated lung
    - Because of this, the DLCO corrected for alveolar ventilation (DLCO/VA) will be similar to the DLCO
  - Patients with obstructive lung disease may have significant areas of unventilated lung such that their TLC measured by He dilution may grossly underestimate their true total lung volume (by liters)
    - Because of this the DLCO/VA will be falsely elevated, and thus it should **not** be routinely used
  - The DLCO/VA may provide useful information in the following scenarios:
    - Correcting for alveolar ventilation may be considered in individuals who have had anatomic lung resection (correcting for the volume of resected lung)
    - A DLCO <50% predicted **and** a DLCO/VA >150% is a pattern associated with obesity (rather than representing a true diffusion limitation)
    - The TLC % predicted obtained by body plethysmography minus the TLC % predicted obtained by He dilution gives the percentage of unventilated lung in an individual (interesting to conceptualize)

BRONCHODILATOR RESPONSIVENESS

- Spirometry in which the FEV_1 or FVC improves by 200 mL **and** 12% qualifies as a significant bronchodilator response (ATS criteria)
  - Importantly, many patients gain a clinical benefit from bronchodilator therapy, despite an "insignificant" response by ATS criteria
- Bronchodilator responsiveness in isolation is of limited utility (remember that asthma is a clinical diagnosis made by eliciting a history of episodic airflow obstruction)
  - Normal spirometry that improves significantly after bronchodilator administration is a normal variant, implying resting airway tone (**not** asthma)
- A significant bronchodilator response in which the FEV_1/FVC ratio normalizes after bronchodilator administration is highly supportive of a reactive airways disease diagnosis (eg, asthma)

RESPIRATORY MUSCLE STRENGTH

- Respiratory muscle strength is traditionally assessed by maximum inspiratory pressure (MIP) and maximum expiratory pressure (MEP) measurements
  - Unfortunately the data sets for "normal values" are very small; thus confidence intervals are large, with the normal range being 60%–140% predicted
- Inspiratory muscle strength assesses diaphragm function
  - An absolute MIP value of < -40 cm H_2O is **always** abnormal, suggesting neuromuscular disease involving the phrenic nerve (eg, spinal cord injury)
  - Patients with significant diaphragmatic muscle weakness will also be restricted
- Expiratory muscle strength assesses extrathoracic muscle health
  - An absolute MEP value of <80 cm H_2O is **always** abnormal, suggesting systemic neuromuscular disease and predicting ineffective cough

PULMONARY FUNCTION TESTING INTERPRETATION (FIGS. 3.7, 3.8, AND 3.9)

- **Obstructive physiology** can be confidently diagnosed when the FEV_1/FVC ratio is $<70\%$ (GOLD criteria)

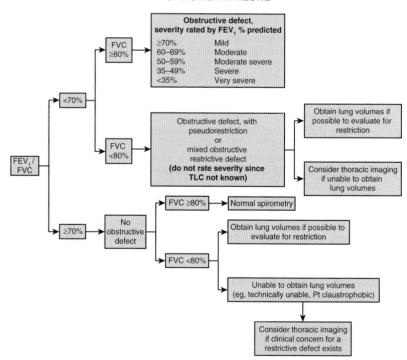

Fig. 3.7 Algorithm for interpreting spirometry. The assessment starts with the forced expiratory volume in 1 second (FEV_1)/ forced vital capacity (FVC) ratio looking for obstruction, followed by the FVC looking for evidence of possible restriction (either pseudo or concomitant). Restriction cannot be confidently diagnosed without a measurement of total lung capacity (TLC) (to separate pseudorestriction from true restriction). If the FVC is $<80\%$, an additional measurement of lung volume (ie, TLC) should be recommended. If a TLC measurement is not possible, diseases that cause restriction (ie, pulmonary fibrosis, pleural disease) may be screened for with thoracic imaging.

SPIROMETRY AND LUNG VOLUMES

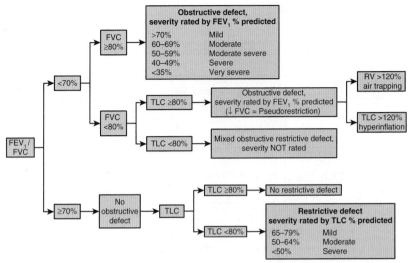

Fig. 3.8 Algorithm for interpreting spirometry and lung volumes. The assessment starts with the forced expiratory volume in 1 second (FEV_1)/forced vital capacity (FVC) ratio looking for obstruction, followed by the FVC looking for evidence of possible restriction (either pseudo or concomitant). If the FEV_1/FVC ratio is <70%, the FVC is <80%, and the total lung capacity (TLC) is ≥80%, the pulmonary function tests (PFTs) show obstruction with pseudorestriction. If the FEV_1/FVC ratio is <70%, the FVC is <80%, and the TLC is <80%, the PFTs show mixed obstructive restrictive disease. The severity of mixed obstructive restrictive disease is assessed clinically and radiographically, not by PFTs. That said, the magnitude of the DLCO reduction often reflects overall disease severity since both processes negatively impact this parameter.

- Defining obstruction as an FEV_1/FVC <70%, rather than an FEV_1/FVC less than the lower limit of normal (<~90% predicted), will tend to:
  - Overcall obstruction in the old
  - Potentially miss obstruction in the young
    - In young individuals whose predicted FEV_1/FVC % is <90% predicted, a diagnosis of obstruction should be considered, especially if:
      - Lung volumes show evidence of air trapping and/or hyperinflation
      - A significant bronchodilator response is also demonstrated
- An FVC >80% predicted rules out a concomitant restrictive defect such that the severity of the obstructive defect can be assessed:
  - Severity of obstruction is rated by the FEV_1 % predicted:
    - >70% Mild
    - 60–69% Moderate
    - 50–59% Moderate to severe
    - 40–49% Severe
    - <35% Very severe
- An FVC <80% predicted suggests a concomitant restrictive defect vs pseudorestriction (from air trapping)
- A TLC <80% predicted confirms concomitant restriction (ie, mixed obstructive restrictive disease)
  - The severity of the mixed obstructive restrictive defect cannot be formally assessed (see the Common Questions section at the end of this chapter)
    - That said, the DLCO is often affected by both processes and thus may give an indication of overall disease severity

DIFFUSING CAPACITY OF THE LUNG FOR CARBON MONOXIDE (DLCO)

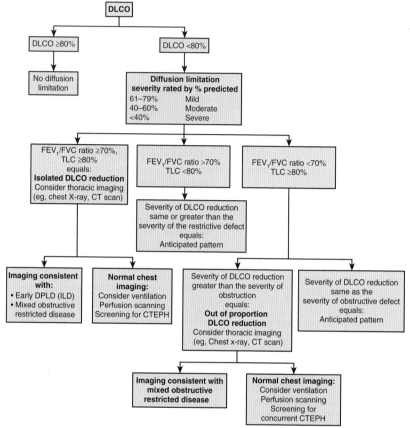

Fig. 3.9 Algorithm for interpreting the DLCO. The key to interpreting the DLCO is to do so in light of the obstructive, restrictive, or mixed obstructive restrictive pattern suggested by spirometry and/or lung volume. In obstructive disease, the severity of the DLCO reduction should mirror the severity of the obstruction. In restrictive disease, any severity of DLCO reduction is anticipated (because extrapleural restriction will not affect the DLCO, and fibrosis often causes a DLCO reduction more severe than the total lung capacity [TLC] reduction). An isolated reduction in DLCO (or an out-of-proportion reduction in obstructive disease) may be seen in mixed obstructive restrictive disease, pulmonary vascular disease, and early diffuse parenchymal lung disease (DPLD). Mixed obstructive restrictive disease should be obvious from thoracic imaging. An isolated reduction in DLCO with normal chest imaging should raise concern for pulmonary vascular disease such that one should consider screening for chronic thromboembolism with ventilation perfusion scanning.

- A TLC >80% predicted rules out concomitant restriction such that an FVC <80% predicted can be attributed to pseudorestriction
  - Air trapping increases the RV by decreasing the VC, yielding a net preserved, or elevated, TLC (ie, hyperinflation)
- The DLCO will typically be preserved or elevated in asthma (and in some phenotypes of COPD) and reduced in other patients with COPD
  - The severity of the DLCO reduction in obstructive disease should mirror the severity of the obstruction
  - A DLCO reduction out of proportion to the degree of obstruction should prompt consideration for concomitant restrictive disease or pulmonary vascular disease
    - Best evaluated by chest imaging and a VQ scan (if chest imaging is **not** suggestive of a concomitant restrictive disease)

- **Restrictive physiology** is suggested by a FVC <80% predicted and be can be confidently diagnosed when the TLC <80% predicted
  - The severity of restriction is rated by the TLC % predicted:
    - 65–79% Mild
    - 50–64% Moderate
    - <50% Severe
  - The DLCO is typically reduced in parenchymal causes of restriction (eg, DPLD) and preserved in extrapleural causes of restriction (eg, pleural scarring)
    - In DPLD the severity of the DLCO reduction may be greater than the severity of the restrictive defect such that **no** additional disease process needs to be screened for
- **Pulmonary vascular loss** is suggested by an isolated reduction in the DLCO (<80% predicted)
  - Severity of diffusion limitation is rated by the DLCO % predicted:
    - 61–79% Mild
    - 40–60% Moderate
    - <40% Severe
  - An **isolated** reduction in DLCO may be seen in:
    - **Mixed obstructive restrictive disease** (Fig. 3.10)
      - Occurs as the obstructed lung (with trapped air) normalizes the lung volume and the fibrotic lung (which resists dynamic airway collapse) normalizes the flow rate

Combined Pulmonary Fibrosis and Emphysema (ie, Mixed Obstructive Restrictive Disease) PFT Pattern

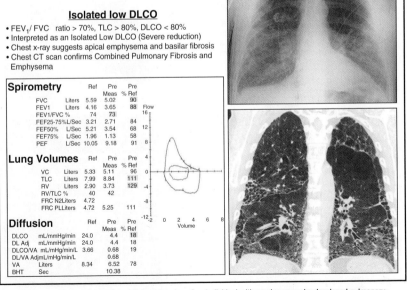

Isolated low DLCO
- FEV_1/FVC ratio > 70%, TLC > 80%, DLCO < 80%
- Interpreted as an Isolated Low DLCO (Severe reduction)
- Chest x-ray suggests apical emphysema and basilar fibrosis
- Chest CT scan confirms Combined Pulmonary Fibrosis and Emphysema

Spirometry

		Ref	Pre Meas	Pre % Ref	
FVC	Liters	5.59	5.02	90	
FEV1	Liters	4.16	3.65	88	
FEV1/FVC %		74	73		
FEF25-75%	L/Sec	3.21	2.71	84	
FEF50%	L/Sec	5.21	3.54	68	
FEF75%	L/Sec	1.96	1.13	58	
PEF	L/Sec	10.05	9.18	91	

Lung Volumes

		Ref	Pre Meas	Pre % Ref
VC	Liters	5.33	5.11	96
TLC	Liters	7.99	8.84	111
RV	Liters	2.90	3.73	129
RV/TLC %		40	42	
FRC N2	Liters	4.72		
FRC PL	Liters	4.72	5.25	111

Diffusion

		Ref	Pre Meas	Pre % Ref
DLCO	mL/mmHg/min	24.0	4.4	18
DL Adj	mL/mmHg/min	24.0	4.4	18
DLCO/VA	mL/mHg/min/L	3.66	0.68	19
DL/VA Adj	mL/mHg/min/L		0.68	
VA	Liters	8.34	6.52	78
BHT	Sec		10.38	

Fig. 3.10 Pulmonary function testing and chest imaging of an individual with emphysema who developed pulmonary fibrosis (a.k.a. combined pulmonary fibrosis and emphysema). The patient's airflow and lung volume are strikingly normal (with the only abnormality being air trapping, suggested by the elevated residual volume). The DLCO of 18% predicted, however, reveals the true severity of the individual's underlying lung disease. Note that the patient's DLCO/alveolar ventilation (VA) is almost normal (78% predicted), highlighting the importance of **not** routinely using this correction for fear of missing a truly significant diffusion impairment. The patient's chest x-ray suggests apical emphysema (L > R) with bibasilar fibrosis (confirmed by chest computed tomography [CT]).

- ◦ **Pulmonary vascular disease**
  - Occurs as blood vessel obstruction decreases the availability of the pulmonary capillary surface area
    - Large vessel obstruction (ie, CTEPH) (Fig. 3.11) is much more common than small vessel obliteration (ie, IPAH)
      - ◦ Because of this, a routine recommendation to consider VQ scanning should be made
- ◦ **Early diffuse DPLD**
  - DPLD may manifest initially as an isolated reduction in DLCO (as interstitial fibrosis impairs diffusion before lung volumes are pathologically reduced)
  - As the disease progresses, lung volumes fall
- Elevated DLCO measurements
  - ◦ The classic teaching is that an elevated DLCO (>120% predicted) may be seen in conditions causing increased pulmonary blood flow (eg, early heart failure or asthma during an exacerbation) or in the setting of diffuse alveolar hemorrhage (where free Hb in the alveolus acts like a sink for CO)
  - ◦ Practically speaking, we do not obtain PFTs in acutely ill individuals
  - ◦ Additionally, PFTs are not designed to screen for these conditions such that a routine suggestion from a PFT interpretation to consider them should not be made
  - ◦ That said, occasionally a case of DAH is disputed, with the typical DDx being DAH vs cardiogenic edema vs inflammatory alveolar infiltrate

Chronic Thromboembolic Pulmonary Hypertension (CTEPH) PFT Pattern

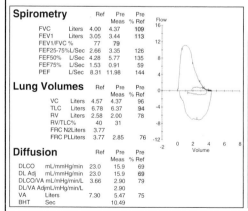
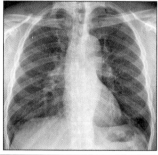
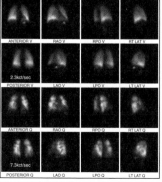

Isolated DLCO Reduction

- FEV_1/ FVC ratio > 70%, TLC > 80%, DLCO < 80%
- Interpreted as an Isolated Low DLCO (Mild reduction)
- Chest x-ray without evidence of parenchymal disease
- VQ scan with multiple segmental and subsegmental perfusion defects consistent with CTEPH

Spirometry

		Ref	Pre Meas	Pre % Ref
FVC	Liters	4.00	4.37	109
FEV1	Liters	3.05	3.44	113
FEV1/FVC %		77	79	
FEF25-75%	L/Sec	2.66	3.35	126
FEF50%	L/Sec	4.28	5.77	135
FEF75%	L/Sec	1.53	0.91	59
PEF	L/Sec	8.31	11.98	144

Lung Volumes

		Ref	Pre Meas	Pre % Ref
VC	Liters	4.57	4.37	96
TLC	Liters	6.78	6.37	94
RV	Liters	2.58	2.00	78
RV/TLC%		40	31	
FRC N2	Liters	3.77		
FRC PL	Liters	3.77	2.85	76

Diffusion

		Ref	Pre Meas	Pre % Ref
DLCO	mL/mmHg/min	23.0	15.9	69
DL Adj	mL/mmHg/min	23.0	15.9	69
DLCO/VA	mL/mmHg/min/L	3.66	2.90	79
DL/VA Adj	mL/mmHg/min/L		2.90	
VA	Liters	7.30	5.47	75
BHT	Sec		10.49	

Fig. 3.11 Pulmonary function testing (PFT) and chest imaging of an individual with chronic thromboembolic pulmonary hypertension. The patient's PFTs are normal except for an isolated reduction in his DLCO. His chest x-ray film was read as normal (despite having the suggestion of enlarged central pulmonary arteries). His VQ scan was grossly abnormal with multiple segmental and subsegmental unmatched perfusion defects.

- In this setting an elevated DLCO strongly points to DAH because the other conditions should reduce DLCO
  - The DLCO is usually >150% predicted in DAH

COMMON QUESTIONS GENERATED BY THIS TEACHING

1. Why is the FVC typically lower than the slow VC?
   Forced exhalation (with higher intrathoracic pressure) provokes airway collapse more than slow exhalation.
2. Why can't the severity of mixed obstructive restrictive disease be rated based on the FEV_1 % predicted and the TLC?
   It is not possible to discern what portion of the FEV_1 reduction is a result of total volume loss (ie, the restrictive disease) vs the obstructive defect. Similarly the lung volume may underestimate the degree of restriction because trapped air from the obstructive defect will elevate the TLC. The DLCO reduction often reflects overall disease severity better than the FEV_1 and/or the TLC.
3. When should I order a methacholine challenge test?
   A methylcholine challenge test should (almost) never be ordered. Methacholine bronchoprovocation testing is of limited clinical utility and is typically reserved for clinical scenarios in which the patient complains of an episodic symptom that is not clearly bronchospasm. Many times these challenging patients have affective components to their complaints that inevitably occur during bronchoprovocation testing, often leading to test termination before meaningful data are obtained.
4. Why shouldn't an evaluation for IPAH (in addition to CTEPH) be routinely recommended for individuals with an isolated low DLCO?
   IPAH is a very rare disease that requires invasive screening. Such that it is not appropriate to routinely suggest that individuals with an isolated low DLCO be evaluated for it.

CHAPTER 4

THE CHEST RADIOGRAPH

COMMON MISCONCEPTIONS AND MISTAKES

- Believing that reading a chest x-ray (CXR) requires advanced training, experience, and/ or a "special eye"
- Declaring a "blunted costophrenic angle" when the entire diaphragm is silhouetted out
- Using a myriad of adjectives to describe an opacity (eg, fuzzy, hazy)
- Missing segmental collapse
- Deciding endobronchial obstruction is the etiology of whole lung atelectasis based on a sharply demarcated cut in the mainstem air column

APPROACH TO THE CHEST RADIOGRAPH

- How we see discrete structures in the chest (eg, heart borders, hemidiaphragms):
  - Borders and outlines are seen on CXR when adjacent structures are of different densities (eg, air and soft tissue)
  - Two adjacent soft tissue densities (eg, the left and right ventricles) will not be visible separately because they lack an air interface
- How we detect pathology (eg, pneumonia, tumor)—the silhouette sign:
  - When a new process occurs in the chest (eg, pneumonia or tumor) it will often opacify or "silhouette out" an expected structure by removing an expected air–soft tissue interface, leading to the loss of an expected line (eg, right middle lobe [RML] pneumonia opacifying the right heart boarder)
  - This area of decreased clarity (or *missing line*) is described as an "opacity"
  - Loss of clarity of a structure (eg, diaphragm, heart border) implies a supervening abnormality
    - Even when the abnormality itself is vague, often just a missing or interrupted line
  - The missing or interrupted line **is the finding** (Fig. 4.1)
  - **Do not** (let your mind and eye) **repair interrupted lines** (natural tendency)
- Screening for opacities:
  - Screening for opacities on the **frontal film** = looking for an interruption or absence of an anticipated line
    - The anticipated lines are:
      - **Right and left**: hemidiaphragm, heart border, main pulmonary artery (PA), and the paratracheal stripe
      - **Left only (the anteroposterior [AP] window)**: ascending and descending aorta, with the top of the left PA
    - Normal hemidiaphragms and heart boarders are **always** sharp
    - Right and left PAs are less distinct (vessels branching in all planes)
      - Should get a sense of left and right main PA and right descending PA (Fig. 4.2)
    - After anticipated lines are identified, screen the remaining lung fields for abnormally increased or decreased attenuation and/or abnormal lines (coarse or fine)

Silhouette Sign

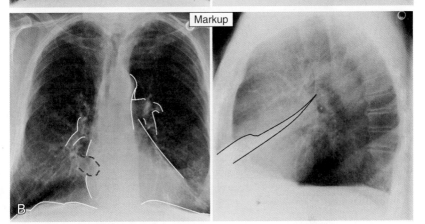

Fig. 4.1 Silhouette sign. (A) Frontal view of the chest shows that the line generated by the right heart boarder is interrupted by a vague, focal, veil-like opacity. The interrupted line is the objective abnormal finding. The lateral film shows a well-circumscribed, wedge-shaped, dense opacity extending from the hilum to the chest wall. Diagnosis: right middle lobe atelectasis. (B) Markup of the same film.

- Screening for opacities on the **lateral film** = looking for an opacified "clear" space
  - The anticipated clear spaces are:
    - Anterior clear space
    - Subcarinal space
    - Base of the spine
  - The hemidiaphragms should also be visualized
    - Note the anterior portion of the left hemidiaphragm is silhouetted out by the apex of the heart (Fig. 4.3)
- Characterizing the opacity:
  - **Dense Consolidation** (soft tissue density / white), implies **complete** alveolar filling or atelectasis
    - Cannot see normal underlying structures (causes complete opacification)
    - DDx: Atelectasis vs. Pneumonia vs. Mass
      - Vague bordered dense consolidation ≈ Pneumonia

Frontal Film Anticipated Structures

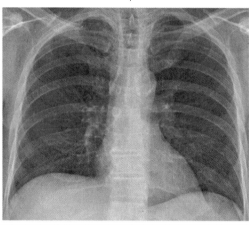

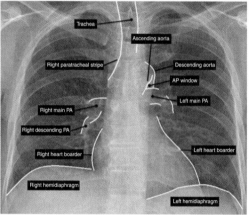

Fig. 4.2 Anticipated lines. The frontal chest radiograph shows the anticipated lines are right and left: paratracheal stripe, main pulmonary artery (PA), heart border, and hemidiaphragm. The anticipated lines of the anteroposterior window are the ascending and descending aorta, with the top of the left PA (forming the floor of the triangle/window). **Note:** normal hemidiaphragms and heart boarders are **always** sharp, where normal pulmonary arteries are less distinct (should get a sense of left and right main PA and right descending PA).

- Well circumscribed dense consolidation:
  - With air bronchograms ≈ Atelectasis
  - Without air bronchograms:
    - With volume loss ≈ Atelectasis with airway obstruction
    - Without volume loss ≈ Mass / Tumor
- **Ground glass** (increased attenuation / gray), implies **partial** alveolar filling or atelectasis
  - Can still see some normal underlying structures (causes incomplete opacification)
  - DDx: Any alveolar filling process (e.g. edema, inflammation, atypical infection, hemorrhage)
- **Fine reticular lines** (lots of fine lines), implies Interstitial edema
  - Normal underlying structures clearly visible, **but** close inspection shows that anticipated lines are **not** sharp, and are instead 'blurry' or 'hazy'
- **Corse reticular lines** (lots of larger lines in lattice like pattern) implies fibrosis

Lateral Film Clear Spaces

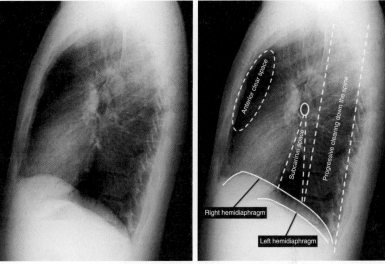

Fig. 4.3 Screening for opacities on the lateral film involves looking for an opacified "clear" space. The anticipated clear spaces are the anterior, and subcarinal spaces and base of the spine. The hemidiaphragms should also be visualized. **Note:** the anterior portion of the left hemidiaphragm is silhouetted out by the apex of the heart.

- **Veil - like** (homogenous increased attenuation / gray) implies effusion (no meniscus anticipated when the patient is supine, or semi supine)
  - Cannot see normal underlying structures (causes complete opacification)
  - Note: Basilar subsegmental atelectasis may appear veil like (indistugusiable from a small effusion)
- Visually isolating areas of the CXR can help (ie, mentally or by zooming in and focusing on just the opacified right hemidiaphragm) (Fig. 4.4)
- Different types of opacities often occur together (Fig. 4.5)
- After an opacity is identified and characterized, decide if it is **focal** or **diffuse**:
  - **If focal**, decide if it is **well-circumscribed** (clearly defined borders) versus **vague** (poorly defined borders)
    - **Well-circumscribed** ≈ segmental atelectasis, lobar PNA, or tumor (note: subsegmental atelectasis may also be well-circumscribed/linear (eg, plate-like atelectasis) (Fig. 4.6)
    - **Vague** ≈ pneumonia or subsegmental atelectasis (note: tumor can also be vague and radiographically indistinguishable from PNA)
  - **If diffuse** (many bilateral structures similarly opacified), decide if the pattern looks acute (eg, pulmonary edema) (Fig. 4.7A–C) or chronic (eg, pulmonary fibrosis, COPD) (Fig. 4.7D)
- Localizing the focal opacity:
  - Midlung opacities obscuring the right heart boarder = process involving the right middle lobe
  - Midlung opacities obscuring the left heart boarder = process involving the lingula
  - Lower lung zone opacities obscuring the right or left hemidiaphragm = right or left lower lobe process respectively
  - Upper lung zone opacities require a lateral film to localize
    - Anterior opacity = upper lobe process
    - Posterior opacity = lower lobe process

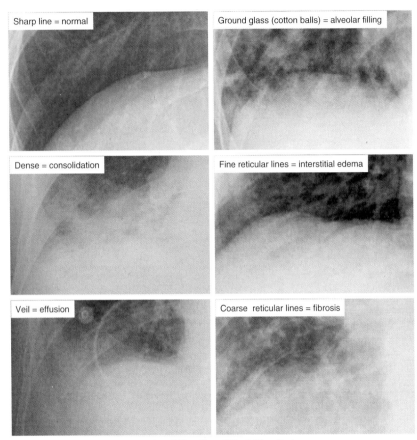

Fig. 4.4 Five basic types of opacities are shown "silhouetting out" the right hemidiaphragm.

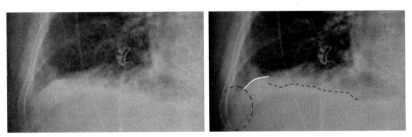

Fig. 4.5 The right hemidiaphragm is nearly completely opacified (white line denotes only remaining visualized portion). It is opacified by both a poorly circumscribed dense consolidation, medially, (with air bronchograms) and a lateral veil. **Note:** this constellation of findings represents either effusion with compressive atelectasis or pneumonia with parapneumonic effusion (clinical correlation required).

- Diaphragm position and shape:
  - Screening for hemidiaphragm elevation and its mimics (eg, eventration and subpulmonic effusion)
    - Normally the right hemidiaphragm sits ≤1.5 cm above the left (because of the liver)
    - When the hemidiaphragm heights appear even, rule out elevation of the left hemidiaphragm (with a lateral film)

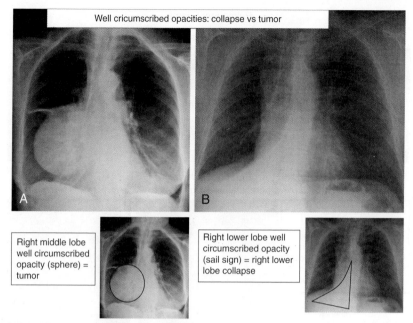

Fig. 4.6 (A) Frontal view of the chest shows a right middle lobe spherical opacity ≈ tumor. **Note:** subsegmental atelectasis (seen at the superior/lateral aspect of the opacity) may also be linear and well-circumscribed (eg, plate-like atelectasis). (B) Frontal view of the chest shows a well-circumscribed, triangular, right lower lobe opacity (a.k.a. **sail sign**) of the right lower lobe segmental collapse/atelectasis (note right sided volume loss).

- When the right hemidiaphragm is >1.5 cm above the left, rule out (or confirm) elevation with a lateral film
- Eventration of the hemidiaphragm refers to an anatomic variant where either the anterior (more common) or posterior portion of the hemidiaphragm focally herniates into the hemithorax
  - The most posterior aspect of the eventrated hemidiaphragm will abut the chest wall in a relatively normal (caudal) position, unlike a truly elevated hemidiaphragm
  - A truly elevated hemidiaphragm is elevated along its entire course such that the most posterior aspect will abut the chest wall in an inappropriately high position (Fig. 4.8)
- Subpulmonic effusion:
  - In some individuals pleural fluid settles in the potential space between the diaphragm and the inferior visceral pleura surface, giving the appearance of an elevated hemidiaphragm
  - An "elevated" hemidiaphragm with a laterally displaced peak should prompt consideration of a subpulmonic effusion
    - The lateral film can rule out eventration but cannot separate a subpulmonic effusion from a truly elevated hemidiaphragm
    - A decubitus film (looking for layering fluid) will differentiate between a truly elevated hemidiaphragm (no layering fluid) from a subpulmonic effusion, in which the fluid layers out along the lateral chest wall
  - Subpulmonic effusions are often significantly larger then they appear on chest x-ray, and can be difficult to tap in the traditional seated position because aerated lung will persist down to the base making the fluid pocket appear small (Fig. 4.9)
- Tenting of the diaphragm:
  - Atelectasis can pull on the diaphragm causing a focal "tent"-like distortion

Pulmonary Edema

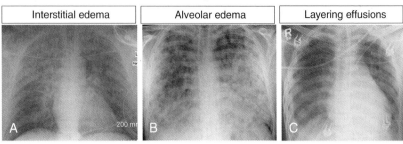

Fig. 4.7 Common radiographic patterns of pulmonary edema (the most common cause of acute diffuse lung disease). (A) Diffuse interstitial edema. (B) Diffuse alveolar edema (either cardiogenic or noncardiogenic). (C) Large layering effusions (no meniscus because the patient is supine). (D) Typical chest radiographs for the two most common chronic lung diseases: pulmonary fibrosis and chronic obstructive pulmonary disease (COPD). **Note:** pulmonary fibrosis and COPD are radiographic (and pathophysiologic) opposites. Fibrosis = small lungs with too many lines, whereas COPD = large lungs, not enough lines.

- Tenting of the diaphragm should prompt increased scrutiny of the x-ray to ensure that an area of atelectasis has not been overlooked (Fig. 4.10)
- Sharp costophrenic angles (CPAs) (Fig. 4.11):
  - Sharp CPAs on a frontal film imply that ≤200 mL of pleural fluid is present, effectively ruling out a moderate or large effusion
  - Sharp CPAs on a lateral film are even more sensitive to ruling out pleural fluid, implying that ≤50 mL of pleural fluid is present
  - Blunted CPAs may be present as a result of basilar pleural scarring (relatively common) or a small pleural effusion

Hemidiaphragm Elevation vs. Eventration

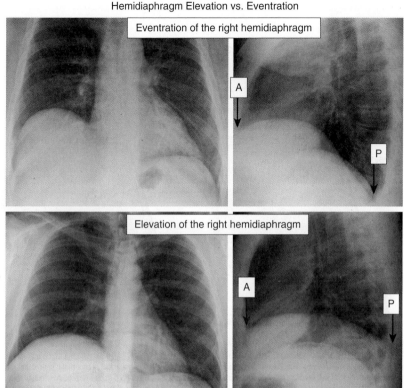

Fig. 4.8 **Eventration of the right hemidiaphragm.** Frontal view suggests an elevated right hemidiaphragm. However, the lateral film instead shows that only the anterior insertion point *(A)* is elevated. The posterior insertion point *(P)* is in the normal position. In contrast, the lateral film of the **elevation of the right hemidiaphragm** shows that both the anterior insertion point *(A)* and the posterior insertion point *(P)* are elevated. In other words, the hemidiaphragm is pathologically high along its entire course. NOTE: Complete eventration (uncommon) may be radiologically indistinguishable form an elevated hemidiaphragm

- **Complete opacification of the hemithorax (a.k.a. whole lung atelectasis, a.k.a. total lung collapse, a.k.a. white-out of the hemithorax):**
  - Complete opacification or "white-out" of a hemithorax **only** occurs when the **entire** lung is atelectatic
    - A unilateral, trilobar pneumonia will not opacify the entire hemithorax because there will always be some aeration (unlike total lung collapse = no aeration)
    - Although the apex of a completely opacified hemithorax always appears more lucent than the base, this lucency **does not** represent apical aeration
      - It occurs because the top of the thorax has less soft tissue than the base
  - Only two processes can cause whole lung atelectasis, leading to hemithorax opacification:
    - Effusion
    - Mainstem airway obstruction
  - Although an expanding pneumothorax can cause whole lung atelectasis (just before tension physiology)
    - The hemithorax appears lucent/black

Subpulmonic Effusion

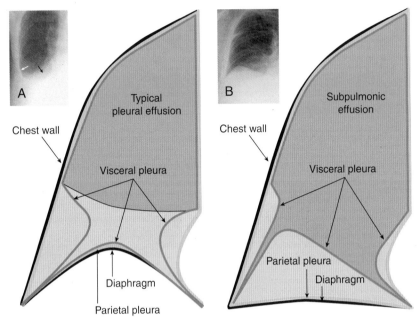

Fig. 4.9 (A) Frontal view of the chest (insert) shows the typical appearance of a right-sided pleural effusion opacifying the right hemidiaphragm (with a meniscus = well-circumscribed superior aspect). Two-dimensional schematic shows that a typical pleural effusion will sit above the visceral pleura along the diaphragm. (B) Upright frontal view of the chest (insert) shows the typical appearance of a right-sided sub pulmonic effusion, where the apex of the right hemidiaphragm appears elevated, laterally displaced, and unusually peaked. This suggests a subpulmonic effusion, where what appears to be the superior aspect of the diaphragm is actually the inferior aspect or the lungs' visceral pleural reflection. Two-dimensional schematic showing that the subpulmonic effusion involves fluid pooling under the lung and above the diaphragm.
Green line, visceral pleura; *yellow line,* parietal pleura; *red line,* diaphragm.

- **Effusion** (exudate or blood) causes whole lung atelectasis by external compression
  - The opacified hemithorax contains the atelectatic lung and the volume of surrounding fluid that caused the compression
    - Therefore the opacified hemithorax appears larger than normal and exhibits signs of volume gain (eg, tracheal deviation away from the opacity and increased rib spacing) (Fig. 4.12)
- **Mainstem airway obstruction** causes whole lung atelectasis by two mechanisms:
  - Mainstem mucus plugs cause rapid whole lung atelectasis by a "ball valve" phenomenon
    - The affected secretion moves proximally on exhalation, allowing air to escape; inhalation seats the mucus plug tightly in the distal airway, preventing air entry
  - Fixed mainstem obstructions (eg, tumor) cause whole lung atelectasis as alveolar air is reabsorbed and not replenished (more gradual)
  - Either way, the opacified hemithorax contains only the atelectatic lung
    - Therefore the opacified hemithorax appears smaller than normal and exhibits signs of volume loss (eg, tracheal deviation toward the opacity and rib crowding) (Fig. 4.13)

Tenting of the Daigphragm

Left upper lobe (ligula) atelectasis
- Frontal view of the left hemithorax demonstrates:
  - Vague, veil-like opacity "silhouetting out" the left heart border
  - Left upper lobe volume loss pulls the hemidiaphragm up
- Giving it a "tented" appearance

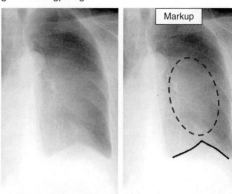

Right upper lobe atelectasis
- Frontal view of the right hemithorax demonstrates:
  - Well circumscribed, veil-like opacity "silhouetting out" the right hilum
  - Right upper lobe volume loss pulls the hemidiaphragm up
- Giving it a "tented" appearance

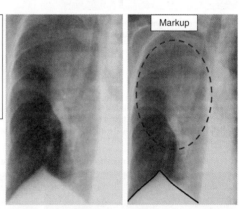

Fig. 4.10 Tenting of the diaphragm. Tenting of a hemidiaphragm should prompt a search for upper and/or middle lobe collapse, or pleural–parenchymal scarring.

Sharp Costophrenic Angles

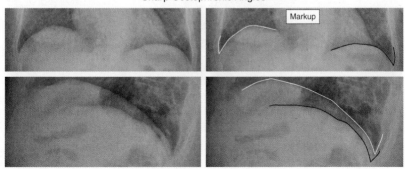

Fig. 4.11 Costophrenic angles. Chest x-ray close-up of the hemidiaphragms (frontal and lateral). Markup traces both the right hemidiaphragm (white line) and the left hemidiaphragm (black line), accentuating the clearly delineated "sharp" costophrenic angles.

White-out of the right hemithorax: Opacified side demonstrates **Volume Gain**

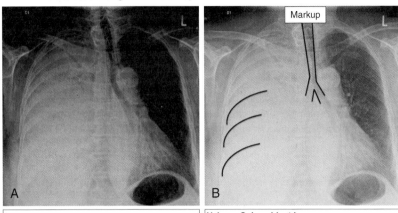

White-out of the right hemithorax with **Volume Gain** (opacified side) = **Pleural Effusion**	**Volume Gain evident by:** • Trachea and carina shifted away from the opacity • Increased rib spacing • Cardiac silhouette shifted to the left (**away** from the opacity)

Fig. 4.12 Complete lung collapse (a.k.a. total lung atelectasis, a.k.a. white-out of the hemithorax) with **volume gain**. (A) Overpenetrated frontal view of the chest demonstrating complete opacification of the right hemithorax with volume gain = right lung collapse from a pleural effusion causing extrinsic compression. (B) Same film with normal penetration and a markup outlining the tracheal shift away from the opacity and increased rib spacing (ie, evidence of volume gain).

White-out of the right hemithorax: Opacified side demonstrates **Volume Loss**

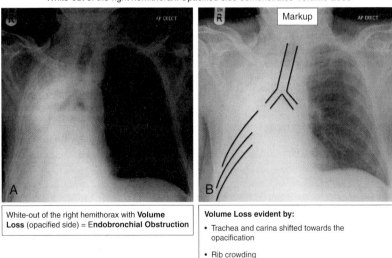

White-out of the right hemithorax with **Volume Loss** (opacified side) = **Endobronchial Obstruction**	**Volume Loss evident by:** • Trachea and carina shifted towards the opacification • Rib crowding • Cardiac silhouette shifted to the right (**towards** the opacity)

Fig. 4.13 Complete lung collapse (a.k.a. total lung atelectasis, a.k.a. white-out of the hemithorax) with **volume loss**. (A) Shows an overpenetrated frontal view of the chest demonstrating complete opacification of the right hemithorax with volume loss = right lung collapse from endobronchial obstruction. (B) Shows the same film with normal penetration and a markup outlining the tracheal shift toward the opacity and rib crowding (ie, evidence of volume loss).

- When whole lung atelectasis occurs acutely, it causes physiologic shunt with severe hypoxemia
- Additionally, when whole lung atelectasis is secondary to compression by an effusion, tension physiology (where high thoracic pressure impairs venous return, thereby decreasing cardiac output) may occur
- Individuals with acute whole lung atelectasis will require an urgent procedure—either:
  - Bronchoscopy to relieve a mainstem airway obstruction, or
  - Thoracentesis to relieve compression
- Determining the etiology hinges on whether the opacified hemithorax exhibits volume loss (mainstem airway obstruction) or volume gain (compression secondary to effusion)
- The mainstem air column of the completely atelectatic lung typically has an abrupt end (in both external compression and airway obstruction)
  - This is often erroneously interpreted as proof of endobronchial obstruction
  - In compression from effusion this represents the point where extrinsic compression is resisted by the cartilaginous rings of the mainstem bronchi
  - In mainstem obstruction this represents the point of airway blockage
- Occasionally the volume of the opacified hemithorax appears normal (no definite shift)
  - When this occurs, caution is warranted as both effusion and obstruction may be present (eg, stage IV lung cancer)
  - A CT scan of the chest (possibly with contrast for better pleural definition) and ultrasound should be considered
  - If advanced imaging still fails to clarify the situation, bronchoscopy should be done first to rule out endobronchial obstruction (before a thoracentesis)
    - If the airway is obstructed, removal of fluid will **not** result in lung re-expansion
    - Instead, thoracentesis may create an "ex vacuo" space, causing pain and possible bronchoplural (BP) fistula formation (see Chapter 17)
- Segmental lung collapse
  - Segmental lung collapse implies airway obstruction and requires investigation, typically with CT scanning and bronchoscopy, to rule out obstructing malignancy, foreign body, or mucus plug
  - Upper lobe collapse is ominous, raising concerning for endobronchial malignancy
    - Upper lobes are preferentially ventilated and thus are disproportionately exposed to inhaled carcinogens
    - Upper lobes are less vulnerable to foreign body aspiration and mucus impaction
  - Lower lobe and middle lobe obstructions are more likely to be benign because these dependent regions are vulnerable to foreign body and mucus impaction
  - Lateral films are essential to confirm or refute collapse concerns
  - Each lung segment collapses in a predictable fashion, giving a classic radiographic pattern, generally:
    - Upper and middle lobes collapse anteriorly; lower lobes collapse posteriorly
    - Right upper, right lower, and left lower lobe collapses result in well-circumscribed opacities on the frontal film (Figs. 4.14–4.16)
    - Right middle and left upper lobes (including the lingula) cause well-circumscribed opacities on the lateral film (Figs. 4.17 and 4.18)

COMMON QUESTIONS GENERATED BY THIS TEACHING

1. Could a trained radiologist see the heart border or diaphragm that I cannot find?
   No. The heart borders and diaphragms should be clear to anyone. The tendency of the neophyte is to create an anticipated line where it actual is not. Zooming in on the line in question can help prevent this error.

Right Upper Lobe Collapse

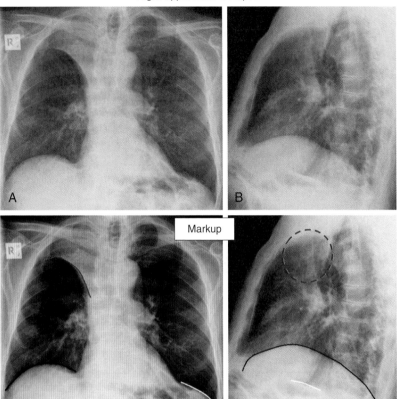

Fig. 4.14 Right upper lobe (RUL) collapse. (A) Frontal film of the chest shows a well-circumscribed, "chalice"-shaped opacity silhouetting out the right paratracheal stripe (and the right apex). The right hemidiaphragm height is >1.5 cm above the left (suggesting elevation). (B) Lateral film shows a vague, veil-like opacity extending from the right apex to the superior aspect of the anterior clear space. Right hemidiaphragm elevation confirmed on the lateral film (posterior insertion point is elevated). **Note:** unrelated to the right upper lobe collapse, this patient has left lower lobe scarring. Frontal film shows retrocardiac linear bands opacifying the medial portion of the left hemidiaphragm. Lateral film shows a vague opacity obscuring the left hemidiaphragm. This demonstrates the "spine sign" (failing to progressively clear toward the base of the spine).
Black line, right hemidiaphragm; *dotted red line,* atelectatic right upper lobe (RUL) (vague in the lateral projection); *solid red line,* minor fissure (concaved and displaced superiorly); *white line,* left hemidiaphragm.

2. **Why is the apex more "aerated" than the base in the completely atelectatic lung?**
   It is not. There is no aeration in a completely atelectatic lung. The apex is more lucent than the base because humans have less soft tissue at the apex of the chest than they do at the base.

3. **How can I tell the difference between subsegmental atelectasis and pneumonia on a CXR film?**
   Unless you are dealing with a linear "plate-like" atelectasis, you cannot. Clinical correlation is required. If the patient has a fever and a cough, it is pneumonia. In the absence of pneumonia symptoms, consider atelectasis.

Right Lower Lobe Collapse

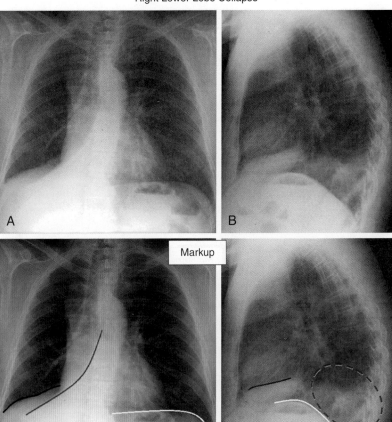

Fig. 4.15 Right lower lobe (RLL) collapse. (A) Frontal view shows a dense, well-circumscribed, "sail" shaped opacity silhouetting out the medial portion of the right hemidiaphragm (the right hemidiaphragm is often completely silhouetted out). The right hemidiaphragm height is >1.5 cm above the left (suggesting elevation). (B) Lateral view shows a vague opacity at the right base, creating the "spine sign" (failing to progressively clear toward the base of the spine). **Note:** right lung volume loss is evident by shifting of the trachea to the right.

Black line, traces the right hemidiaphragm; *red line,* outlines the RLL; *white line,* traces the left hemidiaphragm.

4. **How can I distinguish partial eventration of a hemidiaphragm from true elevation?**
   By examining where the posterior aspect of the diaphragm in question abuts the chest wall on the lateral film. If insertion is normal, you have eventration; if insertion is abnormally high, you have an elevated hemidiaphragm.

5. **When should I get a posteroanterior (PA) and lateral CXR instead of a portable one?**
   Whenever possible, frontal/portable films generate questions that lateral films answer. Only accept a portable film in a patient too sick for a PA and lateral.

6. **What should I do when I find a vague, hard to characterize opacity on a CXR film?**
   Obtain a noncontrast chest CT for better definition. Important lesions (eg, lung cancer) can appear vague on x-ray film.

Left Lower Lobe Collapse

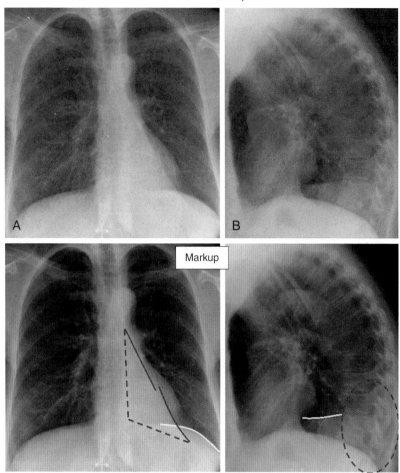

Fig. 4.16 Left lower lobe (LLL) collapse. (A) Frontal view shows a dense, well-circumscribed, triangular opacity in the retrocardiac space, silhouetting out the medial portion of the left hemidiaphragm. The opacity creates the "double left heart boarder" sign. Hemidiaphragm heights appear equal (suggesting elevation of the left). (B) Lateral view shows a vague opacity at the left base, creating the "spine sign" (failing to progressively clear toward the base of the spine). The left hemidiaphragm is elevated and opacified posteriorly. **Note:** though not evident on this film, occasionally LLL volume loss is evident by shifting of the right heart border to the left (behind the spine).

Red lines, outline the LLL; *white line,* traces the visualized portion of the left hemidiaphragm.

Right Middle Lobe Collapse

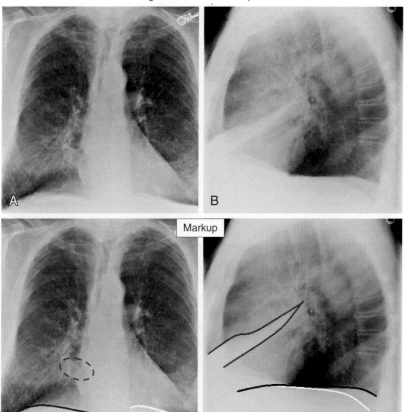

Fig. 4.17 Right middle lobe (RML) collapse. (A) Frontal view shows a vague opacity silhouetting out the right heart border. (B) Lateral film shows a dense, well-circumscribed, wedge shaped opacity sharply demarcating the lower aspect of the anterior clear space. **Note:** the lateral film suggests severe chronic obstructive pulmonary disease with flattened hemidiaphragms and a barrel shaped chest.

Black line, traces the right hemidiaphragm; *red lines,* outline the RML; *white line,* traces the left hemidiaphragm.

Left Upper Lobe and Lingula Collapse

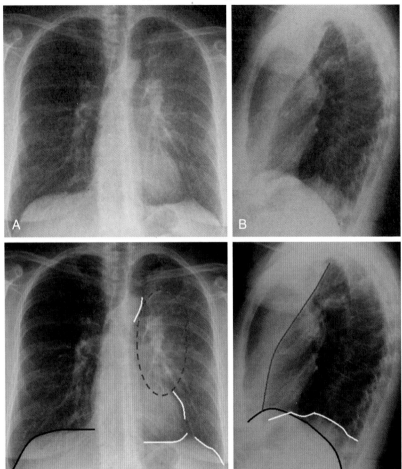

Fig. 4.18 Left upper lobe (LUL) and ligula collapse. (A) Frontal view shows a diffuse veil over the left hemithorax with a vague opacity obscuring the anteroposterior window (descending aorta silhouetted out), and a vascular pattern obscuring the left heart border. Additionally, the left hemidiaphragm is "tented." (B) Lateral view shows a well-circumscribed opacity along the entire anterior chest and an elevated left hemidiaphragm. **Note**: all of the aeration in the left chest is in the hyperexpanded left lower lobe. The arm is not fully raised on the lateral film, causing an additional apical anterior opacity.

Black line, traces the right hemidiaphragm; *red lines,* outline the LUL (and lingula); *white line,* traces the left hemidiaphragm.

DYSPNEA AND EXERCISE LIMITATION

CHAPTER 5

COMMON MISCONCEPTIONS AND MISTAKES

- Hypoxemia is a common cause of dyspnea
- Hypoxemia is a common cause of exercise limitation in patients with chronic obstructive pulmonary disease (COPD)
- Believing that normal exercise is limited by the ability of an individual to blow off CO_2
- Believing that normal exercise is limited by O_2 desaturation and hypoxemia
- Believing that lung disease generates dyspnea solely by gas exchange/ventilation abnormalities (eg, $\uparrow Pco_2$, $\downarrow pH$, $\downarrow Po_2$)
- Failing to treat exertional syncope as a medical emergency

MAJOR MECHANISMS OF DYSPNEA (Fig. 5.1)

- Dyspnea is the **subjective** perception of a **discomfort associated with breathing**
  - Existing on a spectrum ranging from "needing to catch one's breath" after maximal exercise, to shortness of breath, to "air hunger" (ie, a sense of suffocation accompanied by panic)
- Dyspnea is generated (in isolation or in combination) by:
  - **Acidosis** (eg, lactic acid, ketoacid, uncleared organic acids, elevated Pco_2)
  - **Respiratory system neuromechanical dissociation** (especially when paired with a ventilatory stimulus)
  - **Increased cardiovascular pressure** (eg, pulmonary vascular, intracardiac, aortic)
  - **Primary amygdala activation** (eg, anxiety, depression, posttraumatic stress disorder [PTSD], panic disorder)
- **Respiratory system neuromechanical dissociation occurs when the brainstem respiratory center senses a mismatch between breathing effort and return on effort (ie, air movement)**
  - When efferent neurologic output regulating tidal volume (TV) and respiratory rate (RR) fails to achieve the anticipated mechanical result, as sensed by air flow and chest expansion, dyspnea ensues
    - Extreme dyspnea occurs when neuromechanical dissociation is paired with a ventilatory stimulus (eg, hypercarbia, metabolic acidosis, hypoxemia)
    - This is a common cause of ventilator dyssynchrony and patient discomfort in individuals with extremely abnormal pulmonary mechanics who require mechanical ventilation and permissive hypercarbia
- **Dyspnea may also be generated by the cardiovascular system by three major mechanisms** (angina, baroreceptor activation, and cardiogenic pulmonary edema)
  - **Angina** may be perceived as dyspnea (without chest pressure or pain)
    - Dyspnea as an anginal equivalent terminates exercise in an effort to decrease myocardial oxygen demand
  - **Stretch or baroreceptor** activation occurs when cardiac chambers (both right and left) and/or large vessels experience increased pressure (and thus stretch), as occurs during heart failure or increased afterload

MAJOR MECHANISMS OF DYSPNEA

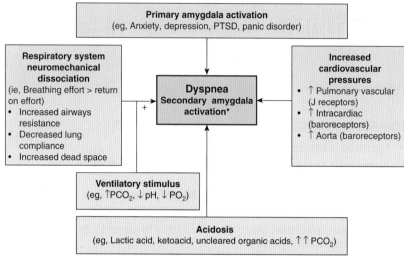

* Secondary to respiratory center activation or increased cardiovascular pressures

Fig. 5.1 Diagram showing the four major mechanisms responsible for the sensation of dyspnea. Ultimately, dyspnea involves activation of the amygdala (responsible for anxiety, discomfort, and panic). This is referred to as secondary amygdala activation because it occurs in response to a stimulus (eg, acidosis) to separate it from the primary anxiety states that cause dyspnea directly (ie, primary amygdala activation). Although a ventilatory stimulus (like hypoxemia) will cause an increased MV, this alone is not enough to cause dyspnea unless it is extreme ($PaO_2 < 50$ mm Hg) or paired with a respiratory system neuromechanical dissociation.

- Baroreceptor activation generates a sense of dyspnea aimed at terminating exercise in an effort to lower cardiovascular pressure
- **Cardiogenic pulmonary edema** may produce extreme dyspnea primarily by decreasing pulmonary compliance, leading to respiratory center neuromechanical dissociation (often paired with hypoxemia as a ventilatory stimulus)
- Primary amygdala activation, as is seen with anxiety, depression, PTSD, and panic disorder may be perceived as dyspnea that occurs intermittently and is **not** associated with an exercise limitation
- Dyspnea generated by the cardiovascular system, the respiratory system, or acidosis is designed to terminate exercise (ie, dyspnea on exertion)
  - Secondary activation of the amygdala occurs to varying degrees based on the magnitude of the acidosis, the neuromechanical dissociation, and/or the cardiovascular pressure increase
- Chronic mild hypoxemia (PaO_2 55–60 mm Hg), most commonly seen with COPD, does not create significant dyspnea or limit exercise and is treated in an effort to extend life and prevent heart failure, not to reduce dyspnea or improve exercise ability (both of which are caused by impaired ventilation, **not** oxygenation)
  - Chronic mild hypoxemia may be asymptomatic or associated with mild cognitive impairment/confusion
- Acute mild hypoxemia may increase minute ventilation via the hypoxic hyperventilation reflex, causing tachypnea, *but* **dyspnea is minimal** if hypoxemia is not coupled with exercise
- Chronic moderate to severe hypoxemia, most commonly seen with pulmonary fibrosis, limits exercise and causes dyspnea by desaturation and hypoxemia

PHYSIOLOGY OF EXERCISE (Table 5.1)

- **Normal exercise** is limited by **cardiac output** and its ability to:
  - Deliver oxygenated blood to exercising muscles
  - Mobilize lactate, generated by skeletal muscle (anaerobic metabolism), to the liver
- Ultimately exercise terminates with symptomatic lactic acidosis (ie, breathlessness, lightheadedness, leg heaviness, nausea)

Table 5.1 Evaluation of Dyspnea

CATEGORY OF EXERCISE LIMITATION (AND ASSOCIATED DISEASES)	ANTICIPATED DERANGEMENTS CARDIAC OUTPUT/ LACTIC ACID/PH/P_{CO_2}	CAUSE OF EXERCISE LIMITATION
Normal exercise limitation	↑↑ Cardiac output, ↑↑ lactic acid, ↓ pH, ↓ P_{CO_2}	Lactic acidosis
Athlete exercise limitation	↑↑↑↑ Cardiac output, ↑↑↑ lactic acid, ↓↓ pH, ↓↓ P_{CO_2}	Lactic acidosis
Deconditioned exercise limitation	↑ Cardiac output, ↑ lactic acid, ↓ pH, ↓ P_{CO_2}	Lactic acidosis
Cardiac exercise limitation LHF (HFpEF/HFrEF/valve disease) Isolated RHF PAH	− Cardiac output, ↑↑ lactic acid, ↓ pH, ↓ P_{CO_2}	Lactic acidosis
Moderate ventilatory exercise limitation Obstructive disease Neuromuscular weakness	↑ Cardiac output, ↑ lactic acid, ↓↓ pH, − P_{CO_2}	Lactic acidosis
Severe ventilatory exercise limitation Obstructive disease Neuromuscular weakness*	↑ Cardiac output, − lactic acid, ↓ pH, ↑ P_{CO_2}	Respiratory acidosis
Exercise induced desaturation Moderate–severe diffuse parenchymal lung disease (and mimics)	↑ Cardiac output, ↑ lactic acid, − pH, ↓↓ P_{CO_2}	Hypoxemia
Dyspnea—cardiovascular origin Hypertension and/or volume overload ↑ Afterload (hypertension) ↑ LVEDP (volume overload) ↑ Pulmonary vascular pressure	↑ Cardiac output, ↑ lactic acid, ↓ pH, ↓ P_{CO_2}	Dyspnea (baroreceptor mediated)
Dyspnea—respiratory origin Mild obstructive disease Mild restrictive disease	↑ Cardiac output, ↑ lactic acid, ↓ pH, ↓ P_{CO_2}	Dyspnea (neuromechanical dissociation and ventilatory stimulus)
Dyspnea/fatigue—metabolic acidosis	↑ Cardiac output, ↑ lactic acid, ↓↓ pH, ↓ P_{CO_2}	Dyspnea (metabolic acidosis)
Dyspnea/fatigue—anemia	↑ Cardiac output, ↑↑ lactic acid, ↓ pH, ↓ P_{CO_2}	Dyspnea (lactic acidosis)

HFpEF, heart failure with preserved ejection fraction; *HFrEF,* heart failure with reduced ejection fraction; *LHF,* left heart failure; *LVEDP,* left ventricular end-diastolic pressure; *PAH,* pulmonary arterial hypertension; *RHF,* right heart failure.
*Although neuromuscular weakness causes restrictive physiology during pulmonary function testing (PFT), it also causes a ventilatory exercise limitation.

- The experience of breathlessness comes from a low pH secondary to lactate (metabolic acidosis)
  - Pco_2 is compensatorily low (ie, pH 7.**32**/Pco_2 **32** mm Hg)
- **Trained athletes** owe their increased exercise capacity to:
  - Trained skeletal muscle, which is more efficient at oxygen uptake
  - The ability to dramatically increase their cardiac output (up to 40 L/min)
  - The ability to tolerate a lower pH
- **Deconditioning** describes the situation in which the normal limitation to exercise, namely cardiac output, oxygen delivery, and lactate mobilization, occur earlier during exercise than normal
  - Atrophied, untrained skeletal muscle enters anaerobic metabolism more quickly

PATHOPHYSIOLOGY OF CARDIAC MEDIATED DYSPNEA ON EXERTION AND EXERCISE LIMITATION (see Table 5.1)

- **Left-sided heart disease limits exercise** primarily by inadequate left ventricular (LV) cardiac output secondary to either:
  - **Decreased LV systolic function** (ie, cardiomyopathy)
  - **Aortic** or **mitral valve stenosis** or **regurgitation**
  - **LV diastolic dysfunction**
    - Exercise-provoked diastolic dysfunction (from ischemia, hypertension, tachyarrhythmia, or hypoxemia) limits exercise, as impaired ventricular filling leads to an inadequate cardiac output (CO) relative to the needs of lactate mobilization and systemic oxygen delivery
      - Exercise terminates early secondary to symptomatic lactic acidosis
- **Decreased LV cardiac output may lead to an increased LVEDP**
- **Increased left ventricular end-diastolic pressure (LVEDP) limits exercise by three major mechanisms:**
  - The biventricular heart failure reflex (triggered at an LVEDP >15 mm Hg) further limits exercise via pulmonary hypertension and decreased right ventricular (RV) cardiac output
  - Additionally, mild increases in LVEDP in the 15 mm Hg to 18 mm Hg range may activate cardiac baroreceptors and pulmonary capillary J receptors, producing dyspnea **before** pulmonary edema
  - Higher LVEDP elevations (>18 mm Hg) cause interstitial and alveolar edema
    - This limits exercise by decreased compliance, increased airway resistance (submucosal edema), and by provoking respiratory system neuromechanical dissociation
    - Pulmonary edema may also cause hypoxemia, further intensifying the sensation of dyspnea (by pairing neuromechanical dissociation with the increased ventilatory drive of hypoxemia)
- **Pulmonary arterial hypertension (PAH)**, as seen in chronic thromboembolic pulmonary hypertension (CTEPH) and idiopathic pulmonary arterial hypertension (IPAH), limits exercise (before right-sided heart failure) by loss of the pulmonary vascular bed cross-sectional area, which leads to increased pulmonary vascular resistance
  - During extreme exercise, CO increases two- to fourfold
  - The systemic circulation handles this increase in blood volume by vasodilatation of resistance arterioles
  - The pulmonary circulation handles this increase in volume by passive distention
    - Vascular obliteration in PAH decreases the capacity of the pulmonary vasculature to distend and accommodate the increased blood volume required by exercise
      - Instead, as the RV attempts to increase CO to handle the increased venous return, pulmonary artery pressure rises, limiting RV CO and underfilling the LV
        - This can lead to exertional syncope (and death), as the vasodilated systemic vasculature fails to receive enough blood return from the failing RV
          - Exertional syncope is a "heralding event," mandating immediate evaluation

- **Isolated right-sided heart failure** (as occurs in decompensated PAH) limits exercise by inadequate RV CO, which leads to an underfilled LV, producing an inadequate CO relative to the needs of lactate mobilization and systemic oxygen delivery
  - Leading to a symptomatic lactic acidosis with minimal exertion (New York Heart Association [NYHA] class III–IV)

PATHOPHYSIOLOGY OF PULMONARY-MEDIATED DYSPNEA ON EXERTION AND EXERCISE LIMITATION (see Table 5.1)

- **Obstructive lung disease** (eg, COPD/emphysema/asthma/bronchial hyperreactivity)
  - **Mild** to **moderate obstruction** causes dyspnea and limits exercise by increasing the work of breathing to a degree that it prevents appropriate respiratory compensation
    - Exercise may terminate prematurely (from a cardiac output standpoint) because of inappropriate respiratory compensation, where a relatively elevated Pco_2, promotes a symptomatic lactic acidosis (ie, pH 7.27/Pco_2 37 mm Hg)
    - Additionally, exercise may terminate prematurely secondary to dyspnea generated by **respiratory system neuromechanical dissociation** (as breathing effort increases with diminishing returns), related to increased airways resistance, dynamic hyperinflation, and intrinsic positive end expiratory pressure (PEEP)
      - Made worse as it is paired with acidosis
  - **Severe obstruction** may cause dyspnea and limit exercise by an inability to increase minute ventilation in response to relatively small amounts of exercise/aerobic metabolism
    - Exercise terminates early (eg, at less than half a flight of stairs) secondary to acidosis as pH falls and Pco_2 increases (producing a threatened or actual respiratory acidosis) before "anaerobic threshold" and significant lactate can be generated
    - Dyspnea from neuromechanical dissociation related to airway resistance, dynamic hyperinflation, and intrinsic-PEEP may further impair exercise, especially when paired with acidosis
  - **Very severe obstruction**, when paired with an intact ventilatory drive (a.k.a. pink puffers) may produce constant dyspnea (even at rest) as the heterogeneously destroyed lung inefficiently scrubs CO_2
    - This inefficient CO_2 removal necessitates an increased resting minute ventilation in an attempt to maintain a normal resting Pco_2
      - Ultimately leading to pulmonary cachexia because of the metabolic demands of persistently increased breathing
    - Individuals with a blunted respiratory drive (a.k.a. blue bloaters) experience less dyspnea, allowing their Pco_2 to rise gradually over time (ultimately causing hypoxemia and heart failure)
- **Restrictive lung disease** (eg, pleural disease, neuromuscular weakness, or diffuse parenchymal lung disease [DPLD])
  - **Pleural disease** alone (eg, pleural thickening, chronic pleural effusion) should not affect exercise or produce a significant restrictive defect
  - **Pleural disease with associated atelectasis** (eg, pleural thickening with lung entrapment) is more likely to produce symptomatic restriction, impairing exercise by increasing the work of breathing and signaling dyspnea through neuromechanical dissociation
  - **Neuromuscular weakness** causes dyspnea via neuromechanical dissociation and restrictive physiology, which limits **ventilatory** ability
    - Dyspnea is worsened by supine positioning, which removes the mechanical advantage of gravity during diaphragmatic excursion
      - Responds well to positive airway pressure (eg, bilevel positive airway pressure)
    - Progressive neuromuscular weakness ultimately leads to hypercarbic respiratory failure
  - **Mild** restriction from **DPLD** may produce dyspnea and limit exercise by neuromechanical dissociation

- **Moderate** to **severe** restriction from **DPLD** may limit exercise by causing profound O_2 desaturations (ie, $PaO_2 < 50$ mm Hg)
  - These individuals experience dramatically improved exercise ability with oxygen supplementation

PATHOPHYSIOLOGY OF ACIDOSIS AND ANEMIA-MEDIATED DYSPNEA ON EXERTION AND EXERCISE LIMITATION (see Table 5.1)

- **Metabolic acidosis:**
  - Patients with an acute metabolic acidosis (eg, ketoacidosis) may present with a chief complaint of dyspnea and/or fatigue (at rest and/or with minimal exertion)
    - Dyspnea is driven by the low pH itself
  - Patients with a chronic metabolic acidosis (eg, chronic kidney disease or end stage renal disease) may have a diminished exercise capacity, as exercise-induced lactic acid adds to the preexisting metabolic acidosis, which further lowers pH, creates dyspnea, and limits exercise by symptomatic acidosis
    - Screen for with a serum HCO_3 and a venous blood gas (VBG) or arterial blood gas (ABG)
    - Increasing the amount of buffer these patients receive either via oral supplementation or at dialysis can help
- **Anemia**:
  - The exact mechanism by which anemia limits exercise is not agreed on, but decreased oxygen-carrying capacity and early lactate generation are probably central
  - The exercise limitation may be described as fatigue more than dyspnea
  - Screen for with a hemoglobin/hematocrit check

PRIMARY ACTIVATION OF THE AYGDALA-MEDIATED DYSPNEA (DYSPNEA WITHOUT AN ACCOMPANYING EXERCISE LIMITATION)

- Dyspnea without an exercise limitation is often caused by primary activation of the amygdala related to untreated or poorly treated depression, anxiety, PTSD, and/or panic disorder
  - **Dyspnea** typically occurs intermittently, often at rest, and is worse during times of stress
  - Individuals may complain of "forgetting to breathe" or dyspnea while speaking
  - Similarly, inadequately treated anxiety and depression intensifies the experience of dyspnea for patients with chronic lung disease
    - Often detectable in a panicked edge to typically routine complaints (eg, "I really felt like I was going to die after being out of breath in the shower")
  - Dyspnea **without** an exercise limitation should be managed with:
    - Reassurance:
      - Providing reassurance may require demonstrating a normal chest x-ray, pulmonary function testing (PFT), and an echocardiogram in some cases (despite normal exercise ability)
    - Depression, anxiety, and PTSD screening
    - Counseling
    - Diagnostic/therapeutic selective serotonin reuptake inhibitor (SSRI) trial can provide dramatic relief/improvement

EVALUATION OF DYSPNEA AND EXERCISE LIMITATION
(Fig. 5.2)

- The first step in the evaluation of dyspnea is to characterize the associated exercise limitation (ie, nonexistent, intermittent or persistent)
- An **intermittent** exercise limitation is unusual in patients with parenchymal lung disease or heart failure and should prompt a screen for:

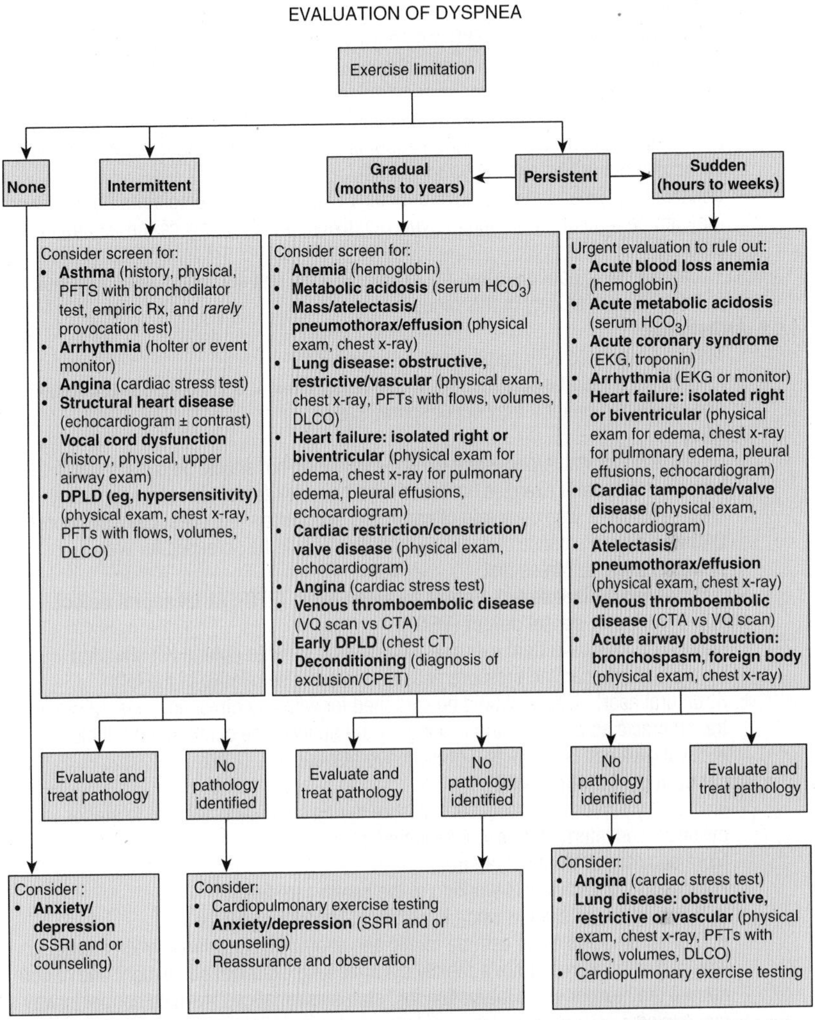

EVALUATION OF DYSPNEA

Fig. 5.2 Schematic diagram outlining the evaluation of dyspnea. The initial step involves characterizing any associated exercise limitation. Absence of an exercise limitation is very suggestive of primary amygdala activation/anxiety as the etiology. An intermittent exercise limitation generates a specific differential. Sudden dyspnea is a red-flag symptom, mandating urgent evaluation to rule out life-threatening cardiopulmonary diseases (eg, ST-elevation myocardial infarction, venous thromboembolism). A sudden exercise limitation is more likely to be of cardiac (rather than pulmonary) origin. A gradual exercise limitation most often represents lung disease (obstructive more common than restrictive). PFTs and echocardiogram should be obtained early in the evaluation of an unexplained exercise limitation.

- **Asthma**:
  - Clinical diagnosis
    - History reveals episodic airflow obstruction/wheezing, often in response to predictable environmental triggers
    - May have personal or family history of atopy and other allergies
    - Diffuse expiratory wheezing during physical examination strongly suggests bronchial hyperreactivity (vs submucosal edema) and, in the right clinical setting, asthma

- PFTs may be normal on a "good day" or obstructed on a "bad day"
- PFTs showing that the FEV_1/FVC ratio **normalizes** after bronchodilator is **very suggestive** of bronchial hyperreactivity and, in the correct clinical setting, asthma (but this finding is not common or required for the diagnosis)
- The suspected diagnosis of asthma should be pursued with a diagnostic/therapeutic trial of a short acting β-agonist (may provide instant relief) or inhaled corticosteroid (ICS) (takes days to weeks)
- Occasionally, when patients have difficulty characterizing complaints (that may or may not be a result of bronchial hyperreactivity), bronchoprovocation testing can be used
  - Unfortunately, patients **often** fail to complete the test secondary to apprehension (high rates of anxiety in this group)
- **Arrhythmia**:
  - May be associated with palpitations
  - Arrhythmia should be screened for with a holter monitor if the episodes are frequent and an event monitor if they occur sporadically
- **Angina**:
  - Often causes a stable/persistent exercise limitation but should be considered in those with an intermittent exercise limitation who have risk factors for coronary artery disease (CAD) or who complain of common associations (eg, chest pain, diaphoresis)
  - CAD as a possible cause of exercise limitation should be screened for with a treadmill exercise stress test
- **Structural heart disease (eg, Patent foramen ovale (PFO), Atrial septal defect (ASD), Ventricular septal defect (VSD))**:
  - May cause an intermittent exercise limitation by variable right to left shunting (if right-sided intracardiac pressure rises during exercise relative to the left)
  - Structural heart disease should be screened for with a contrast (ie, agitated saline) transthoracic echocardiogram looking for the appearance of left-sided bubbles
    - A Valsalva can be used as a provocative maneuver
- **Vocal cord dysfunction (VCD)**:
  - Involuntary paradoxical vocal cord closure during inspiration, leading to stridor, dyspnea, and intermittent exercise limitation
  - More common in women than men
  - Predilection for individuals working in the health care field
  - VCD should be considered when intermittent stridor is detected
  - VCD often presents as an asthma mimic and should be considered when individuals with "asthma" demonstrate a rapidly dynamic lung examination (ie, tight one minute, normal the next) or when intubation for "status asthmaticus" reveals normal airway mechanics
  - VCD may be diagnosed by an upper airway examination demonstrating paradoxical vocal cord motion
  - Treat with speech therapy and reassurance
- **Hypersensitivity lung disease (symptoms may be intermittent related to exposure)**
  - History should attempt to identify triggering exposures (ie, worse at work)
  - Screen for with posteroranterior (PA) and lateral (LAT) chest x-ray and PFTs with flows, volumes and a DLCO measurement
- If the above evaluation for **an intermittent exercise limitation**/dyspnea fails to reveal an etiology, consider:
  - Screening for and/or empirically treating anxiety/depression
  - Reassurance and observation (bad entities have been ruled out)
  - Cardiopulmonary exercise testing (CPET):
    - Allows for the measurement of multiple variables during maximum exercise

- Screens for exercise-induced hypertension, arrhythmia, O_2 desaturation
  - An ABG may be obtained to determine pH and respiratory compensation
- Provides an objective assessment of exercise ability
- Helps exclude less-common etiologies before concluding an individual is deconditioned
- Patients with a **persistent exercise limitation** should be further divided into those whose limitation has occurred **gradually** (over months to years) vs those whose limitation occurred **suddenly** (over hours to weeks)
- A **sudden exercise limitation** (hours to weeks) should prompt an urgent evaluation (ie, emergency room) to screen for:
  - **Acute blood loss anemia** (eg, gastrointestinal bleed) with a hemoglobin and hematocrit
  - **Acute metabolic acidosis** (eg, lactic acidosis, ketoacidosis) with a serum HCO_3
  - **Acute coronary syndrome** (eg, ST-elevation myocardial infarction) with an ECG and serial troponins
  - **Arrhythmia** (eg, atrial fibrillation with rapid ventricular rate) with an ECG or monitor
  - **Heart failure** (eg, biventricular or isolated right) with a physical examination, chest x-ray, and echocardiogram
  - **Cardiac tamponade or valvular heart disease** with a physical examination and an echocardiogram
  - **Atelectasis, pneumothorax, effusion** with a physical examination and a PA and LAT chest x-ray
  - **Venous thromboembolic disease** (eg, acute pulmonary embolism):
    - CT pulmonary angiography (CTA) preferred to ventilation perfusion (VQ) scan for sudden dyspnea/exercise limitation because it may reveal an alternate pathology/explanation
  - **Acute airway obstruction** (eg, bronchospasm, foreign body) with a physical examination and PA and LAT chest x-ray
- If the above emergency room based evaluation for a sudden exercise limitation/dyspnea fails to reveal an etiology, consider additional screening (as an outpatient) for:
  - **Angina** with a cardiac stress test
  - **Lung disease** (ie, obstructive, restrictive, and/or pulmonary vascular disease) with PFT (flows, volumes, and diffusing capacity of the lungs for carbon monoxide [DLCO])
- A **gradual exercise limitation** (years) is more likely to be of pulmonary origin (eg, COPD) and less likely to be a heralding sign of impeding cardiopulmonary catastrophe
- Diagnostic testing focuses on ruling out significant cardiopulmonary disease
- The history, physical examination, and a chest x-ray should guide the initial testing strategy (eg, PFT vs echocardiogram)
  - Both should be obtained if neither heart nor lung is the obvious culprit
- A moderate to severe exercise limitation will usually be associated with an obvious abnormality found on:
  - Physical examination (eg, wheezing, absent breath sounds, new heart murmur, edema)
  - Chest x-ray (eg, mixed emphysema and fibrosis, pulmonary edema, whole lung atelectasis)
  - PFTs (eg, moderate to severe obstruction, restriction, or impaired diffusion)
  - Echocardiogram (ie, heart failure and valvular disease)
- A **gradual** exercise limitation should prompt an evaluation for:
  - **Anemia**:
    - Screen for with a hemoglobin/hematocrit check
  - **Metabolic acidosis**:
    - Screen for with a serum HCO_3 and a VBG or ABG
  - **Mass/atelectasis/pneumothorax/effusion**:
    - Thoracic mass, lobar atelectasis (from pleural disease or airway obstruction), pneumothorax (small and large), and effusion (small or large) may produce dyspnea

and limit exercise by causing neuromechanical dissociation and increasing the work of breathing
- Whole lung atelectasis from mass, effusion, or mainstem airway obstruction causes shunt physiology and may limit exercise by desaturation and hypoxemia
- Large pneumothorax may also limit exercise by decreasing venous return
- Screen for with a physical examination and a PA and LAT chest x-ray

- **Lung disease (obstructive, restrictive, and pulmonary vascular disease):**
  - Most lung disease must be moderate to severe to significantly affect normal daily exertion
  - Mild lung disease may decrease maximum exercise capacity but should not cause impairment in normal activities
    - Be wary attributing a significant exercise limitation to mild PFT abnormalities
      - A concomitant process (eg, heart failure) might be present
  - Screen for with a physical examination and PFT (flows, volumes, DLCO):
    - FEV_1/FVC <70% diagnoses obstruction; the FEV_1 % predicted determines the severity
    - Total lung capacity (TLC) <80% diagnoses restriction; severity based on % predicted
    - FEV_1/FVC <70% with a TLC <80% diagnoses mixed obstructive restrictive disease; severity assessed clinically and radiographically, **not** by FEV_1 or TLC (given pseudonormalization)
    - DLCO <80% diagnoses a diffusion limitation; severity rated based on % predicted
      - An isolated low DLCO (or a DLCO reduced out of proportion to the degree of obstruction) can indicate mixed obstructive restrictive disease, pulmonary vascular disease (PAH), or early DPLD and should prompt consideration for both:
        - Ventilation perfusion scanning to screen for chronic thromboembolic pulmonary hypertension (CTEPH)
        - Noncontrast chest computed tomography (CT) scan looking for early DPLD or radiographically subtle mixed obstructive restrictive disease

- **Heart failure (isolated right or biventricular):**
  - Severity rated clinically (**unlike** lung disease)
    - NYHA class (I = no exercise limitation, II = slight exercise limitation, III = marked exercise limitation, IV = rest symptoms)
    - Screen for with:
      - Physical examination for peripheral and pulmonary edema
      - Chest x-ray looking for pulmonary edema, pleural effusion, and cardiac chamber enlargement
      - Echocardiogram looking at chamber size, ventricular function, and PA systolic pressure
  - Treat with diuresis to euvolemia (no edema, pleural effusion, or ascites remaining)

- **Cardiac restriction/constriction/valve disease:**
  - Physical examination for heart murmur and a pulsus paradoxus
  - Echocardiogram looking for pericardial effusion, thickening, and tamponade physiology

- **Angina:**
  - Screen for with a cardiac stress test (exercise stress preferred to pharmacologic stress)

- **Venous thromboembolic disease:**
  - VQ scan is the modality of choice when screening for CTEPH; alternatively a CT angiography may be used

- **Early DPLD:**
  - Patients with risk factors for DPLD (eg, shipyard worker, bird fancier) or associated signs and symptoms (ie, dry cough, fine rales during examination) may warrant a chest CT scan looking for subtle changes associated with DPLD

- Patients with a significant exercise limitation from DPLD should have a decreased DLCO with or without restriction evident on PFTs
- **Cardiopulmonary exercise testing (CPET)** is used when the above evaluation fails to explain an individual's exercise limitation or dyspnea on exertion
  - CPET allows simultaneous screening of many parameters (ie, blood pressure, heart rate, pH, ventilation, oxygenation)
  - Often reassures the patient and provider that deconditioning is the cause
  - Occasionally reveals exercise-induced arrhythmia, extreme hypertension, O_2 desaturation, or ventilatory limitation
- If the above evaluation for a gradual exercise limitation/dyspnea fails to reveal an etiology, consider:
  - Screening for and/or empirically treating anxiety/depression (SSRIs and counseling)
  - Reassurance and observation (bad entities have been ruled out)
- The majority of patients with unexplained dyspnea on exertion will ultimately be found to have one of the following:
  - Occult left-sided heart failure
  - Deconditioning
  - Mixed obstructive restrictive lung disease
  - CAD and angina
  - PAH (CTEPH much more common than IPAH)
- A pulmonary parenchymal explanation for moderate to severe dyspnea is often obvious during full PFTs; however, patients with **mixed obstructive restrictive lung disease** (eg, combined pulmonary fibrosis and emphysema) may have **pseudonormalization** of flows and volumes, as:
  - Areas of basilar fibrosis exhale pathologically fast masking upper lobe COPD, and
  - Upper lobe air trapping pathologically increases lung volume masking lower lobe restriction
  - Only the diffusing capacity (DLCO) will be significantly reduced (ie, isolated low DLCO)
  - These individuals have grossly abnormal chest imaging
    - This easily differentiates them from PAH and early DPLD (the differential diagnosis for an isolated low DLCO)
- Echocardiography is the initial step in screening for dyspnea of cardiac origin (eg, biventricular heart failure, valvular or pericardial disease, and PAH):
  - Resting cardiac echocardiography is excellent at ruling out **systolic dysfunction** (and thus **heart failure with reduced ejection fraction [HFrEF]**), as well as **valvular** and **pericardial disease**
  - Echocardiography is **much less reliable** at ruling out **heart failure with preserved ejection fraction (HFpEF)** from diastolic dysfunction because:
    - Diastolic dysfunction may be intermittent (ie, occurring only during exercise or sleep)
    - A mild diastolic filling abnormality during a resting echocardiogram may become severe during exercise
      - As heart rate and afterload increase
    - HFpEF from diastolic dysfunction may be inferred from left-sided atrial enlargement (in the absence of mitral valve disease), bilateral pleural effusion, and generalized edema
  - **HFpEF** may be misinterpreted by an echocardiogram as PAH because in the absence of left atrial enlargement, they may be indistinguishable (ie, normal LV function, elevated pulmonary artery systolic pressure, RA enlargement, and reduced RV systolic function)
  - **Early PAH** (before overt right-sided heart failure) requires an exercise right-sided heart catheterization for diagnosis because initially, PA pressures only rise with exercise
- A diagnostic therapeutic/trial of diuresis to euvolemia (no edema, pleural effusion, or ascites remaining) with close clinical follow-up is the most reliable way to rule out HFpEF

COMMON QUESTIONS GENERATED BY THIS TEACHING

1. Why is it OK to attribute moderate to severe HFpEF (NYHA class III) to an individual with only a mild diastolic filling abnormality seen by echocardiogram but it is wrong to attribute a moderate to severe exercise limitation to an individual with only mild PFT abnormalities?

   Because the severity of heart failure is rated clinically (hard to quantify physiologically given many variables), unlike lung disease, which is easier to quantify physiologically (fewer variables).

2. I had a patient with COPD who felt dramatically better with supplemental O_2, but his ambulatory ABG never demonstrated a $PaO_2 < 70$ mm Hg (question implied by tone).

   Some individuals obtain dyspnea relief from supplemental oxygen by a mechanism other than resolving hypoxemia. Oxygen supplementation may improve dyspnea by mechanical air flow sensation (trigeminal nerve), which is also achievable with a fan (mechanism not well established).

3. How can heart failure limit exercise and cause dyspnea during exertion without pulmonary edema?

   Activation of baroreceptors located in the pulmonary vasculature, cardiac chambers, and aorta signal dyspnea (which limits exercise) in response to increased left-sided cardiovascular pressure.

HEART FAILURE FOR THE PULMONARY CRITICAL CARE PHYSICIAN

CHAPTER 6

COMMON MISCONCEPTIONS AND MISTAKES

- Left-sided heart failure (LHF) causes pulmonary hypertension and right-sided heart failure (RHF) as a result of "back pressure"

- Pulmonary hypertension and right ventricle (RV) systolic dysfunction occurring with normal left ventricle (LV) systolic function is synonymous with isolated RHF

- A single hemodynamic assessment demonstrating a mean pulmonary artery pressure > 25 mm Hg, and a pulmonary capillary wedge pressure (PCWP) < 15 mm Hg is sufficient to diagnose isolated RHF (ie, rule out biventricular heart failure [HF])

- Failing to realize that bilateral pleural effusions are virtually pathognomonic for biventricular HF

- Failing to realize that left atrial enlargement, with a normal mitral, valve is pathognomonic for LHF

- Labeling an edematous patient as euvolemic

- Acknowledging that a patient has LHF but deciding that the **severity** of a symptom or sign (eg, pulmonary hypertension, RV failure, exercise limitation) is out of proportion to the pulmonary capillary wedge pressure (PCWP), LVEDP, or the diagnostic filling abnormality seen on echo, **before** a trial of euvolemia

- Confusing failure to diurese (not achieving a negative fluid balance despite loop diuretic administration) with failure of diuresis (achieving a negative fluid balance that unfortunately does not improve the patient's condition)

- Equating renal and serum indices that suggest "prerenal" azotemia (eg, Na$^+$-avid urine, blood urea nitrogen (BUN)/creatinine (CR) >20) with intravascular volume depletion (forgetting they are also produced by cardiorenal physiology) and volume overload

- Considering pulmonary vasodilatior therapy for a patient with LHF because the RV failure is "out of proportion" to the degree of LV failure

- Diagnosing acute respiratory distress syndrome (ARDS) (which requires "no evidence of pulmonary venous hypertension") in a patient with bilateral pleural effusions

HEART FAILURE AND THE PULMONOLOGIST (A.K.A. OCCULT LEFT HEART FAILURE)

- It is the job of the pulmonologist to evaluate and manage unexplained pulmonary hypertension, RHF, and exercise limitation
  - Unexplained means not obvious from pulmonary function tests (PFTS) and/or echocardiogram

- The most common cause of unexplained pulmonary hypertension, RHF, and exercise limitation is "occult left heart failure"

- **Occult left heart failure** describes the situation where other physicians, sometimes cardiologists, have concluded that a patient *is not* suffering from biventricular HF, often despite obvious pathognomonic signs (eg, bilateral pleural effusions, elevated PCWP pressure, left atrial enlargement, and peripheral edema) (Fig. 6.1)

Occult Left Heart Failure

PULMONARY OUTPATIENT CONSULT

HPI:

Mr._____ is a **66** yo M with history of **CKD4, DM, HTN, OSA** poorly compliant with CPAP who was **referred** to pulmonary clinic for **progressive DOE.** For the past year, he has only been able to walk a few blocks limited by SOB. **ROS: + mild lower extremity edema.** No fevers. chills. weight loss, night sweats, cough, chest pain, hemoptysis.

TLC % PRED	63.6
FVC % PRED	69.1
FEV1 % PRED	70.7
FEV1 / FVC	78.00
DLCO % PRED	90.6

PHYSICAL EXAM:
GEN: Obese, NAD
NECK: Supple, no appreciable JVP
CV: Normal S1/S2, no M/R/G, RRR
LUNGS: CTAB, no wheezes or rales appreciated
ABD: SNTND, BS+
EXT: 1+ pitting edema bilaterally
ASSESSMENT/PLAN:

RIGHT HEART CATHETERIZATION
Pressures   (mmHg)
RA mean: 11
RV: 40/17
PA: 40/22, mean 26
PCWP: 16

rt heart cath with elevated **PCWP of 16** and RA pressures, felt most c/w with **biventricular heart failure.** Pt has **no pulmonary edema but notable peripheral edema** and he would benefit from optimization and increased diuretic dosing.
– Lasix 80mg BID
– Metolazone 5mg, Qday 30 mins before AM lasix dose
– Metabolic panel before next appt
Pt seen and discussed with Attending, Dr. Judd Landsberg

Cardiology Attending

Mr._____ is a 67 y.o. with diabetes mellitus, chronic kidney disease, hypertension, hyperlipidemia, OSA. He has had multiple changes in his medications including **increase in Lasix and metolazone to treat peripheral edema, with improved exercise tolerance.**
His cardiac catheterization on 4/10/14 showed pressure (mmHg) in the RA = 11, PCWP 16, PA 40/22, mean 26, SVR 1291, PVR 112 (80 x 1.4 wood units), with cardiac output 7 L/min (thermodilution) and cardiac index 3.1 L/min/m2. These do not indicate marked left or right heart failure, but rather a modest increase RA and PCW pressures, and only modest pulmonary hypertension with a normal PVR and normal ratio of PVR to SVR. This does not indicate marked pulmonary hypertension nor piventricular failure as has been noted elsewhere in the chart.
He may have modest diastolic dysfunction, but not severe enough to explain extreme dyspnea on exertions.

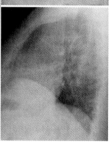

A

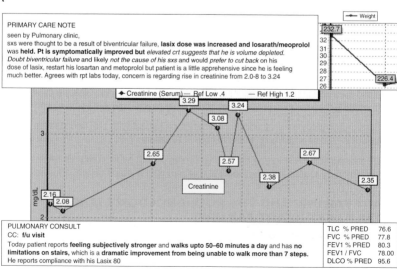

PRIMARY CARE NOTE
seen by Pulmonary clinic,
sxs were thought to be a result of biventricular failure, **lasix dose was increased and losarath/meoprolol was held. Pt is symptomatically improved but** *elevated crt suggests that he is volume depleted. Doubt biventricular failure and likely* not *the cause of his sxs and would* prefer *to cut back on his dose of lasix, restart his losartan and metoprolol but patient is a little apprehensive since he is feeling much better. Agrees with rpt labs today, concern is regarding rise in creatinine from 2.0-8 to 3.24*

PULMONARY CONSULT
CC: f/u visit
Today patient reports **feeling subjectively stronger and walks upto 50–60 minutes a day** and has **no limitations on stairs,** which is a **dramatic improvement from being unable to walk more than 7 steps.**
He reports compliance with his Lasix 80

TLC % PRED	76.6
FVC % PRED	77.8
FEV1 % PRED	80.3
FEV1 / FVC	78.00
DLCO % PRED	95.6

B

Fig. 6.1 See figure legend on opposite page.

- Missed or "occult" LHF is most commonly a phenomenon of **diastolic heart failure (a.k.a. heart failure with a preserved ejection fraction [HFpEF])**
    - Patients with systolic dysfunction are less likely to have their decompensated heart failure "missed" when they present with new or worsening pulmonary hypertension, RHF, and/or exercise limitation
- Occult LHF should be excluded by an empiric trial of euvolemia (which is always indicated) before invasive testing (eg, cardiac catheterization) and/or extensive work up (eg, cardiopulmonary exercise testing)

THE MANY FACES OF BIVENTRICULAR HEART FAILURE SECONDARY TO DIASTOLIC DYSFUNCTION (A.K.A. HFpEF)

- Biventricular HF from diastolic dysfunction mimics a myriad of pulmonary disease presentations; for example:
    - Group I pulmonary arterial hypertension (idiopathic pulmonary arterial hypertension [IPAH]-like "small vessel disease")
        - Patient presents with exercise limitation, increased pulmonary artery systolic (PAS) pressure on echocardiogram, **and** normal LV systolic function
    - Worsening chronic obstructive pulmonary disease (COPD) with cor pulmonale
        - COPD patient presents with increased dyspnea on exertion and increased lower extremity edema
    - Exacerbation of interstitial lung disease (ILD)
        - ILD patient presents with increased interstitial markings, worse oxygenation, more restriction, and increased lower extremity edema
    - Indolent lymphoma
        - Patient presents with fluorodeoxyglucose (FDG)-avid mediastinal adenopathy

- Similarly, biventricular HF from diastolic dysfunction mimics many ICU presentations; for example:
    - Acute pulmonary embolism with RV dysfunction
        - Patient presents with hypotension, new RV dysfunction, **and** normal LV systolic function
    - ARDS
        - Intubated patient develops worsening compliance, oxygenation, and diffuse infiltrates
    - *Ondine's* curse
        - Patient presents with sudden, unexplained central hypoventilation

- Patients with lung disease, preserved LV systolic function, and peripheral edema pose a significant diagnostic challenge:
    - Isolated RHF (from cor pulmonale) vs biventricular HF (from diastolic dysfunction)
    - **The stakes are high** (*hospice for cor pulmonale vs diuretics for LHF*)

Fig. 6.1 Encapsulated case of ***occult left-sided heart failure (LHF).*** (A) Initial pulmonary evaluation for gradually worsening dyspnea on exertion with peripheral edema (NYHA III), revealing moderate restriction on pulmonary function tests (PFTs), a normal chest x-ray, and a right-sided heart catheterization demonstrating LHF (mean pulmonary artery pressure >25 mm Hg with a pulmonary capillary wedge pressure (PCWP) >15 mm Hg). Cardiology mistakenly concludes that the patient's physical limitation is out of proportion to the magnitude of his left and right pressure elevations. This reasoning is flawed because the severity of heart failure is graded clinically and it is not possible to conclude that symptoms are "out of proportion to" a single resting echocardiogram or cardiac catheterization measurement. PCWP systematically underestimates left ventricular end-diastolic pressure (LVEDP), and LVEDP may rise dramatically with exercise in the decompensated individual with heart failure with a preserved ejection fraction (HFpEF). (B) The primary care physician is mistakenly concerned that his rising creatinine-indicated acute kidney injury (AKI), erroneously attributing it to intravascular volume depletion, despite edema. Pulmonary follow-up shows dramatically improved exercise tolerance (NYHA I), improved PFTs and a stable/improving creatinine with only ~6 lbs of net fluid loss. This case also highlights the importance of discontinuing rennin-angiotensin system inhibition during diuresis in patients with significant chronic kidney disease (CKD) (autoregulation already difficult enough for the kidneys in this setting).

- Critically ill hypotensive patients with RV dysfunction and preserved LV systolic function also pose a significant diagnostic challenge:
  - Isolated RHF vs biventricular HF (from LV diastolic dysfunction)
  - Stakes are high (*lytics for presumed massive PE, pulmonary vasodilator therapy for IPAH or diuretics for LHF*)

- Acute and chronic respiratory failure is **always** impacted by LHF, because interstitial edema:
  - Decreases compliance
  - Increases airway resistance (submucosal edema)
  - Worsens obesity-related hypoventilation

HOW LEFT-SIDED HEART FAILURE CAUSES PULMONARY HYPERTENSION AND RIGHT-SIDED HEART FAILURE (THE BIVENTRICULAR HEART FAILURE REFLEX — *NOT BACK PRESSURE*)

- Definition of LHF:
  - LHF is synonymous with biventricular HF
    - Isolated LHF does not exist (not compatible with human physiology)
  - LHF is **defined** as an **LVEDP >15 mm Hg** (normal <12 mm Hg) regardless of the mechanism:
    - Primary cardiac causes (eg, myocardial infarction [MI], arrhythmia) or volume overload (eg, anuric renal failure)
  - LHF, regardless of the mechanism, ultimately involves:
    - Decreased LV cardiac output (CO) leading to increased pressure in the left ventricle at the end of diastole, or an elevated LVEDP

- LHF occurs as a consequence of either **systolic** or **diastolic** dysfunction:
  - **Systolic dysfunction** equals impaired LV squeeze (a.k.a. heart failure with reduced ejection fraction [HFrEF])
    - Systolic dysfunction occurs in people with a cardiomyopathy, most commonly from ischemic heart disease, hypertension (HTN), alcohol, and viral or idiopathic disease
  - **Diastolic dysfunction** equals impaired LV filling, despite a normal or high ejection fraction (a.k.a. HFpEF)
    - Diastolic dysfunction occurs in people experiencing poor ventricular compliance (eg, stiff ventricle) as seen with LVH and hypertensive heart disease, and shortened diastole (ie, filling time) as seen in tachycardia
    - Diastolic dysfunction represents a functional, dynamic failure that can occur in any normal heart if appropriately stressed
    - Diastolic dysfunction is often provoked, unmasked, or exacerbated by:
      - Hypoxia (stiffens the ventricle and causes tachycardia)
      - Tachycardia (shortens diastole, ie, the time allowed for ventricular filling)
      - Hypertension (stiffens the ventricle (LVH) and decreases CO directly by afterload)
      - Total body volume overload (increased preload)
        - Total body volume overload is commonly caused by:
          - Impaired natriuresis (as in chronic kidney disease [CKD] or acute kidney injury [AKI])
          - Intravenous sodium loading (as occurs during resuscitation)

- Regardless of the mechanism of the LHF (ie, systolic or diastolic dysfunction), RHF occurs via a neurohormonal reflex (a.k.a. the **biventricular HF reflex**) (Fig. 6.2):
  - Increased LVEDP causes an increase in left atrial (LA) pressure and pulmonary venous (PV) pressure directly, via "back pressure"

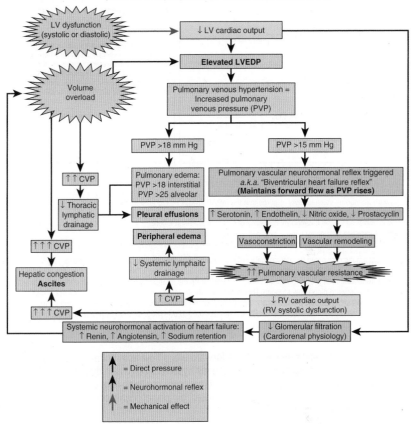

Fig. 6.2 Flow diagram depicting the pathophysiology of biventricular heart failure (HF) (heart failure with preserved ejection fraction [HFpEF] and heart failure with reduced ejection fraction [HFrEF]), where black arrows denote direct "back pressure," blue arrow denote "mechanical effect," and red arrows denote "neurohormonal signaling." The **biventricular HF reflex** describes the pulmonary vascular aspect of the neurohormonal signaling that is responsible for pulmonary hypertension and right-sided heart failure (RHF). The diagram shows that transudative pleural effusions are pathognomonic for biventricular HF (ie, do not occur with isolated RHF) by requiring both an elevated pulmonary venous pressure (causing pulmonary edema that weeps into the pleural space) and an elevated central venous pressure (CVP) (to prevent thoracic lymphatic drainage of the fluid). The diagram highlights that individuals whose heart failure leaves them with LVEDP values in the 15–18 mm Hg range will be clinically and radiographically indistinguishable from patients with pulmonary vascular disease and isolated RHF (ie, pulmonary hypertension, peripheral edema, and exercise limitation).

- Increased PV pressure triggers a neurohormonal reflex that causes pulmonary artery vasoconstriction leading to an increase in PA pressure, ensuring and maintaining forward blood flow through the lungs (Fig. 6.3)
- Increased PA pressure then increases right ventricular end-diastolic pressure (RVEDP) directly (via increased afterload), causing right heart failure
- Increased RVEDP leads to an increased right atrial pressure (RAP) and central venous pressure (CVP) directly, via "back pressure," leading to peripheral edema and pleural effusions

FORWARD PULMONARY VASCULAR FLOW REQUIRES THAT THE mPAP PRESSURE ALWAYS BE HIGHER THAN THE 'WATERFALL' PRESSURE

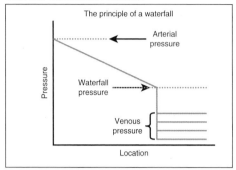

The "starling resistor" or "waterfall" hypothesis of pulmonary vascular flow:

Pulmonary blood flow is determined by the proximal arterial, minus the distal waterfall pressure. If the venous pressure where able to rise above the waterfall pressure, forward blood flow would stop. This **DOES NOT** occur. Therefore pulmonary artery pressure must always be higher then pulmonary venous pressure.

- The pulmonary artery "waterfall pressure" is a difficult to measure value between mean pulmonary artery pressure (mPAP) and left ventricular end-diastolic pressure (LVEDP)
- Forward pulmonary vascular flow requires that the mPAP always be higher than the "water fall pressure," which is always higher then LVEDP
- This is achieved via the neurohormonal reflex of biventricular heart failure
- Where increased pulmonary venous pressure reflexively triggers an increase in mPAP
- Some individuals have a blunted reflex and others have a robust or exaggerated reflex

Fig. 6.3 Schematic describing the determinants of pulmonary blood flow via the "waterfall hypothesis." Said differently, the distensible nature of the pulmonary vasculature, behaving like a "starling resistor," means that direct, backward transmission of pressure (a.k.a. "back pressure") from the pulmonary veins to the pulmonary arteries would only occur after forward blood flow stopped. This is not compatible with human physiology (and does not occur). The only time left sided cardiac pressures are directly and rapidly transmitted to the right side is during tamponade physiology. *(Adapted from Westerhof N et al. Physiol Rev 2006;86:1263–1308. © 2006 by American Physiological Society.)*

- This neurohormonal reflex maintains forward blood flow from pulmonary arteries to pulmonary veins **despite** pulmonary venous hypertension (which threatens to stop forward flow by removing the right-to-left pressure gradient) (Fig. 6.4)
  - This reflex also ensures that, as LVEDP rises, peripheral edema occurs before (and preferentially to) pulmonary edema
- The biventricular HF reflex is the mechanism by which LV diastolic dysfunction gives rise to RV systolic dysfunction, an echocardiogram finding often misconstrued as pathognomonic for pulmonary vascular disease (Fig. 6.5)

THE MISLEADING NATURE OF THE TRANSPULMONARY GRADIENT AND "PASSIVE," "REACTIVE," AND "OUT OF PROPORTION" PULMONARY HYPERTENSION

- The biventricular HF reflex maintains forward flow **and** is protective against pulmonary edema in the face of LVEDP elevations
- As LVEDP rises, left atrial and pulmonary venous pressure rise via "back pressure," leading to pulmonary edema
- If increased pulmonary venous pressure were then directly transmitted to the pulmonary arteries in a continued "back pressure" fashion, the pulmonary vascular pressure gradient from right to left would disappear and blood would **not** flow forward (this does not occur)
- Instead, an increase in pulmonary venous pressure reflexively triggers an increase in pulmonary artery tone (either a little or a lot) via a neurohormonal reflex

EXPERIMENTAL DEMONSTRATION OF THE BIVENTRICULAR HEART FAILURE REFLEX

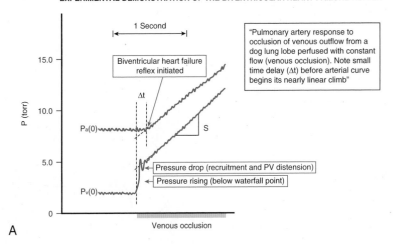

A

EQUILIBRATED PRESSURE AFTER OCCLUSION OF BOTH Pv AND Pa IS ABOVE THAT WHICH IS PREDICTED BY "BACK PRESSURE"

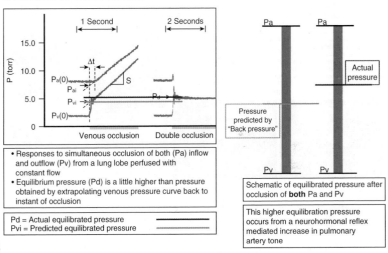

B

Fig. 6.4 (A) Neurohormonal reflex of biventricular heart failure (HF) demonstrated in an isolated perfused dog lung lobe. In this model, left ventricular end-diastolic pressure (LVEDP) increase is simulated by pulmonary venous occlusion, which leads to a nearly instantaneous linear rise in pulmonary artery pressure. (B) The same experimental model as in *A* after simultaneous occlusion of both the pulmonary vein and artery to obtain an equilibration pressure. A model where the pulmonary artery and vein behave like a solid conduit (ie, back pressure model) predicts that the equilibrated pressure, after simultaneous occlusion of both pulmonary artery and vein, should equal the pulmonary venous pressure at the time of occlusion (obtained by backward extrapolation). Instead, the actual equilibrated pressure is higher than predicted because of pulmonary arterial tone generated by the biventricular HF reflex. *(Adapted from Linehan, JH, Dawson CA, Rickaby DA. Distribution of vascular resistance and compliance in a dog lung lobe. J Applied Physio: Respir, Enviro and Exer Physio 53(1):158–68, 1982.)*

RV Systolic Dysfunction from LV Diastolic Dysfunction

- 75 yo with HTN admitted to cardiology with new Afib, RVR, HFpEF, SOB, and peripheral edema
- Patient improved with diuretics and nodal blockers
- Anticoagulated for stroke prevention
- Transferred to ICU service after echocardiogram raised concern for PE because of new RV systolic dysfunction
- ICU team decides the echocardiogram is consistent with biventricular heart failure and the patient with treated with continued diuresis
- Repeat Echo (with improving, but still persistent volume overload volume overloaded) showed resolution of RV systolic dysfunction

Echocardiogram, chest x-ray, vital signs and exam on the day of transfer for possible acute pulmonary embolism

There is **normal left ventricular systolic function** with no wall motion abnormalities.
Mild concentric **left ventricular hypertrophy** is observed.
The **left atrium is severely dilated.**
The **right ventricle is moderately dilated.**
The **right ventricular function is hypodynamic.**
The right atrial cavity size is severely dilated.
There is mild aortic regurgitation.
There is moderate aortic stenosis.
There is mild to moderate mitral regurgitation.
There is mild to moderate mitral stenosis.
There is mild to moderate tricuspid regurgitation.
There is **moderate to severe pulmonary hypertension** noted.
A trivial pericardial effusion is visualized.

99.7 97/57 80's 96% 4L NC **–1.7 L o/n**
Neck: **+ JVP 10cm**
Lungs: **Crackles at L base, decreased BS R base**
CV: irregularly irregular
Extrem: **1+ pitting of LE**

A

Echocardiogram, chest x-ray, vital signs and exam, 5 days later with diuresis but NOT euvolemia, evident by bilateral pleural effusions on chest CT (same day)

There is normal left ventricular systolic function with no wall motion abnormalities.
The right ventricle is moderately dilated.
The right ventricular global systolic function is normal.
There is mild aortic regurgitation.
There is mild to moderate mitral regurgitation.
There is mild tricuspid regurgitation.
Mild pulmonary hypertension is noted.

No Pulmonary Embolism

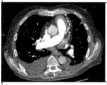 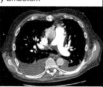

S: Pt reports feeling much better than previous days.
O: VS Tm98.9 HR 85–145 BP 80–120/40–60 R 17–27 I/O=803/1490
Neck: No JVD
CV: tachycardic, regular rhythm, no m/r/g appreciated
Resp: fine bibasilar crackles
Extr: no LE edema

Important Points

- RV systolic dysfunction is common (and expected) in HF from diastolic dysfunction
- Peripheral edema resolves BEFORE pleural effusions

B

Fig. 6.5 Encapsulated case showing new right ventricle (RV) systolic dysfunction misinterpreted as acute pulmonary embolism in a patient admitted with heart failure with preserved ejection fraction (HFpEF). Repeat studies were obtained 5 days later because the patient was deemed to be euvolemic (by the absence of peripheral edema). His chest x-ray and computed tomography (CT) scan demonstrate persistent bilateral pulmonary embolisms pleural effusions, illustrating the point that that peripheral edema resolves before pleural fluid during diuresis. A lateral film with close inspection of the costophrenic angles is the simplest screen for euvolemia (after peripheral edema resolves) in a patient with biventricular heart failure. **Note**: CT angiography was ultimately obtained by the medicine SVC, after transfer from the intensive care unit, given persistent (but unfounded) concerns for pulmonary embolism based on the original echocardiogram finding and the disbelief that RV systolic function could be caused by left ventricle (LV) diastolic dysfunction (which is actually quite common).

- Traditionally, if the increase in mPAP is just enough to overcome the increase in LVEDP and maintain forward flow, the patient is said to have "passive pulmonary hypertension"
  - Where the transpulmonary gradient (mPAP-LVEDP) is ≤12 mm Hg

- Conversely, if the mPAP is significantly elevated, the patient is said to have "out-of-proportion" or "reactive" pulmonary hypertension
  - Where the transpulmonary gradient (mPAP-LVEDP) >12 mm Hg

- Thus the "passive" vs "reactive" designation given to the pulmonary hypertension seen with LHF is arbitrary and **not** physiologic as implied
  - So-called passive patients have a more blunted biventricular HF reflex
    - Making them prone to pulmonary edema
  - So-called reactive patients have a more robust biventricular HF reflex
    - Making them prone to excessive peripheral edema and ascites (RHF symptoms) protecting them against pulmonary edema (Fig. 6.6)

- The passive vs reactive designation has **no** implications on management

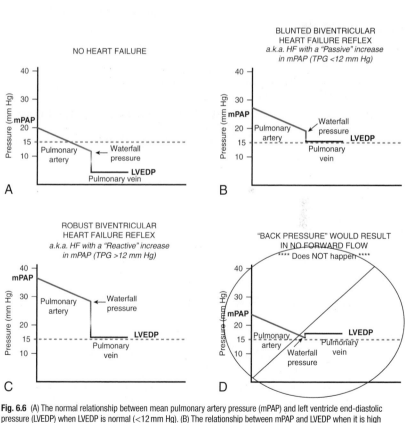

Fig. 6.6 (A) The normal relationship between mean pulmonary artery pressure (mPAP) and left ventricle end-diastolic pressure (LVEDP) when LVEDP is normal (<12 mm Hg). (B) The relationship between mPAP and LVEDP when it is high (>15 mm Hg) in individuals with a "blunted" or "passive" biventricular HF reflex, resulting in a modest elevation in mPAP, just enough to keep it above the waterfall point ensuring forward flow. (C) The relationship between mPAP and LVEDP when LVEDP is high (>15 mm Hg) in individuals with a "robust" or "reactive" biventricular HF reflex, resulting in a large elevation in mPAP, keeping it well above the "waterfall point." (D) The fictitious scenario known as "back pressure," where LVEDP rises above the waterfall point such that it can directly affect pulmonary artery pressure (doing so only after forward flow stops).

- Additionally, the terms cause significant confusion:
  - "Passive" is misconstrued as "back pressure"
  - "Reactive" is misconstrued as "vasoreactive"
  - "Out of proportion" is misconstrued to imply a need for specific pulmonary vasodilator therapy (actually contraindicated)

INDIVIDUAL VARIABILITY IN THE BIVENTRICULAR HEART FAILURE REFLEX CHALLENGES THE CONCEPT OF OUT-OF-PROPORTION PH

- Scatter plot below, shows that a PCWP of 25 may generate a pulmonary artery systolic (PAS) pressure anywhere from ~38 mm Hg to ~99 mm Hg Fig. 6.7
- The range in PAS pressures among people is explained by individual variability in the biventricular HF reflex—**not** small vessel vascular remodeling, hypoxic vasoconstriction, or back pressure
  - This variability makes the designation "out of proportion" impossible to make

PATHOPHYSIOLOGY OF BIVENTRICULAR HEART FAILURE (THE NUMBERS)

- Normal LVEDP is 3–8 mm Hg (<12 mm Hg)
- When LVEDP and pulmonary venous pressure (PVP) rise to >15 mm Hg, the biventricular HF reflex is triggered, increasing mPAP by vasoconstriction, and to varying degrees, vascular remodeling
- Elevated mPAP leads to an increased RVEDP (often with RV systolic dysfunction) and subsequently right atrial pressure (RAP) and CVP

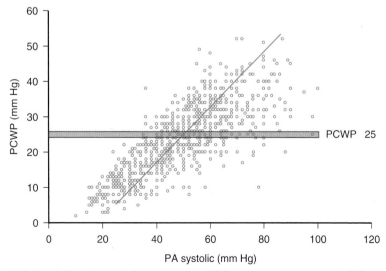

Fig. 6.7 Scatterplot of the pulmonary capillary wedge pressure (PCWP) and the pulmonary artery systolic (PAS) pressure of 1000 patients with left-sided heart failure. The data demonstrate the enormous individual variability in pulmonary artery pressure for any given PCWP (*or* left ventricle end-diastolic pressure [LVEDP]) (ie, enormous variability in the biventricular heart failure reflex). *(Adapted from Drazner et al. J Heart and Lung Transplant 18:11.)*

- Ensuring continued right-to-left pulmonary blood flow
- Causing peripheral edema before pulmonary edema

- When LVEDP and PVP rise >18 mm Hg, interstitial edema ensues

- When LVEDP and PVP rise >25 mm Hg, alveolar edema occurs

- When sustained elevations of both CVP and PVP occur, **bilateral pleural effusions** accumulate

- When biventricular HF continues, further sustained elevations of CVP lead to accumulation of ascites

LVEDP (mm Hg)	Physiologic Consequence
3–12	None (normal)
15	Pulmonary hypertension, right-sided heart failure, peripheral edema
18	Pulmonary interstitial edema
25	Pulmonary alveolar edema

PATHOPHYSIOLOGY OF BIVENTRICULAR HEART FAILURE (THE PROCESS)

- The biventricular HF reflex, though poorly characterized, occurs when elevated LVEDP (>15 mm Hg) causes pulmonary venous hypertension, which triggers both:
  - An instantaneous increase in mPAP involving PA vasoconstriction (likely via serotonergic neurons) and
  - A sustained increase in mPAP, likely driven by hormonal changes in pulmonary artery endothelial cells such as:
    - Increased endothelin synthesis, decreased nitric oxide synthesis, and decreased prostacyclin synthesis

- These hormonal changes act on pulmonary artery smooth muscle cells, causing:
  - Hypertrophy, hyperplasia, and increased tone
  - Together these changes lead to varying degrees of pulmonary vascular (small vessel) remodeling with luminal narrowing and complete occlusion

- The instantaneous (vasoconstrictive) increase in pulmonary artery tone seen in biventricular HF is vulnerable to reversal with pulmonary vasodilators (eg, IV prostacyclin)
  - Causing sudden pulmonary edema, failure of forward blood flow through the heart, and death

RESIDUAL SMALL VESSEL DISEASE

- The small vessel remodeling seen with long-standing elevations in PVP may be reversible over weeks to months **if** sustained reductions in PVP and/or LVEDP are achieved

- However, in some this remodeling remains fixed, leading to "group I pulmonary arterial hypertension (PAH)" type pathologic vascular changes (a.k.a. **residual small vessel disease**)

- Individuals with residual small vessel disease are clinically **very** different from people with IPAH
  - Residual small vessel disease is **not** progressive and does **not** require specific therapy (>95% of the time)
  - Unlike IPAH, where progressive vascular remodeling leads to RHF and death if specific therapy is not employed

- Pulmonary vasodilation/antiremodeling therapy aimed at residual small vessel disease is **rarely** indicated
- Should only be entertained in patients able to maintain sustained reductions in LVEDP (months to years) who **still** complain of an exercise limitation possibly attributable to increased PA afterload from vascular remodeling leading to symptomatic isolated RHF **with** exercise
- **Remember:**
- Most of these patients **actually** have an exercise limitation based on persistent, often occult, ongoing elevated LVEDP physiology
- All of the edematous ones
    - Before vasodilatior therapy, an exercise right-sided heart catheterization should be considered to ensure LVEDP remains low during exercise
        - Only at this point can one cautiously entertain a trial of PDE_5 inhibitors to improve exercise ability (because this class of drugs is the safest if LVEDP becomes elevated again)
    - LHF patients treated with pulmonary vasodilators should be screened closely for the development of new or worsening pulmonary edema, left atrial stretch, and/or atrial tachyarrhythmias—any of which should prompt urgent discontinuation of therapy
- Therapy for residual small vessel disease **never** needs to be started urgently in the hospital or ICU, unlike therapy for IPAH
    - Even though this is (inappropriately) often considered

BIVENTRICULAR HEART FAILURE: REFLEX, NOT BACK PRESSURE ... SO WHAT?

- The *false* belief that LV failure causes PH and RV failure by **back pressure** leads to **three critically flawed** assumptions:
    1. *Patients with edema and no obvious thoracic fluid likely have isolated RHF*
        a. **As LVEDP and PV pressure rise, pulmonary hypertension and biventricular HF occur before the development of pulmonary edema**
    2. *A single, simultaneous, hemodynamic measurement of right- and left-sided pressure can rule out biventricular HF*
        a. **Intermittent LVEDP elevations lead to sustained PAP elevations (via the biventricular heart failure reflex), and a sustained reduction in LVEDP may be required for normalization of PAP**
    3. *The degree of pulmonary artery pressure elevation should be tightly linked to the degree of LVEDP elevation*
        a. **Enormous variability exists in the degree of PAP elevation for any given LVEDP**

PITFALLS IN SCREENING FOR HFPEF (A.K.A. BIVENTRICULAR HEART FAILURE FROM DIASTOLIC DYSFUNCTION)

- Inappropriate focus on identifying and rating the severity of the diastolic filling abnormality on an echocardiogram
- Echocardiograms often mislead, suggesting isolated RHF by demonstrating:
    - Pulmonary hypertension
    - Euvolemia (>50% inferior vena cava (IVC) collapse with respiration)
        - Normal LV function and mild or **no** diastolic filling abnormality
    - Normal left atrial size *or* volume

- Echocardiogram suggestions of a low LVEDP are **far *less* sensitive** than physical findings of LVEDP elevation (eg, **bilateral pleural effusions [*no matter how small*]**)
  - Transudative pleural effusions are physiologic evidence of biventricular HF, requiring both an elevated LVEDP and RVEDP to form
  - LA enlargement (without mitral disease) is also physiologic evidence of elevated LVEDP and thus biventricular HF

- The clinical syndrome associated with diastolic dysfunction referred to as HFpEF, **cannot be ruled out by:**
  - **Echocardiogram:** diastolic dysfunction is a dynamic process and thus is often Intermittent
  - **Low B-type natriuretic peptide (BNP) values:** Left ventricular chamber stretch is **not** a feature of diastolic dysfunction
  - Right-heart catheterization (RHC) with PCWP estimation, for two reasons:
    - **PCWP is a poor predictor of LVEDP**
    - Halpern's pivotal 2009 *Chest* publication studying nearly 4000 patients, titled "Misclassification of Pulmonary Hypertension Due to Reliance on Pulmonary Capillary Wedge Pressure Rather Than Left Ventricular End-Diastolic Pressure," demonstrated that:
      - Nonexpert RHC is **misleading** the **majority** of the time
        - **85%** of patients who received an RHC in a nonvascular center (nonexpert) were **misclassified** as having PAH when they actually had biventricular HF
        - Halpern's data further showed that **expert RHC was misleading *half*** of the time
        - **53%** of patients who received an **expert RHC would have been misclassified** as having PAH (PCWP <15 mm Hg), when they actually had biventricular HF (LVEDP >15 mm Hg), if they had not had a simultaneous left heart catheterization with direct LVEDP measurement (gold standard) (Fig. 6.8)
      - The data also demonstrate that PCWP systematically underestimates LVEDP:
        - On average, by ~3 mm Hg
        - 40% of the time, by >5 mm Hg
        - 10% of the time, by >10 mm Hg
    - **LVEDP elevations** may be **intermittent** (not occurring at the time as cardiac evaluation)
      - Biventricular HF from diastolic dysfunction is often misinterpreted as isolated RHF because it represents a dynamic process in which LVEDP elevations may be intermittent; for example, occurring during sleep (untreated apneas) or with exercise (which can provoke hypertension and arrhythmia)
        - **Intermittent** episodes of LV diastolic dysfunction may lead to the sustained clinical syndrome of biventricular HF (a.k.a. HFpEF), said differently
        - **Intermittent** LVEDP elevations over time (eg, occurring at night from untreated apneas) may trigger a sustained increase in mPAP and RHF via activation of the neurohormonal biventricular HF reflex

- Biventricular HF often has to be inferred by the physiologic proof of elevated LVEDP physiology—namely pulmonary edema, pleural effusions, and left atrial enlargement (LAE)

- Furthermore, biventricular HF should be suspected in those with peripheral edema and significant risk factors (eg, CKD stage III, HTN, obesity)

- Exclude biventricular HF from diastolic dysfunction by **empiric treatment**, not by advanced testing (eg, RHC)

- **Empiric treatment** equals a *trial of euvolemia,* not RHC (Fig. 6.9)

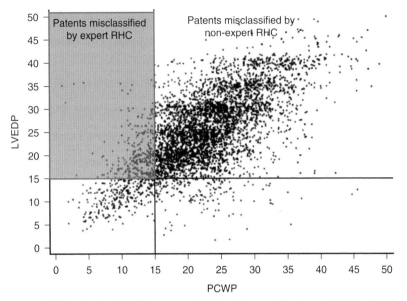

Fig. 6.8 Scatterplot of PCWP and LVEDP among 3926 patients referred for evaluation of possible PAH based on a "nonexpert" RHC at their local institution showing a mean pulmonary artery pressure >25 mm Hg with a PCWP <15 mm Hg. Repeat "expert" RHC revealed that **85% of the referrals actually had a PCWP >15 mm Hg**, showing the dangerously misleading nature of "nonexpert" RHC. Additionally, of the remaining 310 patients whose expert RHC had a PCWP <15 mm Hg, **53% actually had an LVEDP >15 mm Hg**, on left-sided heart catheterization, showing how poorly PCWP estimates LVEDP. *(Adapted from Halpern SD, Taichman DB. Chest: 136(1), 2009.)*

- **Diuresis to euvolemia is always indicated**, regardless of the pathophysiology driving the Na⁺-avid state (ie, LHF, isolated RHF, cirrhosis, or CKD) making this the obvious approach

BILATERAL PLEURAL EFFUSIONS: THE PHYSIOLOGIC PROOF OF BIVENTRICULAR HEART FAILURE

- Bilateral pleural effusions can be assumed to be transudative the majority of the time
  - 99.9% of the time if they are large and layering
  - Only a handful of rare diseases (eg, lymphangiomatosis) or unusual presentations give bilateral exudates
  - Bilateral transudative pleural effusions often have an exudative or loculated appearance (not free flowing) in patients with parenchymal lung disease and pleural scarring
    - May be unilateral:
      - As occurs when one lung has been effectively pleurodesed or
      - When imaging occurs during active diuresis

- Transudative pleural effusions are **pathognomonic** for **biventricular HF** (requiring both increased LVDEP and increased RVEDP):
  - Increased LVDEP (≥18 mm Hg) causes PV hypertension significant enough to cause fluid to leak from the pulmonary capillaries into the interstitium of the lung (interstitial edema)
    - This fluid readily enters the pleural space and is **rapidly drained** by large thoracic **lymphatic channels** embedded **in the parietal pleura** that drain directly into the SVC

The Misleading Nature of RHC

> 68 yo with HFpEF, AS (mild to moderate), OSA, CKD IV
> - Admitted 3 months prior, for abscess debridement, getting wound care and physical therapy
> - Cardiology consulted for persistent edema
> - Primary team notes 'diuresis limited by hypotension and AKI'
> - Echo with "... increasing RVSP (now 91) and RV/RA enlargement... despite unchanged EF and AS"
> - Admitted from rehab floor to CCU for management of edema and worsening pulmonary hypertension and right heart failure

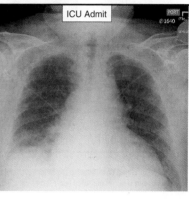

PHYSICAL EXAM
Tc 97.5 BP 100/66 HR 02sat 95% 4 L NC
Wt 268# (dry weight ~245#)
I/0 2260/550+BPP (previous day 1680/770)
GEN- morbidly obese, anasarcic, speaking full sentences
HEENT-unable to assess JVP given body habitus, dry MMM
CV-distant heart sounds, faint SEM
PULM-CTAB anteriorly, **mildly decreased BS throughout**
ABS-obese, faint BS, nontender
EXTR-2-3+ pitting edema to proximal thighs B/L with e/p chronic stasis

ICU Admit

Echocardiogram Prompting ICU Transfer

Normal left ventricular ejection fraction with wall motion abnormalites.
Septal and basal-mid inferior wall appear hyokinetic.
The septum is flattened systole and siastole consistend with
right ventricular pressure and volume overload.
Mild diastolic dvsfunction.
The left atrial chamber size normal.
The right ventricle severely dilated.
The right ventricular function is hypodynamic.
The right atrial cavity size is severely dilated.
No atral septal defect is demonstrated by color Doppler and saline contrast.
There is mild aortic stenosis.
There is mild mitral regurgitation.
There is mild tricuspid regurgitation.
The estimated right atrial pressure is greater than 20 mmHg.
Severe pulmonary hypertension is noted.

A

CCU CARDIOLOGY ATTENDING NOTE:
The patient was **transfered** to the **CCU service** because of **anasarca,**
He has a history of **severe OSA.** He has a **severely elevated** PA
pressure of 91 mmHg. *This pressure is much higher than one usually sees with left sided heart failure.* Diuresis has been difficult because of poor kidney
function. *He has clinical characteristics of cor pulmonale.* He has moderate As,
with only mild MR which cannot explain the severely elevated pulmonary artery
pressures. Swan-Ganz catheter in the cath lab would help clarify his his left
pressures and help us determine if severe pulmonay hypertension derives
severe left sided pressure elevation or if it is intrinsic to the lunqs.

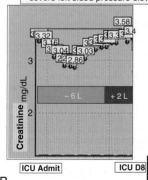

Diuresis stopped because of increasing Cr (despite 3+ edema). Team aims for positive fluid balance) because of rising Cr and a RHC performed ...

RIGHT HEART CATHETERIZATION
Pressures (mmHg)
RA mean: 23
RV: 60/11
PA: 60/11, mean 44 Pulmonary vascular resistance: 8.2
PCWP: 13
CI (Thermodilution) : 1.7 L/m
CI (Fick) : 1.6 L/min/m2
FINAL DIAGNOSIS
1) **Moderately elevated R** and **mildly elevated L heart filling filling pressures.**
2) **Severe pulmonary hypertension.**

 # PULMONARY HTN: seen on right heart cath today; has Swan-Ganz in place, and started sildenafil as potential treatment option. will monitor his response with catheter in place for the next few days.
- Pulmonary consult for Primary pulmonaray HTN

- **Pulmonary Consult:** RHC concerning for group II PH, therefore DIURESIS and inotropic support (as necessary to support BP given low cardiac index ~1.7)
- **No role for pulmonary vasodilators**

B

Fig. 6.9 See figure Legend on next page.

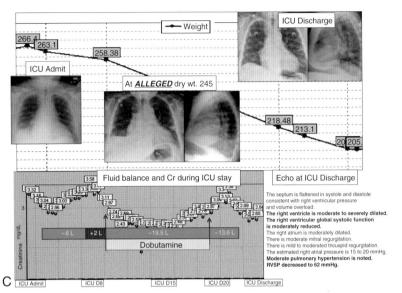

Fig. 6.9 Encapsulated case showing the potential misleading nature of right-sided heart catheterization (RHC) in a patient with known decompensated heart failure with preserved ejection fraction (HFpEF). (A) The transfer of a patient from the rehab floor to the CCU because of gross volume overload and daily positive fluid balance, despite diuretics. His echocardiogram suggests worsening isolated right-sided heart failure (RHF) (concerning for pulmonary hypertension [PAH], a new disease in this individual), but his chest x-ray results refute this, confirming instead decompensation of his known disease, HFpEF, as evidenced by bilateral pleural effusions (R > L) and interstitial edema. Use of the term "anasarca" implies that his edema is caused by **non**hydrostatic forces (as in nephrotic syndrome), making it potentially undiureseable. This is not true of the generalized edema seen in HF. (B) Cardiology decides to pursue an RHC, despite decompensated left-sided heart failure (LHF) (patient at >20 lbs above alleged dry weight), because of three flawed assumptions:

1. Echocardiogram suggestions of isolated RHF are more sensitive than bilateral pleural effusions (the pathognomonic "footprint" of biventricular heart failure [HF]). **You cannot make a diagnosis of cor pulmonale (isolated RHF) in the presence of decompensated LHF.**
2. A rising creatinine-indicated acute kidney injury (AKI), secondary to intravascular volume depletion (despite **obvious** total body volume overload **and** no response to 2 L of volume). **In actuality, one anticipates a sine wave–like fluctuation of glomerular filtration rate (GFR) (and thus Cr) to occur while diuresing a patient with intrinsic renal disease and impaired renal autoregulation. It is *not* possible to cause AKI while diuresing an edematous patient in HF.**
3. The magnitude of the right-sided heart pressure elevation should be tightly linked to the magnitude of the left-sided pressure elevation (implying a "back pressure" mechanism), **when in in actuality there is enormous variability in the biventricular HF reflex.** Additionally, the assertion that right-sided pressures were "out of proportion to the degree of diastolic dysfunction seen on the echocardiogram" **fails to recognize that ECHO pressure estimates are just that, estimates (and often way off).**

The "nonexpert" RHC showed a pulmonary capillary wedge pressure (PCWP) of 13 mm Hg (normal <12 mm Hg) still <15 mm Hg (definition of LHF). Failure to acknowledge that PCWP systematically underestimates left ventricular end-diastolic pressure (LVEDP) (Halpern's data) leads to an erroneous (and potentially dangerous) new diagnosis of PAH. In doing so, cardiology starts pulmonary vasodilation therapy, threatening to inhibit the normal and **necessary** reflex of biventricular HF. The remainder of the nearly month-long intensive care unit (ICU) stay. **Note:** The patient's alleged dry weight is >40 lbs off. Serial chest x-ray results show improved but persistent pulmonary edema with small bilateral pleural effusions still evident upon ICU discharge. Repeat echocardiogram, unfortunately before euvolemia, shows improved pulmonary hypertension and right ventricle (RV) function. The patient was placed on dobutamine **not** because of symptomatic cardiogenic shock but rather because of a number, his CI (calculated at RHC), thereby becoming a "dobutamine hostage" until his central venous O₂ saturation improved. Seen again (as always) serum Cr fluctuates in a sine wave–like fashion, reflecting impaired renal autoregulation. Interestingly this process seemed to be blunted by dobutamine, perhaps because of renal vascular β2 dilatory effects.

- Increased RVEDP from the biventricular HF reflex causes increased CVP, removing the hydrostatic gradient favoring thoracic lymphatic drainage
- This results in cessation of thoracic lymphatic drainage and fluid accumulation in the pleural space (ie, bilateral pleural effusions)

- Isolated RHF (elevated RVEDP alone) **does not** cause bilateral pleural effusions (Fig. 6.10)

**Bilateral Pleural Effusions are Physiologic Proof of Biventricular
Heart Failure (no matter how small)**

33 yo with quadriparesis (MVA 10 years PTA) and autonomic instability presenting with AFIB, complaining of 3 +
pitting edema associated with worsening SOB and increased BiPAP use occurring gradually over the past year. An
echocardiogram suggested isolated RHF from pulmonary hypertension (i.e. normal LV function and normal LA size
with severe PH and RV failure), possibly Cor Pulmonale from end stage restrictive lung disease secondary to
neuromuscular weakness or undiagnosed pulmonary vascular disease. CT scan suggested biventricular heart failure
(despite small LA size) given bilateral pleural effusions.

There is **normal left ventricular systolic function** with no wall motion abnormalities.
Flattened septum is noted, consistant with **right ventricular overload.**
Unable to assess diastolic function, no apical views available.
The **right ventricle** is moderately **dilated** and mildly **hypodynamic.**
No atrial septal defect or persistant superior vena cava are demonstrated by color Doppler
and agitated saline contrast. Four separate bubble studies were performed.
The **left atrial** chamber **size** is **normal.** or **small in size.**
The inferior vena cave is dilated without inspirational collapse.
Severe pulmonary hypertension is noted. RVSP=106.5 mmHg.

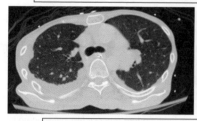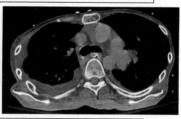

Swan floated at 1830: **WEDGE 19,**
CO/CI/SVR **4.3/2. 29/1283, CVP 17,** and **PAS/PAD 64-72/35-45,** MDs are aware.

RHC confirms biventricular heart failure with an LVEDP estimated to be ~22 (applying the correction suggested
by Halpern's data)

Fig. 6.10 Encapsulated case of an individual with quadriparesis (C4-C5 partial), presenting with a year of gradually worsening
edema and respiratory failure associated with new atrial fibrillation (AFIB). Although his echocardiogram suggested pulmonary
hypertension and isolated right-sided heart failure (RHF), his computed tomography scan showed small bilateral pleural
effusions, the "footprint" of biventricular heart failure (HF). confirmed by right-sided heart catheterization (RHC) likely triggered
by respiratory failure (a common provocateur of diastolic dysfunction via intermittent hypoxia and tachycardia). The edema
and effusions resolved with initiation of mechanical ventilation and a small daily diuretic dose.

MANAGEMENT OF BIVENTRICULAR HEART FAILURE FROM DIASTOLIC DYSFUNCTION (TRIAL OF EUVOLEMIA)

- The cause of elevated LVEDP physiology in patients with diastolic heart failure (HFpEF)
  is often a combination of **total body volume overload** and factors that provoke a
  diastolic filling abnormality—namely:
  - Obesity and obstructive sleep apnea (OSA)
  - Renal insufficiency (impaired natriuresis)
  - HTN and tachyarrhythmia (eg, AFIB)
  - Severe parenchymal lung disease (often with hypoxemia)
- The cornerstone of management is **euvolemia** *and* **management** of provocative
  factors (eg, Na$^+$ intake, OSA, hypoxemia, tachycardia, and HTN)

FLUID "SPACES" AND THE ANTICIPATED SEQUENCE OF FLUID ACCUMULATION AND MOBILIZATION IN BIVENTRICULAR HEART FAILURE (HEpEF AND HFrEF)

- Definitions:
  - First space refers to fluid in the vasculature
  - Second space refers to fluid in the systemic interstitium (ie, peripheral edema) and
    pulmonary interstitium (ie, interstitial edema)

- Second and a half space refers to fluid in the pleural space (ie, pleural effusions)
- Third space refers to fluid in the abdomen (ie, ascites)

- Sequential order of fluid **accumulation** in biventricular HF as LVEDP and PVP rise **gradually** (typical of decompensated HFpEF):
  - Systemic interstitium, before pulmonary interstitium, before pleural space, before abdomen
    - The alveolus, though not traditionally considered a space for fluid accumulation (very poorly tolerated), requires the highest LVEDP to occur (>25 mm Hg); therefore, if the LHF is gradual, the alveolus fills last

- Sequential order of fluid **accumulation** in biventricular HF as LVEDP and PVP rise **suddenly** (a.k.a. flash pulmonary edema):
  - Alveolar edema and pulmonary interstitium, before systemic interstitium, before pleural space, before abdomen

- Sequential order of fluid **mobilization** in biventricular HF as LVEDP and PVP fall (quickly or slowly):
  - Alveolar edema, followed by pulmonary interstitium, followed by systemic interstitium, followed by pleural space, followed by abdomen

- Peripheral edema resolves after interstitial edema **but** before pleural effusions
  - Failure to understand this order leads to two common problems:
    - A premature euvolemia assessment the first day the peripheral edema resolves
    - The desire to work up pleural fluid as an independent process (eg, parapneumonic or malignant) because the fluid remains despite the resolution of peripheral edema

- Pleural fluid will resolve **after** peripheral edema but **before** ascites

- Ascites accumulates last and resolves last (if at all)
  - Fluid absorption only occurs across the serosal membrane of the abdomen (no capillary bed or significant lymphatic drainage channels), and thus is limited to ~1200 mL every 24 hours

- With adequate renal function (intrinsic **or** renal replacement therapy) **everyone** can be diuresed, free of **all** second spaced fluid (interstitial edema) and pleural effusions, but **not** third spaced fluid (ascites)

- Hepatic hydrothorax behaves like ascites (because it is) and will not mobilize as quickly as the effusions seen in heart failure
  - Once peripheral edema resolves in the cirrhotic, diuresis goals should be reduced from the normal 1–2 L daily to 500 mL–1 L daily

SEPARATING DECOMPENSATED HEART FAILURE FROM END STAGE HEART FAILURE

- **Decompensated heart failure** presents with second- and third-spaced fluid
  - Compensation requires diuresis to euvolemia (no more second- or third-spaced fluid)
  - Second-spaced fluid can **always** be removed (by urination or ultrafiltration)

- **End stage heart failure** (and cirrhosis for that matter) are defined by undiuresable third-spaced fluid (ascites)
  - Occurs when central venous pressure is so high, and hepatic congestion so great, that more than ~1.2 L of ascites is generated in a 24-hour period
  - 1.2 L per 24 hours represents the maximum amount of fluid that can be reabsorbed across the serosal surface of the abdomen in an individual being diuresed
    - Further attempts at diuresis at this point lead to vascular volume depletion despite ascites

- No such "24-hour fluid removal limit" exists for second-spaced fluid because of the near perfect equilibrium that exists between the vasculature and the interstitium, nor dose it exist for pleural fluid because of thoracic lymphatics (hence the 2 and half space designation)
- End stage heart failure requires intermittent, large-volume paracentesis and/or organ transplant
- Hypoalbuminemia does **not** cause undiuresable interstitial edema
- Three classic diseases that are complicated by chronic generalized edema and low albumin are responsible for the **false** suggestion that, via poor oncotic pull, **hypoalbuminemia** causes edema: (1) nephrotic syndrome, (2) protein losing enteropathy, and (3) Kwashiorkor malnutrition
  - Now disproven, microcapillary studies demonstrate a preserved oncotic gradient in all of the above conditions, implicating instead increased capillary permeability
  - As albumin levels fall, interstitial and capillary albumin concentrations decrease proportionately
    - Maintaining an oncotic gradient favoring fluid return despite hypoalbuminemia
  - Profound hypoalbuminemia **may** decrease oncotic pull, hastening fluid accumulation and slowing mobilization
    - **But** hypoalbuminemia alone does **not** cause generalized edema or pulmonary edema in critically ill patients
      - **Sodium** (and thus volume) overload does

EFFECTIVE DIURESIS (IE, ACHIEVING A SIGNIFICANT NET NEGATIVE FLUID BALANCE)

- How to dose loop diuretics
  - Loop diuretics have 3 dose ranges; below threshold, above threshold (BUT below ceiling), and above ceiling
  - Step 1, establish '**above ceiling dose**':
    - Low GFR and /or chronic loop diuretic user, start higher dose
    - IV furosemide is twice as potent as PO, therefore 20 mg IV equals 40 mg PO
    - IV butanamide has the same potency as PO therefore 1 mg IV equals 1 mg PO
  - For those naive to loop diuretics start 40 – 80 mg of furosemide, or 1-2 mg of butanamide (based on the urgency of the diuresis)
  - Establish the ceiling dose by doubling the dose and repeating administration until dramatic urine output occurs
  - Ceiling dose IV furosemide and butanamide should start working in 30 min and last 2 hours, while PO has its effect 1-2 hours after administration, and lasts 4-6 hours
  - Once the (above) ceiling dose has been established, increase the interval from once daily to every 2 hours, based on the magnitude of the diuresis required (ie, the liters of urine that need to be made in 24 hours to established the desired net negative fluid balance)
- When the ceiling dose exceeds 80 mg of furosemide (or 2 mg of bumetanide) consider adding a thiazide diuretic to mitigate distal convoluted tubule Na^+ reabsorption (which is upregulated in the setting of chronic loop diuretic use)
  - Give metolazone 5 mg PO or Chlorthalidone 500 mg IV, 30 min before the loop diuretic (q 12 hours)
- Attempt to stay under 320 mg Q 24 hours (to avoid ototoxicity- case reports)
  - Ototoxicity has not been reported with butanamide
- Minimize Salt Input (<2gm daily)
- Furosemide is both filtered and secreted into the tubule
- Butanamide is nearly 100% filtered therefore is action depends entirely on an adequate GFR

PERCEIVED (BUT *NOT* ACTUAL) STUMBLING BLOCKS ENCOUNTERED WHILE DIURESING EDEMATOUS LEFT-SIDED HEART FAILURE PATIENTS TO EUVOLEMIA

- Hypotension:
  - Often iatrogenic, secondary to antihypertensive dugs and/or afterload reducing agents
    - Hold all antihypertensive drugs and afterload reducing agents until the patient is euvolemic
  - Patients with LV or RV systolic dysfunction will have an improvement in CO and MAP with euvolemia
    - Diuresis improves RV and/or LV starling curve forces; therefore diurese despite hypotension, to improve hypotension
      - Must explain to nursing or they will always hold the diuretic
  - Volume-overloaded intubated patients taking sedatives often need SVR support to allow for diuresis
    - A more appropriate strategy than preload for the volume overloaded

- Progressive azotemia and threatened renal failure:
  - Often iatrogenic secondary to ACE and angiotensin receptor block (ARB) (inappropriate before euvolemia)
  - It is **not possible** to cause AKI while diuresing an edematous patient
    - Loop diuretics are **not** nephrotoxins
      - They **do not** decrease renal blood flow
      - Loop diuretics (especially Bumetanide) must be filtered to function; when GFR approaches zero (as occurs with intravascular volume depletion) no medication is filtered and the drug has no effect
        - Erroneous administration of loop diuretics to a dehydrated individual has no effect (unlike erroneous fluid administration to a volume overloaded patient)
  - Overdiuresis presents as volume depletion (orthostasis, decreased urination, thirst), **not** shock or acute tubular necrosis (ATN)
    - ATN occurs with additional insults, such as ARB, ACE, or NSAID
  - Kidney injury is caused by volume overload, **not** its resolution
  - Renal function and serum Cr will either improve with diuresis (eg, cardiorenal physiology) **or**:
    - In a patient with intrinsic renal disease (most of them) the Cr will oscillate in a sine wave fashion
      - Between a "high" and "low" value reflecting impaired renal autoregulation
      - **Tolerate the rise, anticipate the fall, and continue to diurese**
  - If renal failure occurs while diuresing an edematous patient, **work it up**
    - Edematous patients with profoundly worsening renal insufficiency during diuresis **are not** simply hypovolemic or "a little intravascularly dry"
      - Start an evaluation of acute renal failure (eg, obstructive uropathy, ATN, AIN) (Fig. 6.11)
  - **Tolerate** fluctuations **in serum creatinine** and asymptomatic elevations in BUN **to attain euvolemia**

- Irrational fear of preload dependent physiology:
  - Manifests as a hesitation or refusal to diurese an edematous patient, concerned specifically that they may actually be suffering from PAH and isolated RHF, not PH from LHF
    - Fortunately, the management of decompensated, isolated, RHF in edematous patients is **also** diuresis
    - Even when they are hypotensive (assuming no other acute pathophysiology present eg, sepsis or hemorrhage)
      - Patients with isolated RHF who have edema and hypotension are "off" of their RV starling **curve and thus will have improved CO with diuresis**
  - Decompensated IPAH patients presenting with edema and hypotension **always** need diuresis

- Erroneous administration of fluid to decompensated, isolated RHF is **much** more **dangerous** than erroneous administration of diuretics
  - IV fluid administration (as little as 500 mL) to a decompensated IPAH patient may be **fatal**
    - Causing further RV stretch, which increases RV wall tension, decreasing RV perfusion, leading to RV infract and death
- Sudden death attributable to preload-dependent physiology is a phenomenon involving volume-depleted **outpatients** who suffer a fatal episode of **exertional** syncope
  - Occurring because the systemic circulation is vasodilated during exercise to accommodate the an increased CO
  - When RV CO cannot match LV CO because of a remodeled pulmonary vasculature (as seen in IPAH), a sudden decrease in CO can occur, causing syncope or death
    - Does not happen to inpatients, supine in a monitored bed (unless they are receiving general anesthesia, which is capable of producing a similar hemodynamic profile)
- Preload-dependent physiology is neither subtle nor unstable in monitored, hospitalized patients, manifesting as fluid responsive tachycardia and hypotension (despite volume overload)
- Furthermore, if you are wrong about filling pressures or in need of increased filling pressures (as in RV infarct or acute PE), you can always give fluid faster than any human can urinate
- **Empiric diuresis is always safer than empiric IV fluids** in patients who may have decompensated heart failure (right- or left-sided)

Pitfalls in Diuresis

HD # 1	73 y/o male with DM, HTN, CHF (last EF 23% 10/2011 mild conc LVH), scrotal edema and 3+ pitting edema up to thighs bilaterally

HD # 6	improving LE edema but worsened pulmonary edema that is concerning hold lasix due to contraction alkalosis for now Consult pulm

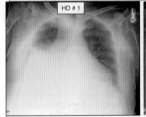 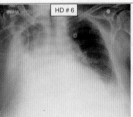 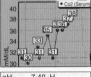

pH	7.49	H	
PCO2	52	H	mmHG
PO2	84		mmHG
HC03	39.6	H	mmol/L

Pulmonary Critical Care Medicine
– **Aggressive diuresis with a goal of net negative fluid balance 1–2 L every day**
– **Add diamox for metabolic alkalosis along with furosemide**

- 73 yo with DM, HTN, HF from systolic dysfunction (HFrEF) admitted with volume overload, did well until HD# 6
- Pulmonary consulted for persistent (asymptomatic) effusion "despite diuresis and contraction alkalosis"
- Pulmonary recommends continued diuresis with addition of acetazolamide. No indication for thoracentesis

A

Fig. 6.11 Encapsulated case showing an individual admitted with obvious decompensated heart failure with reduced ejection fraction (HFrEF), illustrating common real and *perceived* stumbling blocks encountered while diuresing an individual to euvolemia. (A) After a week of 1–2 L daily negative fluid balance, the patient develops a significant contraction alkalosis, causing a compensatory respiratory acidosis. If this process were allowed to continue, HCO_3 and PCO_2 would continue to gradually increase, ultimately causing CO_2 narcosis. The alkalosis occurs because of diuresis induced hypochloremia which prevents the kidney from alkalizing the urine. Fortunately this process is easy to screen for (daily HCO_3) and is easy to mitigate with potassium chloride repletion and acetazolamide. A contraction alkalosis occurring during diuresis should not prevent continued diuresis, nor should it be treated with volume expansion (the typical treatment for a contraction alkalosis occurring in dry individuals). Interpreting the chest x-ray film as "worsening pulmonary edema" likely reflects positional change and fluid shift from the right-sided hemithorax.

(Continued)

HD #12	# CFF: improving LE edema and pulmonary edema. Hold Lasix 20mg IV BID given AKI. # AKI Cr Baseline at I but currently >2 which is likely 2/2 intense diuresis. He is likely intravascularly dry causing AKI given BUN: Cr ration >20. Will hold diuresis during the day and f/u BID chem to monitor renal fxn. # **Pleural effusion:** Chronic and likely transudative, though not resolving with diuresis. **Given AKI, patient likely intravascularly dry and since only mild improvement in pleural effusion,** will consider further imaging and possible thoracentesis

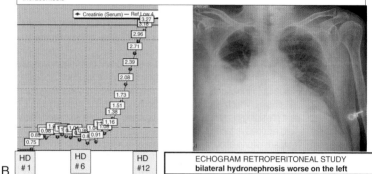

B

ECHOGRAM RETROPERITONEAL STUDY
bilateral hydronephrosis worse on the left

- Patient develops AKI wrongly attributed to diuresis and "intravascular volume depletion despite total body volume overload". Because he is deemed intravascularly volume depleted, and his pleural effusion persists, the primary team again asks pulmonary to consider thoracentesis (looking for an explanation other then HF).
- Pulmonary and Renal recommend working up the AKI (not attributable to diuresis), which reveals bladder outlet obstruction (patient wearing a condom catheter). Still no indication for thoracentesis.
- After Foley catheter placed AKI resolves and the patient continues to diurese, loosing 63 lbs of water weight

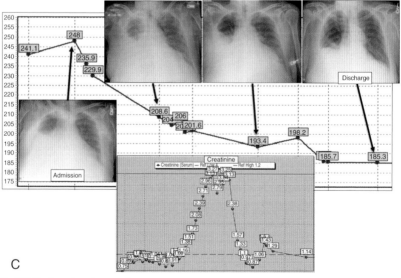

C

Fig. 6.11 See figure legend on opposite page.

REAL PROBLEMS ENCOUNTERED WHILE DIURESING THE EDEMATOUS PATIENT

- Contraction alkalosis:
  - Attempt to avoid a significant contraction alkalosis because of the compensatory respiratory acidosis (and risk of CO_2 narcosis)
  - Give intermittent acetazolamide (eg, 250–500 mg daily, prn HCO_3 > baseline)
  - Aggressively replete chloride with KCL

- Diuretic resistance:
  - After a patient becomes resistant to >80 mg furosemide (2 mg of bumetanide), add thiazide to address compensatory increased DCT sodium retention (metolazone or chlorthalidone)

- Hypernatremia (hypervolemic hypernatremia):
  - Hypernatremia, occurring in the setting of total body volume overload, implies a free water deficit with ongoing free H_2O loss, as seen in diarrhea, fever, or glycosuria
  - Treat the cause of excessive H_2O water loss, replete free H_2O as usual, **and** attempt to make the patient **net negative despite the increased free water**
    - That said, it is reasonable to leave the free H_2O repletion (for hypernatremia) out of the daily "in-and-out" total because the water is expanding in the intracellular space (**not** the interstitium)

HEART FAILURE—IMPORTANT REVIEW POINTS

- Interstitial edema can affect pulmonary function and exercise tolerance without radiographic change (Fig. 6.12)

- Edematous patients should not be **condemned** as **"ventilator dependent"** (Fig. 6.13)

- Biventricular HF can cause pulmonary hypertension and limit exercise before pulmonary edema occurs
  - As LVEDP is elevated in the 15–18 mm Hg range
  - Peripheral edema may be the only sign of symptomatic LHF

- A trial of diuresis *is not* equal to a trial of euvolemia
  - Because intermittent LVEDP elevations lead to manifestations of biventricular HF, **sustained reductions in LVEDP are required for resolution**

- Occasionally, mediastinal lymph nodes swell (with fluorodeoxy glucose (FDG)-avidity) in decompensated heart failure
  - Normalizing their size **only** after sustained resolution of heart failure (Fig. 6.14)

- Euvolemia first
  - Patients in decompensated congestive heart failure should **not** be given β-blockers until they are euvolemic (compensated)

Fig. 6.11, cont'd (B) The patient develops acute kidney injury (AKI) with a rapid, steep Cr increase (suggesting obstruction), which the primary team erroneously attributes to fictitious physiology (ie, "total body volume overload with intravascular volume depletion"). The false belief that the diuresis of an individual with decompensated heart failure (HF) itself could result in AKI threatened to delay definitive diagnosis (renal ultrasound) and treatment (Foley). (C) Chest x-ray films, weight measurements, and serum creatinine values for the remainder of the hospital stay. The medicine team was repeatedly concerned by the right-sided pleural effusion based on the magnitude of the R > L asymmetry (not that unusual) and its failure to improve significantly despite 40 lbs of fluid being removed (asking us to consider a right-sided thoracentesis a total of three times). In doing so, they were failing to acknowledge that all the peripheral edema must be mobilized first. This individual still had bilateral pleural effusions (R > L) on discharge, indicating persistent (though improved) decompensated HF. **Note**: AKI episode aside, this individual displayed the typical sine wave–like fluctuations in glomerular filtration rate (GFR) during diuresis because of impaired renal autoregulation (as they all do). His CR fluctuated between ~0.8–1.0 before his episode of AKI and ~0.8–1.5 after. **Note**: The patient gained weight late in the hospital stay (193–198 lbs), and diuresis was needlessly put on hold because of an increase in Cr.

70 yo with mild COPD evaluated for new DOE occurring over weeks, with a new mixed obstructive restrictive defect, and a mildly decreased DLCO on lung function testing. PFTs show BOTH FEV1 and FVC decreased (by ~ 1L). He endorsed weight gain, orthopnea and was found to have peripheral edema and basilar crackles on exam. His chest Xray showed NO evidence of pulmonary edema or effusions.

CC:	**70 yo man referred to the pulmonary clinic for** evaluation of a **decrease in his FEV1 on his PFTs.**

Vitals: T 98.3 P 60 BP 132/71 Sa02 96% (RA)
General: Obese adult male
Cardiac: JVP 8 cm H20. Regular rate and rhythm with I/VI systolic murmur at the LSB without radiation. **2 mm pitting edema to the mid-shins bilaterally.**
Chest: **Fine bibasilar rales that do not clear with repeated deep inspiration.**

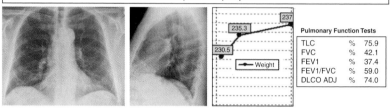

Pulmonary Function Tests

TLC	%	75.9
FVC	%	42.1
FEV1	%	37.4
FEV1/FVC	%	59.0
DLCO ADJ	%	74.0

A

At the last visit, he c/o increased LE edema and 45 degree angle orthopnea **Since the last visit, he feels his symptoms have greatly improved.** He responds well to each lasix dose and **notes a dramatic decrease in LE edema and improvement in exercise ability.**

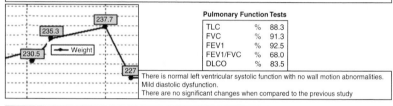

Pulmonary Function Tests

TLC	%	88.3
FVC	%	91.3
FEV1	%	92.5
FEV1/FVC	%	68.0
DLCO	%	83.5

There is normal left ventricular systolic function with no wall motion abnormalities. Mild diastolic dysfunction.
There are no significant changes when compared to the previous study

He was treated with diuresis which resolved his dyspnea, edema and his restrictive PFT pattern. His echocardiogram showed mild diastolic dysfunction.

B

Fig. 6.12 Encapsulated case showing an individual with mild COPD presenting with decompensated heart failure with preserved ejection fraction (HFpEF) manifesting as an exercise limitation, edema, and restrictive physiology, despite an x-ray without *obvious* edema, or effusions. (A) Clear chest x-ray, weight gain, and pulmonary function tests (PFTs) demonstrating a mixed obstructive (FEV$_1$/FVC percent ration <70) and restrictive defect (total lung capacity [TLC] <80%) with a mildly decreased diffusing capacity of lung for carbon monoxide (DLCO). (B) The individual's symptoms and PFT abnormalities completely resolved with diuresis to euvolemia. This episode of HFpEF was triggered by significant dietary Na$^+$ intake.

- Patients in decompensated congestive heart failure **without** profound left ventricular systolic dysfunction should not be afterload reduced until they are euvolemic

- Bilateral pleural effusions rule out isolated RHF and/or cor pulmonale

- Pleural effusions resolve after peripheral edema and before ascites

- Patients with edema are not euvolemic or at DRY weight

- You **cannot** cause AKI while diuresing an edematous patient with HF

- PCWP <15 mm Hg is unreliable at ruling out LVEDP >15 mm Hg

- Total body volume overload and intravascular volume depletion is **not** normal physiology
  - **Only** occurs in a handful of catastrophes:
    - Sudden hemorrhage, sepsis, adrenal crisis, systemic allergic reaction, and burns

78 yo with **severe COPD (FEV$_1$ 33%, DLCO 49%)**, admitted with small bowel obstruction requiring an exploratory laparotomy, revealing no etiologic cause, treated with bowel rest. Postoperative course was complicated by both urosepsis and line sepsis requiring reintubation. The patient defervesced and came off of pressors, **But was unable to wean from the ventilator** (despite no thoracic or pulmonary insult during his hospitalization). The patient receives a tracheostomy and the team and family prepare for transfer to a long term acute care (**LTAC**) facility. Until, HD # 56 when a change of attendings leads to the **diagnosis of decompensated HFpEF** from volume overload (a.k.a heart failure) based on the presence of generalized edema and pleural effusions. Plan for LTAC transfer changed to **Diuresis to Euvolemia**, which was complicated initially by contraction alkalosis and iatrogenic hypotension. Ultimately the patient is easily diuresed (i.e. **NET negative 1–2 L daily**) and liberated **8 days later**. He was then decanulated, sent to the rehabilitation floor, and was **discharged to home** ~4wks later.

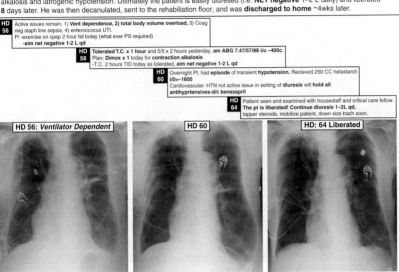

HD 56 Active issues remain, 1) **Vent dependence, 2) total body volume overload**, 3) Coag neg staph line sepsis, 4) enteroccocus UTI.
P/ -exercise on cpap 2 hour tid today (what ever PS required)
-aim net negative 1-2 L qd

HD 58 Tolerated T.C. x 1 hour and 5/5 x 2 hours yesterday, **am ABG 7.47/57/88 i/o –400c.**
Plan: Dimox x 1 today for contraction alkalosis
-T.C. 2 hours TID today as tolerated, aim net negative 1-2 L qd

HD 60 Overnight Pt. had **episode of transient hypotension.** Recieved 250 CC hetastarch i/0=−1600
Cardiovascular: HTN not active issue in setting of **diuresis will hold all antihypertensives-d/c benazapril**

HD 64 Patient seen and examined with housestaff and critical care fellow.
The pt is liberated! Continue diuresis 1–2L qd, tapper steroids, mobilize patient, down size trach soon.

HD 56: Ventilator Dependent | **HD 60** | **HD: 64 Liberated**

Fig. 6.13 Encapsulated case of an individual with severe chronic obstructive pulmonary disease (COPD) who is admitted to the hospital and intubated for noncardiopulmonary disease and is deemed ventilator dependent (based on COPD and deconditioning) when in actuality he was suffering from decompensated heart failure (HF) (heart failure with preserved ejection fraction [HFpEF]) caused by gross volume overload alone (ie, no history of HF). His HF was missed because (1) his edema was erroneously attributed to hypoalbuminemia and (2) radiology underread his chest x-ray results with regard to pulmonary edema, erroneously attributing both the fluid in his superior accessory fissure on the left (the dense, well-circumscribed, curved opacity extending from the left hilum superiorly) and his left-sided pleural effusion as chronic scarring. His HF occurred because he was allowed to "autoregulate" his volume status, leading to a daily positive fluid balance and volume overload (obvious on physical examination and chest x-ray). Positive pressure ventilation alone, by decreasing cardiac output (CO) causes sodium avidity. Additionally, hospitalization entails significant IV sodium infusions (via medications, drips, and fluids), further perpetuating volume overload. This patient had been prescribed his home ACE inhibitor (full dose) because of hypertension (actually caused by volume overload). The patient went from only tolerating a tracheostomy collar for 1 hour a day to liberation from mechanical ventilation in just 8 days as his HF and pulmonary edema resolved. HF decreases compliance, increases airway resistance, and impairs oxygenation such that patients should not be condemned as ventilator dependent while volume overloaded

This case also illustrates two common *perceived* and real stumbling blocks to diuresis: (1) The patient suffered a real contraction alkalosis, which is common during diuresis and discussed in detail in Fig. 6.11. Again, this is easy to mitigate with acetazolamide and should **not** hinder ongoing diuresis. (2) He suffered iatrogenic hypotension during diuresis, secondary to an ACE inhibitor given for essential hypertension (HTN). Significant hypotension is **not** anticipated while diuresing an edematous patient and should prompt a search for antihypertensive medications vs a new pathophysiology (eg, bleeding or sepsis). It also illustrates the point that basilar pleural scarring in COPD, especially with flattened diaphragms, can be difficult to distinguish from pleural fluid (misread by radiology in this case—until it resolved).

- And third-spacing physiologic states:
  - Pancreatitis, cirrhosis, and S/P large intraabdominal surgery
- **Very** uncommon in outpatients

- Hypoalbuminemia does **not** cause edema

- Do not fear preload dependent physiology, fear volume overload

- Patients with **parenchymal lung disease** or long-standing LVEDP elevations may have **subtle or absent pleural fluid**, *despite* biventricular HF:

66 yo with interstitial lung disease (ILD) and biventricular HF from systolic dysfunction (HFrEF) referred to pulmonary for enlarging, PET avid mediastinal and hilar adenopathy found on chest CT. Pulmonary, noting pleural effusions, increases diuretic regimen, and plans a repeat CT when euvolemic.

PULMONARY - OUTPATIENT   Reason For Request:

Other: **mediastinal lymphadenopathy, PET +, with ILD, repeat Chest CT shows enlargening lymphadenopathy, eval for possible EBUS.**

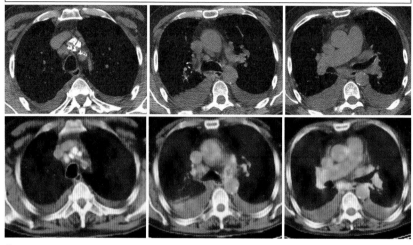

A

Repeat Chest CT 2 months later (6 lbs lighter) shows persistent adenopathy and improved (but still present) pleural effusions. Pulmonary plans EBUS to rule out lymphoma and / or sarcoidosis. The patient *'no shows'* for the EBUS procedure, and is lost to follow up for a year. He represents, 12 lbs lighter, without edema and has a repeat CT scan with no effusions and all lymph nodes normal in size

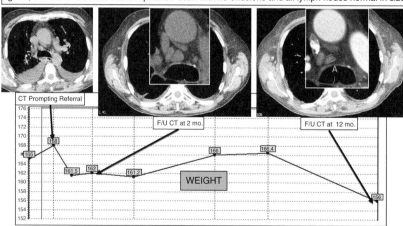

B

Fig. 6.14 See figure legend on opposite page.

- Pleural scarring can produce effective pleurodesis
- Longstanding LVEDP elevations can lead to increased lymphatic drainage (compensatory)

- **Common HF mistakes, by level of training:**
  - House staff:
    - *"Maintenance IV fluid"* given to the patient with generalized edema
    - Repetitive sub-ceiling loop diuretic dosing, called "failed diuresis"
    - Daily positive fluid balance in edematous patients **not** being intentionally resuscitated
      - Presuming "autoregulation" of volume
    - Missing dependent edema (eg, sacral edema, scrotal edema)
  - Fellows:
    - Failing to mention the left atrial size when reporting an echocardiogram "suggesting PAH"
    - Labeling a volume overloaded patient as "ventilator dependent"
    - Labeling a volume overloaded patient as having "ARDS"
    - Assuming peripheral edema in a patient with severe lung disease represents cor pulmonale
  - Attendings:
    - Believing echocardiographic signs suggesting isolated RHF are more sensitive than the physical findings of biventricular HF (eg, pleural effusions—no matter how small)
    - Believing that patients with decompensated LHF might be suffering from out-of-portion RHF, requiring pulmonary vasodilator therapy
    - Believing that a PCWP <15 mm Hg is reliable at ruling out an LVEDP >15 mm Hg

COMMON QUESTIONS GENERATED BY THIS TEACHING

1. **How does LHF cause pulmonary hypertension and RHF?**
   Via a neurohormonal reflex, **not** back pressure.

2. **What if all the peripheral edema in my patient is from isolated RHF (no obvious thoracic edema)?**
   Edematous patients with isolated RHF **also** need diuresis to euvolemia. The failing RV is vulnerable to overdistension ("falling off of its starling curve")

3. **How can my patient have severe biventricular HF when the diastolic filling abnormality seen on an echocardiogram is only mild?**
   The severity of heart failure is rated clinically (eg, NYHA class). The severity of the abnormal filling pattern routinely observed on an echocardiogram "underestimates" the severity of the disease because the provocative factors of diastolic dysfunction (eg, volume

Fig. 6.14 Encapsulated case of an individual referred for endobronchial ultrasound–mediated biopsy of growing, fluorodeoxy glucose (FDG)–avid mediastinal and hilar adenopathy. (A) Computed tomography (CT) and positron emission tomography scan images with multiple, "hot," slightly enlarged mediastinal and hilar lymph nodes bilaterally and symmetrically. Additionally, the patient had bilateral pleural effusions (ie, biventricular heart failure [HF]) with small focal areas of pleural-based FDG avidity. Given the relatively benign appearance of the thorax, combined with the evidence of decompensated HF, the plan was made to reimage after diuresis to euvolemia. (B) Three CT scan images over a year, overlaid against weight. The follow-up CT scan obtained 2 months after initial evaluation and significant diuresis (but not euvolemia, as evidenced by small effusions) showed persistent adenopathy. At this point it was considered reasonable to offer an endobronchial ultrasound (EBUS) to rule out lymphoma and/or sarcoidosis. Unfortunately for us (fortunately for him), the patient was lost to follow-up for a year, returning euvolemic with repeat imaging demonstrating resolution of both effusions and adenopathy. This case highlights that euvolemia may take time to achieve in outpatients and that diuresis with resolving HF is **not** the same as euvolemia. Furthermore, long-standing manifestations of HF (like pulmonary hypertension, effusions, and ascites) may take both time and euvolemia to resolve. It should also be noted that attributing mediastinal and/or hilar adenopathy to HF is a diagnosis of exclusion. That said, an EBUS (or any procedure) is safer when HF is compensated, making diuresis to euvolemia a reasonable first step (assuming imaging is not ominous, ie, obvious malignancy).

status, hypoxia, tachycardia and blood pressure) may vary widely throughout the day and over time.

4. **In my patient with known LHF and pulmonary hypertension how can I separate out the proportion of the pulmonary hypertension that is a result of the biventricular HF reflex (group II disease), and how much is secondary to vascular remodeling (group I disease), the trans pulmonary gradient?**
   No. It is not possible, nor is it a worthwhile pursuit. The management of group II PH involves reducing and maintaining a low LVEDP. Only after a sustained reduction in LVEDP has been achieved can one assess the pulmonary vasculature for "primary" small vessel disease. Pulmonary vasodilators are contraindicated in group II disease.

5. **In hospitalized patients with decompensated biventricular HF and severe RV systolic dysfunction (hypokinesis), when should I use pulmonary vasodilators to "unload the RV?"**
   Never. Despite how dysfunctional the RV looks, compared to the LV on an echocardiogram, pulmonary vasodilators are **never** needed to compensate for decompensated biventricular HF; in fact they are **contraindicated**. Diuresis with inotropic support (if needed) is the therapy.

EVALUATION AND TREATMENT OF PULMONARY HYPERTENSION

CHAPTER 7

COMMON MISCONCEPTIONS AND MISTAKES

- Believing that the most common cause of pulmonary hypertension (PH) in patients with severe lung disease is group 3
- Obtaining an nonexpert right-sided heart catheterization (RHC) to rule out World Health Organization (WHO) group 2 disease
- Believing that WHO group 2 patients with "out-of-proportion PH" require pulmonary vasodilator/antiremodeling therapy
- Thinking that chronic thromboembolic pulmonary hypertension (CTEPH) represents the accumulation of multiple untreated pulmonary emboli over time
- Believing that patients with isolated right-sided heart failure (RHF) are not safe to diurese to euvolemia because of preload-dependent physiology

PULMONARY HYPERTENSION

- PH is defined as a **mean pulmonary artery pressure (mPAP)** >25 mm Hg and is grouped by cause/category
- The diagnosis of PH is most commonly suggested by an elevated pulmonary artery systolic (PAS) pressure, as estimated by transthoracic echocardiogram
  - Requires tricuspid regurgitation, which is common when the pulmonary artery (PA) is high
    - PAS pressure is estimated from the maximum velocity of the tricuspid regurgitant jet
  - Echocardiography may overestimate, underestimate, or entirely miss PH
- A definitive diagnosis of PH and an accurate severity assessment requires an RHC, with direct measurement of PA pressure and an assessment of cardiac output and pulmonary vascular resistance
  - Pulmonary vascular resistance is superior to mPAP in the assessment of pulmonary vascular disease because as right ventricular cardiac output (RV CO) decreases, mPAP goes **down**
    - Pulmonary vascular resistance, on the other hand, increases (by taking CO into account), reflecting the worsening pulmonary vascular disease (despite a lower mPAP)
  - Pulmonary vascular resistance (in dyn-sec-cm^{-5}) = (mPAP − left-ventricular end-diastolic pressure [LVEDP])/cardiac output × 80
  - Because pulmonary capillary wedge pressure (PCWP) systematically underestimates LVEDP, LVEDP may need to be measured directly by left-sided heart catheterization
- This invasive approach should be reserved for patients with proven or **strongly** suspected group 1 disease (eg, idiopathic pulmonary arterial hypertension [IPAH])
- PCWP measurement (even in expert hands) is a poor predictor of LVEDP, making RHC generally **unhelpful** in excluding left-sided heart failure (LHF) as the etiology of PH (ie, group 2)

- Most PH (>90%) can be easily attributed to LHF or underlying lung disease based on clinical assessment using the patient history, physical examination, imaging, pulmonary function testing (PFT), echocardiogram, **and response to diuresis**
- The evaluation of PH hinges on an approach that presumes (and thus works hard to exclude) LHF (group 2 disease) as the etiology, because this is the cause the vast majority of the time **(Fig. 7.1)**
- Sudden severe PH, without shock from acute RHF **(Fig. 7.2)**, and intermittent PH (Fig. 7.3) are common in individuals with LHF and rare or unheard of in individuals with primary pulmonary vascular disease (eg, chronic thromboembolic pulmonary hypertension [CTEPH], idiopathic pulmonary arterial hypertension [IPAH]), or PH related to lung disease

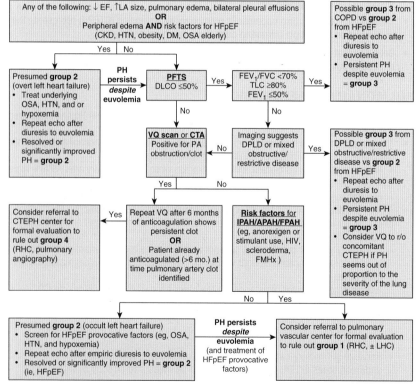

EVALUATION OF PULMONARY HYPERTENSION
(ELEVATED PULMONARY ARTERY SYSTOLIC PRESSURE ON ECHO)

Fig. 7.1 Flow diagram outlining the evaluation of suspected pulmonary hypertension (ie, elevated PAS pressure suggested by an echocardiogram). Approach hinges on excluding left-sided heart failure by diuresis to euvolemia. Pulmonary function testing (PFT) and a ventilation-perfusion (VQ) scan should be done relatively early for individuals without obvious left-sided heart failure. Diuresis to euvolemia is indicated in both decompensated isolated right-sided heart failure and biventricular heart failure. In cases of isolated right-sided heart failure, diuresis will improve CO (via improved starling forces) but will not significantly reduce pulmonary artery (PA) pressures. In cases of biventricular heart failure, diuresis to euvolemia will significantly improve or resolve the pulmonary hypertension (PH) (pathognomonic for group 2 disease).

Sudden Severe Pulmonary Hypertension

PULMONARY - OUTPATIENT consult request
Provisional diagnosis: Pulmonary hypertension
Reason for request: 48 yo male admitted with volume overload, pt improved with diuresis, found to have **PAP 72 on TTE in house new since 2 mo.** Prior with nml EF, PE protocol CT neg

Echo 7 years prior to consult

Normal study, except:
Left ventricle has concentric hypertrophy.
No previous study available for comparison.

Echo 1 year prior to consult

Left ventricular systolic function is normal.
The left ventricle has concentric hypertrophy.
Left ventricular diastolic function is abnormal.
Compared to the prior study: Abnormal diastolic function is now present.

Echo 2 months prior to consult

The left atrium is enlarged.
Left ventricular systolic function is normal.
The left ventricle has concentric hypertrophy.
Left ventricular diastolic function is abnormal.

Echo prompting the consult

Left ventricular systolic function is normal.
Severe pulmonary hypertension is present.
Regurgitation of the tricuspid valve (s) is present.
Compared to the prior study: Severe pulmonary hypertension, and an increase in tricuspid regurgitation gradient are now present.

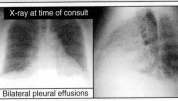
X-ray at time of consult
Bilateral pleural effusions

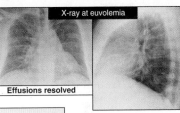
X-ray at euvolemia
Effusions resolved

Consult DISCONTINUED LANDSBERG, JUDD
Please repeat echo when pt euvolemic and refer if sig pulm HTN persists (doubt)

Euvolemic echo

There is normal left ventricular systolic function with no wall motion abnormalities.
Abnormal left venticular diastolic function is observed.
No evidence of pulmonary hypertension.

Fig. 7.2 Encapsulated case illustrating pulmonary hypertension (PH) secondary to overt or obvious left-sided heart failure. At the point the patient is admitted with volume overload (decompensated heart failure with preserved ejection fraction [HFpEF]), he has 7 years of echocardiograms showing the gradual development of HFpEF: echo 1, LVH; echo 2, diastolic filling abnormality; echo 3, left atrial enlargement; and finally echo 4, severe PH. Even without serial echocardiograms, the patient's PH and volume overload can be confidently attributed to biventricular heart failure from the presence of bilateral pleural effusion and left atrial enlargement, seen on the echocardiogram that prompted the pulmonary consult. Ruling out pulmonary embolism should only have been pursued if the patient had failed to improve with euvolemia.

PATHOPHYSIOLOGY, EVALUATION, AND TREATMENT OF PULMONARY HYPERTENSION BY GROUP (Table 7.1):

- **Step 1: rule out group 2 disease**
  - Exclude (or more likely confirm) LHF **by reassessment after diuresis to euvolemia**
- **PH secondary to LHF (WHO group 2):**
  - The vast majority of PH is group 2, related to the biventricular heart failure reflex, because LHF is a **very** common disease
  - Many group 2 patients have **overt LHF** (most commonly heart failure with reduced ejection fraction [HFrEF]) and pose no diagnostic challenge
  - Others have **occult or "missed" LHF** (most commonly heart failure with preserved ejection fraction [HFpEF]), often leading to needless subspecialty referral, invasive advance testing, and erroneous administration of contraindicated medications (ie, pulmonary vasodilators)

Intermittent Pulmonary Hypertension

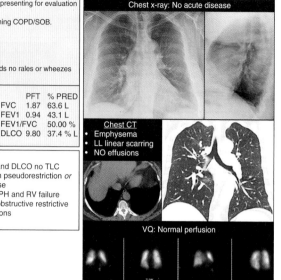

58 year old FEMALE w/ COPD and HTN presenting for evaluation of 2 mo. increased DOE
Pt reports she is concerned about worsening COPD/SOB.
gen: out of breath when walking
Weight: 251.4 lb
PE: BP: 138/78
CV: RRR, no MRG
Lungs: extremely decreased breath sounds no rales or wheezes
Ext: 1+ b/1 LEE

Plan:
- Continue inahlers
- CT non-contrast to evaluate for CPFE
- VQ scan, to evaluate for CTEPH
- Start lasix 20 mg po qam
- f/u ECHO, done today

	PFT	% PRED
FVC	1.87	63.6 L
FEV1	0.94	43.1 L
FEV1/FVC	50.00 %	
DLCO	9.80	37.4 % L

- **Chest x-ray:** Normal
- **PFT:** Obstruction with a low FVC and DLCO no TLC available, either severe COPD with pseudorestriction *or* mixed obstructive restrictive disease
- **Echo:** Normal LA and LV EF with PH and RV failure
- **Chest CT:** No evidence of mixed obstructive restrictive disease, interstitial edema or effusions
- **VQ scan:** Normal perfusion

Chest x-ray: No acute disease

Chest CT
- Emphysema
- LL linear scarring
- NO effusions

VQ: Normal perfusion

ANT Q   POST Q   RAO Q   LPO Q
LAO Q   LPO Q   LLAT Q   LLAT Q

A

Fig. 7.3 Panel A shows the encapsulated case of an obese woman with severe chronic obstructive pulmonary disease (COPD) presenting with heart failure with preserved ejection fraction (despite no obvious thoracic fluid) illustrating the point that pulmonary hypertension (PH) and peripheral edema may be the only objective signs of biventricular heart failure. This occurs in individuals whose left ventricular end-diastolic pressure (LVEDP) remains in the 16 to 17 mm Hg range (not high enough to cause interstitial edema, which is required for pleural effusion formation). Panel B shows the same individual demonstrating intermittent pulmonary hypertension over several years, occurring with repeated episodes of decompensated LHF Resolving and remitting PH is *only* seen with group 2 disease. Note how unhelpful assessment of inferior vena cava (IVC) collapse is with regard to determination of total body volume status.

- LHF causes PH via the biventricular heart failure reflex:
  - Where elevated LVEDP causes increased PVP via back pressure, and
  - Increased PVP triggers an increase in PAP, via a neurohormonal reflex (**not** backpressure)
- Ensuring that PAP is always greater then PVP
  - This pressure gradient is required to maintain forward flow through the pulmonary vasculature (waterfall/reservoir mechanism)
- Enormous individual variability exists in the biventricular heart failure reflex (ie, an LVEDP of 25 may trigger a PAS pressure anywhere from 35 to 99 mm Hg [see CH 6])
- Unfortunately, group 2 has been further subdivided (descriptively/deceptively) into three (misleading) categories based on the magnitude of the biventricular heart failure reflex (ie, comparing the magnitude of the mPAP elevation to the LVEDP elevation)
  - Passive PH is defined as an mPAP-LVEDP ≤ 12
  - Reactive PH is defined as an mPAP-LVEDP ≥ 12
  - Out-of-proportion PH is defined as an mPAP-LVEDP ≥ 12 and LVEDP ≤ 25

One month follow-up after diuresis (9 lbs lighter), DOE improved, pulmonary hypertension resolved

58 year old woman with PMH of COPD here for f/u after PH evaluation reveled HFpEF. Started on lasix last month feeling much better with much improved exercise tolerance. Will plan to repeat echo to ensure pulmonary hypertension improved

Echocardiograms over the next 3.5 years show intermittent pulmonary hypertension occurring as a consequence of episodic HFpEF exacerbations (ie, tracking closely with the patients weight which is reflective of her volume status)

#1 Echo: Normal LV,LA, moderate PH, RV failure	#3 Echo (2 years later): Moderate PH, RV failure
There is normal left ventricular systolic function with no wall motion abnormalities.	There is normal left ventricular systolic function with no wall motion abnormalities.
Abnormal left ventricular diastolic function is observed.	Mild diastolic dysfunction.
The left atrial chamber size is normal.	The left atrial chamber size is normal.
The right atrial cavity size is normal.	The right ventricle is mildly dilated with normal systolic function.
The right ventricle appears mildly dilated in some views though with normal systolic function.	The right atrium is mildly dilated.
There is mild tricuspid regurgitation.	There is mild dilatation of the ascending aorta.
The inferior vena cava is dilated.	The inferior vena cava appears normal in size. The estimated right atrial pressure is normal. There is a greater than 50% respiratory change in the inferior vena cava dimension. Moderate pulmonary hypertension is noted.
There is less than 50% respiratory change in the inferior vena cava dimension.	When compared to the previous study performed on mild right ventricular enlargement, mild right atrial enlargement, mild ascending aortic dilation, and moderate pulmonary hypertension are now present.
Moderate pulmonary hypertension is noted.	
No previous study available for comparison.	

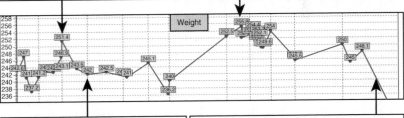

#2 Repeat echo (2 mo. later): No PH, nl RA/RV	#4 Echo (3.5 years later): No PH, nl RA/RV
Compared to the prior study: **the right ventricle no longer appears mildly enlarged, the right atrial pressure is now within normal range, moderate pulmonary hypertension has decreased to within normal range, and mild pulmonic insufficiency and tricuspid regurgitation have decreased to trace.**	There is normal left ventricular systolic function with no wall motion abnormalities.
	Mild diastolic dysfunction.
	No significant valvular disease.
	When compared to the prior study: **RV and RA sizes are normal now.**
	Pulmonary pressure have decreased from 49 mmHg to 21 mmHg.

B

Fig. 7.3, Cont'd

- The terms are misconstrued such that "passive" is interpreted as back pressure and "out of proportion" is interpreted as a remodeled vasculature requiring pulmonary vasodilator/antiremodeling therapy
- Instead the terms are descriptive only and have no physiologic basis or implications with regard to management
- Out-of-proportion PH is the most dangerous because it suggests the need for pulmonary vasodilator therapy in individuals with known LVEDP elevation, which is a **contraindication**
  - These patients are typically referred for PH or exercise limitation thought to be "out of proportion" to the perceived degree of left-sided dysfunction, **or** a RHC showing an mPAP-PCWP $\geq$12 and PCWP $\leq$25

Table 7.1 Pathophysiology, Evaluation, and Treatment of Pulmonary Hypertension by World Health Organization (WHO) Grouping Group

WHO GROUP (ESTIMATED PREVALENCE)	UNDERLYING DISEASE STATE(S)	MECHANISM	TREATMENT AND RATIONALE
Group 2 (~80%)	**Left-sided heart failure (overt)** • Most commonly HFrEF (cardiomyopathy from CAD, MI, HTN, valvular disease, alcohol, viral, idiopathic) **Left-sided heart failure (occult*)** • Most commonly HFpEF (diastolic dysfunction and volume overload from CKD, OSA/OHS, HTN, DM, end-stage lung disease, age >65 years)	**Biventricular heart failure reflex** • Increased LVEDP increases PVP (via back pressure) • Increased PVP triggers a neurohormonal reflex that increases PAP	**Diuresis to euvolemia** • Decreases LVEDP, RVEDP • Improves CO • Resolves (or significantly improves) PH **Treatment of HFpEF provocative factors (eg, OSA, HTN, sodium intake)** • Improves diastolic filling/CO • Prevents volume overload
Group 3 (~15%)	**Severe parenchymal lung disease** Emphysema Diffuse parenchymal lung disease Mixed obstructive restrictive disease (eg, combined pulmonary fibrosis and emphysema)	**Loss of small- to medium-sized pulmonary arteries from parenchymal destruction** Decreasing vascular cross-sectional area Increasing pulmonary vascular resistance	**Oxygen for the hypoxemic** Improves survival in COPD Improves exercise in DPLD Prevents diastolic dysfunction and HFpEF Does **not** significantly improve PH (itself) **Diuresis to euvolemia** Improves RV starling forces, increasing RV cardiac output Lowers LVEDP, preventing concomitant HFpEF
	Severe sleep disordered breathing and hypoventilation • Obstructive sleep apnea • Obesity-related hypoventilation	**Hypoxemia and HFpEF** • Hypoxic pulmonary vasoconstriction (minor role only, PA pressure does not rapidly drop with oxygen administration) • Occult left-sided heart failure (ie, actually group 2)	**Positive airway pressure and oxygen for the hypoxemic** • Prevents desaturations improving diastolic filling • Prevents the systemic adrenergic response to apneas improving diastolic filling **Diuresis to euvolemia** • Lowers LVEDP

Group 4 (~4%)	**Chronic thromboembolic pulmonary hypertension**	**Large vessel occlusion with chronic clot** • Decreasing vascular cross-sectional area • Increasing pulmonary vascular resistance **Progressive small vessel vascular remodeling** • Decreasing vascular cross-sectional area • Increasing pulmonary vascular resistance	**Pulmonary endarterectomy** • Improves RV CO and resolves (or significantly improves) PH **Lifelong anticoagulation** • Prevents recurrent CTEPH and sudden death from recurrent emboli **IVC filter placement** • Prevents recurrent embolism **Antiremodeling/pulmonary vasodilator therapy for nonsurgical candidates (minority)** • Prevents progressive small vessel vascular remodeling **Diuresis to euvolemia** • Improves RV starling forces, increasing RV cardiac output
Group 1 (~1%)	**Idiopathic, associated, and familial pulmonary arterial hypertension** • **IPAH** (idiopathic) • **APAH** (associated with scleroderma, HIV, portal HTN, anorexigen/stimulant use) • **FPAH** (inherited)	**Remodeling of small- to medium-sized pulmonary arteries** • Muscularization, luminal narrowing, and in situ thrombosis leading to vascular obliteration • Decreasing vascular cross-sectional area • Increasing pulmonary vascular resistance	**Antiremodeling/pulmonary vasodilator therapy** • Prevents progressive small-vessel vascular remodeling • Improves RV CO and improves PAH **Lifelong anticoagulation** • Prevents small-vessel in situ thrombosis **Oxygen for the hypoxemic** • Improves exercise ability • Prevents hypoxemic PA vasoconstriction **Diuresis to euvolemia** • Improves RV starling forces, increasing RV cardiac output

APAH, Associated pulmonary hypertension; *CAD*, coronary artery disease; *CKD*, chronic kidney disease; *CO*, cardiac output; *COPD*, chronic obstructive pulmonary disease; *CTEPH*, chronic thromboembolic pulmonary hypertension; *DM*, diabetes mellitus; *FPAH*, familial pulmonary arterial hypertension; *HFpEF*, heart failure with preserved ejection fraction; *HFrEF*, heart failure with reduced ejection fraction; *HTN*, hypertension; *IPAH*, idiopathic pulmonary arterial hypertension; *IVC*, inferior vena cava; *LVEDP*, left-ventricular end-diastolic pressure; *MI*, myocardial infarction; *OHS*, obesity hypoventilation syndrome; *OSA*, obstructive sleep apnea; *PA*, pulmonary artery; *PAH*, pulmonary arterial hypertension; *PAP*, pulmonary artery pressure; *PH*, pulmonary hypertension; *PVP*, pulmonary venous pressure; *RV CO*, right ventricular cardiac output; *RVEDP*, right ventricular end-diastolic pressure.

- The cornerstone of management of these patients is euvolemia and optimization of LHF (eg, treatment of HFpEF provocative factors)
- Worsening PH in these patients is an indication of increasing LVEDP, **not** progressive vascular remodeling
- **Group 2** disease should be the **presumed cause of PH** in:
  - Individuals with systolic dysfunction, increased left atrial (LA) size (without mitral valve disease), pulmonary edema, and/or pleural effusion
    - Because these conditions are virtually pathognomonic for LHF
  - Edematous patients with risk factors for HFpEF, such as chronic kidney disease (CKD), hypertension (HTN), obesity, obstructive sleep apnea (OSA), diabetes mellitus (DM), and age >65 years
    - Because these are the most common conditions associated with occult LHF, a very common disease
- Traditional teaching suggests that **group 2 PH** should be differentiated from **group 1** via RHC with PCWP (a.k.a. pulmonary artery occlusion pressure) measurement, demonstrating an mPAP >25 mm Hg occurring with a PCWP <15 mm Hg
  - This approach fails for two reasons:
    1. PCWP is a poor predictor of LVEDP (mischaracterizing PH 50%–85% of the time, depending on the expertise of the RHC operator)
    2. Intermittent LVEDP elevations may lead to sustained elevations in mPAP (such that a single, resting pressure measurement is **not** adequate at ruling out the clinical syndrome of HFpEF)
- A more robust, practical strategy involves a reassessment of PA pressure **after** diuresis to euvolemia
  - PH that improves significantly (or resolves) with diuresis is pathognomonic for **group 2** disease (ie, secondary to LHF)
- **Diuresis to euvolemia is critical to the management of *both* group 2 and group 1 disease, making this the obvious approach**
- Even though longstanding elevations of LVEDP may cause areas of IPAH-like remodeling, there is almost **no role for pulmonary vasodilators**/antiremodeling agents in these patients
  - Pulmonary vasodilators should only be considered in patients with LHF who:
    - Demonstrate the ability to maintain outpatient euvolemia for months to years:
      - No pleural effusion, no peripheral edema
      and
    - Still have an exercise limitation believed to be secondary to RV afterload from a remodeled vasculature, from previous longstanding LVEDP elevation
  - Theses patients may be trialed on a phosphodiesterase 5 inhibitor with significant risk/benefit counseling regarding possible worsening LVEDP physiology
    - Endothelin receptor antagonists and prostacyclins are contraindicated because they may dramatically worsen left-sided heart failure, causing arrhythmia; flash pulmonary edema and death
      - Use of these medications with known LHF requires referral to an IPAH center of excellence (and likely LVEDP measurement by left-sided heart catheterization) before initiation
- **Step 2: rule out group 3 disease**
  - Individuals without obvious signs of LHF or risk factors for HFpEF, or individuals whose PH does not improve/resolve with diuresis, should have PFTs obtained (flows, volumes, and diffusion capacity of the lungs for carbon monoxide [DLCO]) to rule out group 3 disease
- **PH secondary to end-stage parenchymal lung disease and severe OSA/obesity hypoventilation syndrome (OHS) (WHO group 3):**
  - Group 3 represents the next largest category because lung disease and sleep-disordered breathing/hypoventilation are common

- **Group 3 PH, from severe parenchymal lung disease,** occurs in patients with:
  - Emphysema, diffuse parenchymal lung disease (DPLD), and/or combined pulmonary fibrosis and emphysema (CPFE)—a.k.a. mixed obstructive restrictive disease
    - Usually obvious from the patient history, physical examination, imaging, and PFTs
  - **PH secondary to end-stage parenchymal lung disease** is caused by parenchymal destruction, with its accompanying loss of small–medium sized blood vessels
    - Decreasing the cross-sectional area available to receive RV CO, increasing pulmonary arterial resistance
  - Normally the DLCO needs to be $\leq$50% predicted (ie, over half of the vasculature destroyed) to cause PH at rest
  - If the DLCO is $\leq$50%, the forced expiratory volume 1 (FEV_1)/forced vital capacity (FVC) ratio is <70%, FEV_1 is $\leq$50%, and the total lung capacity (TLC) is $\geq$80%, a diagnosis of cor pulmonale, secondary to emphysema (the most common cause), may be considered if diuresis to euvolemia fails to resolve the PH
  - If the DLCO is $\leq$50%, but either the the TLC is < 80%, or the FEV1/FVC ratio is > 70, then the differential diagnosis becomes group 4 disease (CTEPH) vs group 3 PH secondary to severe mixed obstructive restrictive disease (eg, **CPFE**), or MUCH less likely group 1 disease (eg, IPAH)
    - Individuals with CPFE may demonstrate pseudonormalization of air flows (from restricted areas) and volumes (from obstructive areas) leading to an apparent 'isolated low DLCO' on PFT testing
    - However, the physical examination and chest imaging are **not** subtle for severe mixed obstructive restrictive disease, often making the distinction easy
    - Patients with mixed obstructive restrictive disease (eg, CPFE) often warrant a ventilation-perfusion (VQ) scan because disease severity may be more challenging to establish, potentially allowing severe PH to be erroneously attributed to moderate mixed disease (missing concomitant CTEPH, a relatively common comorbid condition)
  - **Group 2 PH is *more* common in patients with end-stage lung disease than group 3**
    - Lung disease, with its associated tachycardia and hypoxemia, is a common provocateur of LHF, causing diastolic dysfunction, leading to concomitant HFpEF
  - Because of this, edematous patients with severe parenchymal lung disease **should have concomitant group 2 PH excluded by a trial of euvolemia** before a diagnosis of cor pulmonale is made (Fig. 7.4)
    - **Euvolemia is also indicated in group 3 disease** to maintain optimal RV starling forces and myocardial perfusion (both jeopardized by RV overdistension), making this the obvious approach
  - Oxygen therapy for hypoxemic patients with group 3 PH is important **but** does not significantly lower their PA pressures (because the mechanism responsible for PH is **not** hypoxemic vasoconstriction)
    - It improves survival (when worn >18 hours a day) and prevents HFpEF
  - **Group 3 patients typically experience a pulmonary exercise limitation, either ventilatory** (emphysema) or, less commonly, from exercise-induced **hypoxemia** (DPLD or CPFE), not PH and RHF
  - There is **no role** (theoretical or otherwise) for pulmonary vasodilators/antiremodeling agents in these patients
  - Worsening PH is typically an indication of worsening lung function, inadequately treated hypoxemia, or superimposed HFpEF (provoked by tachycardia and hypoxemia)
  - Treat group 3 PH secondary to severe parenchymal lung disease by optimization of lung function, smoking cessation, oxygen for the hypoxemic, workup and treatment of DPLD (if present), and **euvolemia**
- **Group 3 PH, PH secondary to OSA, and OHS** are included in this category because they are associated with alveolar hypoventilation and subsequent hypoxemia
  - Hypoxemia is capable of causing mild PH via diffuse PA vasoconstriction, which rapidly reverses with oxygen administration

Decompensated Group 2 Disease Masquerading as End-stage Group 3 Disease

56 yo with severe COPD presenting with a 3 month decline in exercise ability, and new peripheral edema. Baseline echo, CXR and PFTS suggest group 3 PH, making his current deterioration concerning for decompensated / end-stage **cor pulmonale**

Spirometry		Ref	Pre Meas	Pre %Ref
FVC	Liters	3.93	2.32	59
FEV1	Liters	2.86	0.66	**23**
FEV1/FVC	%	73		**28**

Lung volumes		Ref	Pre Meas	Pre %Ref
VC	Liters	3.93	2.57	65
TLC	Liters	5.50	6.80	**124**
RV	Liters	1.99	4.23	212

Diffusion		Ref	Pre Meas	Pre %Ref
DLCO	mL/mmHg/min	22.7	13.5	**59**

Flow 4 2 0 −2 −4 −6 −1 0 1 2 Volume

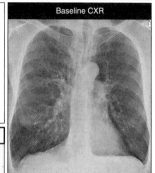

Baseline CXR

Repeat CXR

Baseline echo: Moderate PH

The left ventricle is normal in size.
Left ventricular diastolic function is abnormal as evidenced by decreased E/A ratio.
The left atrium is normal in size.
The right atrium is normal in size.
The right ventricle is normal in size.
The right ventricular systolic function is normal.
The aortic root is normal in size.
The pulmonary artery is dilated.
Moderate pulmonary hypertension is present.

Repeat echo to evaluate deterioration: LA,RA, and RV enlargement

The left ventricle is normal in size.
Left ventricular systolic function is normal.
The left atrium is mildly enlarged.
The right atrium is mildly enlarged.
The right ventricle is moderately enlarged.
The pulmonary artery is dilated.
The inferior vena cava is dilated but does not collapse on inspiration suggesting elevated central venous pressure, estimated between 10 to 15 mmHg.

Repeat chest x-ray and echocardiogram instead suggest that the clinical deterioration and new RV failure, are related to concomitant HFpEF and group 2 PH (note subtle bilateral pleural effusions and left atrial enlargement). The patient returned to baseline with diuresis.

Fig. 7.4 Encapsulated case of an individual with severe chronic obstructive pulmonary disease (COPD) evaluated for a decline in exercise tolerance and peripheral edema. The patient's symptoms were initially concerning for cor pulmonale given his severe lung disease and baseline echocardiogram, showing moderate PH with a normal LA size, suggesting group 3 disease. However, a repeat chest x-ray and echocardiogram instead show left-sided heart failure (bilateral pleural effusion and left atrial enlargement), giving the patient a diagnosis of concomitant heart failure with preserved ejection fraction (significantly better prognosis). HFpEF is the most common mimic of cor pulmonale, making its exclusion essential.

- Rapid reversal of PH is **not** observed clinically in OSA/OHS patients given supplemental oxygen, making hypoxic pulmonary vasoconstriction an unsatisfying pathophysiologic explanation
- In actuality, most of these individuals have (occult) LHF from diastolic dysfunction provoked by untreated sleep-disordered breathing, made worse by daytime hypoventilation and hypoxemia (see CH 8) and thus would be more appropriately classified as group 2 PH (secondary to HFpEF)
  - This explains their slow response to therapy (weeks to months), timing compatible with resolution of HFpEF (not hypoxemic vasoconstriction)
- Euvolemia is challenging to establish in the obese:
  - Chest x-ray sensitivity for pulmonary edema is decreased by low lung volumes which increase interstitial markings, and adipose tissue, that creates a veil that is hard to distinguish from pleural fluid

- The physical examination for generalized edema also loses sensitivity in obese patients, as adipose makes peripheral edema more difficult to detect
- Empiric diuresis should always be attempted in these individuals
- **Step 3: rule out group 4 disease with VQ scan or computed tomography angiography (CTA)**
  - Individuals without LHF or parenchymal lung disease should have a VQ scan or CTA preformed to exclude CTEPH
- **PH secondary to chronic thromboembolic pulmonary hypertension (CTEPH) (WHO group 4):**
  - **CTEPH** occurs when an acute thromboembolism fails to resolve and instead organizes and grows distally (ie, chronic clot)
  - Chronic clot causes:
    - Loss of pulmonary vascular bed (beyond the chronic clot)
    - Progressive PH (without new perfusion defects)
      - From secondary, small-vessel (IPAH-like), progressive vascular remodeling (incompletely understood)
      - Resulting in isolated RHF and death if not treated
  - Individuals with CTEPH may have an isolated low DLCO or a restrictive pattern on PFTs
    - Restriction may be a result of decreased large vessel vascular compliance, as well as parenchymal scarring associated with infarction
  - A screening VQ scan or CTA should be considered early in the workup of PH when patients have a history of VTE or when:
    - Left-sided heart disease has been excluded by diuresis to euvolemia
    - Severe parenchymal lung disease has been excluded by patient history, physical examination, PFTs, and imaging
  - Individuals with CTEPH typically have grossly abnormal perfusion scans, revealing multiple segmental unmatched perfusion defects (Fig. 7.5 A)
  - CTA may reveal signs specific to CTEPH by implying chronicity—ie, right ventricular enlargement, mosaic attenuation (Fig. 7.5 B), **and** linear intraluminal thromboembolic material (Fig. 7.5 C)
  - CTEPH affects up to 4% of individuals who survive a (diagnosed) acute pulmonary embolism
    - 70% have a clinical history of acute pulmonary embolism, 50% have lower-extremity ultrasound findings of chronic/prior lower-extremity deep vein thrombosis
    - Remainder of individuals likely suffered a silent or misdiagnosed acute pulmonary embolism
  - Patients with possible/probable CTEPH require referral to a CTEPH center of excellence (eg, the University of California San Diego), where they may receive:
    - Angiography to confirm the disease and assess surgical accessibility of the clot
    - Followed by (potentially curative) pulmonary thromboendarterectomy (PTE) if they are deemed to have surgically accessible disease (Fig. 7.5 D)
  - Patients with CTEPH have a lifelong thromboembolic recurrence risk, mandating lifelong anticoagulation
    - Individuals who discontinue anticoagulation after successful endarterectomy, have a high rate of recurrence
  - Most CTEPH centers place inferior vena cava (IVC) filters in all patients undergoing pulmonary endarterectomy, in case anticoagulation is interrupted
  - PTE surgery requires sternotomy, cardiopulmonary bypass/circulatory arrest, and deep hypothermia
    - It represents an endarterectomy, not embolectomy (Fig. 7.5 E)
  - Complications after PTE surgery include:
    - Reperfusion lung injury:

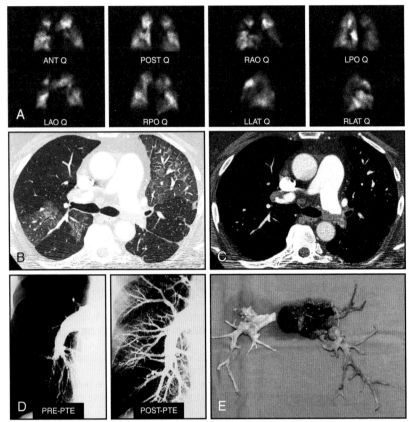

Fig. 7.5 (A) Grossly abnormal perfusion scan of a patient with chronic thromboembolic pulmonary hypertension (CTEPH) (ie, multiple segmental defects bilaterally). (B) Computed tomography (CT) scan of a patient with CTEPH. Lung windows demonstrate mosaicism representing differential perfusion where the low attenuation areas are oligemic and the high attenuation areas are hyperemic. (C) Mediastinal windows (same scan) demonstrating a linear thrombus in the central pulmonary arteries bilaterally. (D) Pre- and postoperative pulmonary angiography (different patient). (E) Endarterectomy material (different patient).

- Focal capillary leak with inflammatory infiltrate (neutrophils)
- Confined to endarterectomized segments
- Occurs in the first 72 hours postoperatively
- Leads to hypoxemia and poor compliance, prolonging the need for mechanical ventilation
  - Persistent PH after PTE (pulmonary vascular resistance [PVR] >500 dynes-sec-cm^{-5}) may cause postoperative death from refractory RHF
    - Particularly when combined with reperfusion lung injury
  - It is common for post-PTE patients to require oxygen for weeks as lung VQ relationships normalize and reperfusion injury resolves
- **Pulmonary arterial hypertension (PAH) from progressive pulmonary vascular remodeling (WHO group 1):**
  - PAH is an **extremely rare** diagnosis of exclusion and should **only** be considered in patients who "pass" the screening previously outlined for LHF (obvious and occult), lung disease, and CTEPH

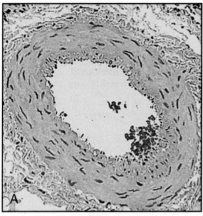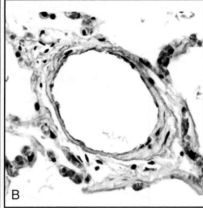

Fig. 7.6 (A) Typical histopathology of small-vessel vascular remodeling. The medial layer of the vessel has multiple layers of smooth muscle cells. The endothelial cells lining the intima have an abnormally large cytoplasm, indicating their activated state. (B) A normal small-vessel pulmonary artery where the medial layer is one smooth muscle cell layer thick; the cytoplasm of the endothelial cells are scant/normal.

- PAH occurs when small- to medium-sized pulmonary arterioles undergo pathologic vascular remodeling consisting of:
  - Muscularization (medial hypertrophy), where layers of PA smooth muscle cells narrow the vascular lumen (Fig. 7.6)
  - Upregulated abnormal PA endothelial cells, which line the lumen and promote smooth muscle cell growth and platelet activation (causing in situ thrombosis)
  - Ultimately both processes lead to obliteration of the vessel
- **Pulmonary vascular remodeling** in PAH is progressive, leading to RHF and death if untreated
- PAH occurs idiopathically (ie, **IPAH**), hereditarily (ie, **familial pulmonary arterial hypertension [FPAH]**), and in association (ie, **associated pulmonary hypertension [APAH]**) with drugs and toxins (eg, anorexigens, central stimulants) or conditions/diseases (eg, HIV, portal hypertension, scleroderma/mixed connective tissue disease)
- Because group 1 PAH is so rare and group 2 PH is so common, **most** (>90%) individuals evaluated for group 1 disease will ultimately be found to have group 2 disease
- Most individuals with PAH are young and have a well-known associated condition or exposure
- Formal IPAH evaluation requires an **expert** RHC, demonstrating:
  - Mean PAP >25 (PH) with an PCWP <15 mm Hg
    - Typically, PCWP is low (<8 mm Hg), as is the cardiac index (<2.0)
  - Patients with a history concerning for LHF (eg, HTN, CKD) may deserve direct LVEDP measurement because PCWP can appear low, despite elevated LVEDP (~50% of the time, despite expert RHC)
- IPAH treatment should be initiated and supervised by a pulmonary vascular center/expert
  - Patients **must** be evaluated over time with serial RHC so that the cardiac index can be followed
  - Echocardiograms can be misleading and suggest disease improvement, as PAS pressure falls, when it actually represents end-stage disease reflecting a decreased RV cardiac output (Fig. 7.7)
- **PH secondary to diseases with unknown or multiple mechanisms (WHO group 5):**
  - Heterogeneous set of disorders (eg, sarcoidosis, pulmonary langerhans cell histiocytosis, Gaucher's disease) that are associated with PH by either unclear or multifactorial mechanisms

THE NATURAL HISTORY OF GROUP 1 PAH AND GROUP 4 CTEPH
Importance of RHC (CO determination and PVR calculation) over echocardiogram (PAP estimation alone)

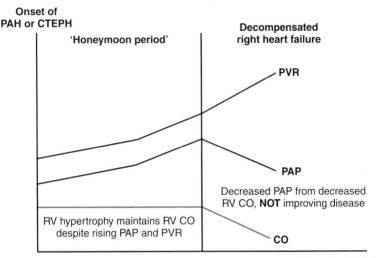

Fig. 7.7 Diagram illustrating the natural history of both group 1 and 4 disease (ie, progressive pulmonary hypertension). As pulmonary artery (PA) pressure increases gradually over time, right ventricular hypertrophy allows CO to be maintained (up to a point). Right-sided heart catheterization is required to follow disease progression and assess response to therapy by allowing for CO determination and pulmonary vascular resistance calculation. PA pressure assessment alone (ie, echocardiogram) may be misleading because a falling PA pressure can mean either improving *or* worsening disease.

- Diseases in this category most commonly cause PH by:
  - Main PA external compression (eg, fibrosing mediastinitis), or
  - IPAH-like vascular remodeling (eg, Gaucher's disease)
- This group is complicated by the fact that a disease like sarcoidosis may cause PH by multiple mechanisms simultaneously (eg, stage 2 sarcoidosis causing severe parenchymal lung disease and main PA compression from hilar adenopathy)
- Additional diseases in this category are strongly associated with occult LHF and thus may actually represent group 2 disease (eg, end-stage renal disease on hemodialysis)

COMMON QUESTIONS GENERATED BY THIS TEACHING

1. What if my edematous patient has isolated RHF and is preload-dependent such that diuresis is not safe?
   Edematous patients with isolated RHF also require diuresis to euvolemia (ie, no edema).
2. When the IVC demonstrates >50% respiratory variation, does it mean that the patient is not volume overloaded?
   No, when the IVC fails to collapse with respiration, it suggests that CVP is high. An IVC that collapses with respiration is unhelpful in the assessment of total body volume status in edematous patients with heart failure.
3. I was taught that isolated RHF occasionally causes a right-sided transudative pleural effusion (question implied by tone).
   Isolated RHF with ascites may cause a hepatic hydrothorax (uncommon).

CHAPTER 8

EXACERBATION OF OBESITY HYPOVENTILATION SYNDROME

COMMON MISCONCEPTIONS AND MISTAKES

- Attempting to force awake patients with central hypoventilation and no increased work of breathing to use bilevel positive airway pressure (BiPAP)
- Diagnosing a chronic obstructive pulmonary disease (COPD) patient with end-stage COPD because they present with a compensated severe respiratory acidosis (failing to notice that it developed over weeks to months)
- Failing to work up an elevated serum HCO_3 with an arterial blood gas (ABG) (instead assuming it represents a primary metabolic alkalosis)

OBESITY HYPOVENTILATION SYNDROME

- Obesity is a common cause of blunted ventilatory drive (unknown mechanism) and thus chronic hypoventilation
  - Individuals typically experience mild-moderate hypoventilation, with Pco_2 values in the 45–55 mm Hg range
  - This leads to renal compensation and serum HCO_3 elevations in the 30–34 mmol/L range
    - Assuming no renal tubular acidosis (RTA) or end-stage renal disease (ESRD)
  - Patients with RTA or ESRD may have an uncompensated respiratory acidosis (despite chronicity), giving them an ABG with the appearance of acute hypercarbic respiratory failure
    - Clinically they have no acute respiratory complaints, which:
      - Distinguishes them from patients with true acute hypercarbic respiratory failure, and
      - Demonstrates their tolerance to acidosis, with regards to dyspnea (ie, blunted ventilatory drive), and hypercarbia, with regard to CO_2 narcosis
- Patients obese enough to suffer from hypoventilation almost always have concomitant obstructive sleep apnea (OSA)
- Hypoventilation is always worse during sleep; therefore poorly treated OSA exacerbates chronic hypoventilation

EXACERBATION OF OBESITY HYPOVENTILATION SYNDROME

- An exacerbation of obesity hypoventilation syndrome (OHS) describes a subacute presentation in which patients gradually retain CO_2 (20–40 mm Hg) over weeks to months, allowing for renal compensation and central tolerance to CO_2 narcosis
- Ultimately they present complaining of shortness of breath and/or worsening exercise limitation
- Occasionally they present with lethargy secondary to symptomatic CO_2 narcosis (because of the absolute magnitude of the Pco_2 elevation or the rapidity of its rise)
- The syndrome often presents as a "cor pulmonale" mimic, with:
  - Severe, chronic, compensated respiratory acidosis (Pco_2 often >60 mm Hg)
  - Peripheral edema
  - Cardiac echo cardiogram suggesting pulmonary hypertension and isolated right-sided heart failure (ie, preserved left-ventricular (LV) function ± normal left artery (LA) size)
  - Profound exercise limitation

- Unlike true cor pulmonale, the phenomena are potentially reversible in weeks to months with diuresis to euvolemia, supplemental O_2 use, and OSA treatment (nocturnal positive airway pressure therapy)
- The chest x-ray (especially portable) is often difficult to interpret, given obesity:
  - Soft tissue veil may represent effusion **or** adipose
  - Increased interstitial markings with hilar fullness may represent cardiogenic edema **or** low lung volumes
- Decompensated heart failure (commonly heart failure with a preserved ejection fraction [HFpEF]), with gross total body volume overload (>15 L/30 lbs), is central to the pathophysiology of the OHS exacerbation:
  - Volume overload (pulmonary edema and pleural effusion) decrease compliance, increasing the work of breathing required to maintain the patient's baseline P_{CO_2}
  - Individuals with blunted ventilation choose, instead, to maintain the same work of breathing, hypoventilating (gradually) and allowing their P_{CO_2} to rise, thereby triggering both renal and central compensation
- A viscous cycle ensues where Hypoventilation and pulmonary edema cause hypoxemia, which worsens diastolic dysfunction leading to decompensated HFpEF, pulmonary edema, worse compliance, and further hypoventilation (worse during sleep)
- When looked at over time, HCO_3 levels and patient weight can be seen to increase and decrease together, as episodes of heart failure (as evidenced by fluid mediated weight gain), provoke episodes of hypoventilation (as evidenced by HCO_3 rise) OHS (Fig. 8.1).

61 year old with obesity (BMI 39), chronic obstructive pulmonary disease (COPD), heart failure with reduced ejection fraction (HFrEF) admitted three times in 1 year with acute on chronic mixed hypoxemic, hypercarbic respiratory failure showing weight (from volume overload) and HCO_3 (from renal compensation for hypoventilation) track closely during obesity hypoventilation syndome (OHS) exacerbations

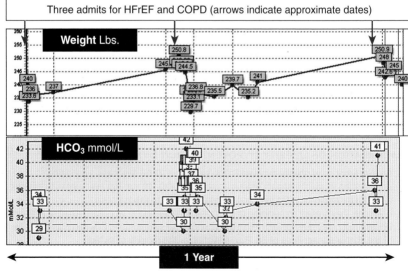

Fig. 8.1 Graphical display of an obese individual's weight and HCO_3 values over a 1-year period, showing three points in time *(red arrows)* when they were admitted with acute respiratory failure secondary to chronic obstructive pulmonary disease (COPD) and heart failure (HF). The episodic dramatic elevations in weight reflect heart failure and volume overload, whereas the elevation of HCO_3 reflects renal compensation for subacute hypoventilation. This pattern is typical of patients with obesity hypoventilation syndrome and HF.

- Patients present on a **spectrum of acuity:**
  - **Worsening exercise limitation and dyspnea on exertion** (Fig. 8.2)
    - ABG suggests chronic hypercapnic respiratory failure
      - Acidic pH in the normal range (7.35–7.39) and a severe respiratory acidosis
  - **Acute on chronic hypercapnic failure with shortness of breath** (often with no increased work of breathing)
    - ABG suggests acute on chronic hypercapnic respiratory failure
      - Acidotic pH (<7.35) and a mostly compensated severe respiratory acidosis
  - **Lethargy to obtundation (symptomatic CO$_2$ narcosis)** with no increased work of breathing
    - ABG shows either an extremely high Pco$_2$ (>90 mm Hg) or a mostly uncompensated severe respiratory acidosis (ie, evidence of rapid Pco$_2$ rise)
  - **Acute hypoxemic respiratory failure from hypoventilation and alveolar edema** (often with increased work of breathing)
    - ABG suggests mixed hypoxemic hypercapnic respiratory failure with at least a partially compensated severe respiratory acidosis

51-year-old male with heart failure with a preserved ejection fraction (HFpEF), chronic kidney disease 3, obesity (BMI 40) and obstructive sleep apnea admitted with decompensated heart failure

- Physical shows 2+ LE edema
- Admission HCO$_3$ 42 mmol/L
- HCO$_3$ 27 mmol/L one month prior
- Arterial blood gas (ABG) obtained showing chronic compensated respiratory acidosis
- Pulmonary function tests restricted with a low diffusing capacity of the lung for carbon monoxide
- Echo shows HFpEF
- VQ scan low probability
- Patient diuresed ~ 17 L
- Discharge ABG shows resolution of the chronic respiratory acidosis, HCO$_3$ 24 mmol/L

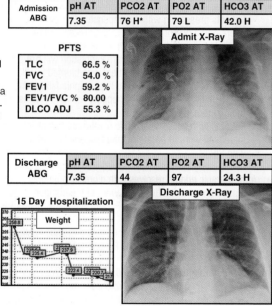

Admission ABG	pH AT	PCO2 AT	PO2 AT	HCO3 AT
	7.35	76 H*	79 L	42.0 H

Admit X-Ray

PFTS

TLC	66.5 %
FVC	54.0 %
FEV1	59.2 %
FEV1/FVC %	80.00
DLCO ADJ	55.3 %

Discharge ABG	pH AT	PCO2 AT	PO2 AT	HCO3 AT
	7.35	44	97	24.3 H

Discharge X-Ray

15 Day Hospitalization

Weight

Fig. 8.2 Encapsulated case of a patient with obesity, obstructive sleep apnea, chronic kidney disease 3, and heart failure with preserved ejection fraction (HFpEF) who presented complaining of shortness of breath and diminished exercise capacity and was admitted for an exacerbation of HFpEF. His echocardiogram showed normal systolic function, an increased pulmonary artery systolic with right-arterial dilation, and right-ventricular hypokinesis, but his chest x-ray showed interstitial edema with probable bilateral pleural effusion. He had a VQ scan that was low probability for pulmonary embolism (PE). His admission chemistry was notable for a HCO$_3$ of 42 mmol, which had been normal 1 month prior. His arterial blood gas (ABG) showed a chronic compensated respiratory acidosis with a Pco$_2$ of 76 mm Hg, occurring over the past month based on his last normal HCO$_3$. His preadmission (baseline) pulmonary function tests (PFTs) showed a restrictive pattern (likely from cardiogenic pulmonary edema). The patient was supported with oxygen, nocturnal bilevel positive airway pressure (BiPAP) (though poorly compliant), and diuresis with loop diuretics and intermittent acetazolamide (on any day that his pH was alkalotic). After diuresis of 17 L, he left the hospital 2 weeks later with a near normalization of his ventilation. This case illustrates how individuals with blunted ventilation, like the morbidly obese, may suffer subacute hypoventilation when they experience worsening respiratory mechanics, such as the decreased compliance associated with cardiogenic pulmonary edema. Ventilation returns to normal as the pulmonary edema resolves and respiratory mechanics return to baseline. The patient was not taking narcotics, sedatives, or other centrally acting medications or drugs (urine toxicology screen negative).

- Recent history shows weight gain (often 15–30 lbs of fluid weight)
- Physical examination reveals peripheral edema, often with pulmonary edema (ie, crackles and diminished basilar breath sounds with dullness to percussion)
- Serum chemistry shows a dramatically elevated serum HCO_3
  - Prior laboratory results show serum HCO_3 close to normal (or normal) in the recent past, before the onset of volume overload
- Chest x-ray shows interstitial edema, pleural effusion, and varying degrees of alveolar edema
- Narcotics and sedatives (often poorly cleared in the setting of decompensated HF with cardiorenal physiology) may complicate the picture, worsening hypoventilation
- Underlying COPD and baseline CO_2 retention also increase the propensity for hypoventilation
  - Doctors may erroneously attribute these patients' severe respiratory acidosis to progression of their obstructive lung disease, labeling them as end-stage COPD with cor pulmonale
    - This happens despite the fact that their CO_2 retention occurred over weeks to months, not years as is the case with COPD (Fig. 8.3)
    - This mistake can lead to misguided patient counseling regarding intubation and code status
- A mainstay of therapy is diuresis and oxygen support with or without BiPAP
  - Patients presenting with a compensated respiratory acidosis and no increased work of breathing do not need, tolerate, or receive significant benefit from noninvasive ventilatory support (eg, BiPAP) while awake
    - Noninvasive positive pressure ventilation will **not** significantly increase the minute ventilation of an awake patient with blunted ventilatory drive
  - Patients with acute on chronic hypercapnic failure and shortness of breath may benefit from noninvasive ventilatory support with BiPAP to assist them with the acute aspect of their hypercapnic failure
  - Patients with acute hypoxemic respiratory failure from cardiogenic edema often have increased work of breathing and typically benefit from noninvasive ventilatory support with BiPAP
  - Occasionally, brief intubation is required because of obtundation or flash pulmonary edema
- After thoracic edema resolves with diuresis, pulmonary compliance returns to normal
- The patient maintains the same work of breathing, minute ventilation increases (because compliance has improved), and P_{CO_2} falls quickly toward the patient's true baseline (within days)
  - ABGs obtained during this time show a metabolic alkalemia (posthypercapnic)
    - This happens because the kidneys take time to spill HCO_3 after the respiratory acidosis resolves
    - Acetazolamide can be used to speed up this process
      - Given on a daily basis, whenever the patient's pH is >7.40
    - Chloride infusion is also helpful, allowing the kidneys to alkalize the urine
      - Potassium chloride is preferred since sodium chloride is a step backwards for recently diuresed individuals
- Treatment of sleep-disordered breathing is crucial to facilitate diuresis and resolve the subacute respiratory acidosis
  - Even individuals who are noncompliant with PAP therapy for OSA as outpatients can usually be convinced to use a BiPAP machine in the acute setting (at least initially) while sleeping

COMMON QUESTIONS GENERATED BY THIS TEACHING

1. What happens when you use BiPAP for central hypercapnic respiratory failure?
   Very little. Patients may take larger breaths, but they decrease their respiratory rate, maintaining an almost identical minute ventilation.

58-year-old with severe chronic obstructive pulmonary disease (COPD), obesity, obstructive sleep apnea, and heart failure with preserved ejection fraction (HFpEF), presented complaining of shortness of breath admitted for a COPD exacerbation and decompensated heart failure

- Physical showed 2+ LE edema
- Admission HCO$_3$ 48 mmol/L **up from 29 mmol/L four months prior**
- Arterial blood gas (ABG) showed a chronic compensated respiratory acidosis
- Pulmonary function tests demonstrated severe obstruction with a low diffusing capacity of the lung for carbon monoxide
- Echo showed HFpEF
- Computed tomography angiogram was negative for pulmonary embolism
- Patient diuresed ~ 14 L
- Discharge ABG shows near resolution of the chronic respiratory acidosis

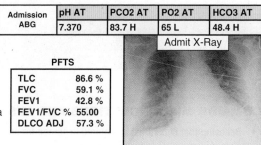

Admission ABG	pH AT	PCO2 AT	PO2 AT	HCO3 AT
	7.370	83.7 H	65 L	48.4 H

Admit X-Ray

PFTS

TLC	86.6 %
FVC	59.1 %
FEV1	42.8 %
FEV1/FVC %	55.00
DLCO ADJ	57.3 %

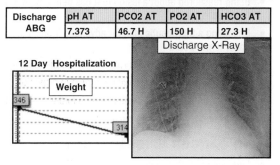

Discharge ABG	pH AT	PCO2 AT	PO2 AT	HCO3 AT
	7.373	46.7 H	150 H	27.3 H

Discharge X-Ray

12 Day Hospitalization

Weight

346

314

Fig. 8.3 Encapsulated case of a patient with severe chronic obstructive pulmonary disease (COPD), obesity, obstructive sleep apnea, and heart failure with preserved ejection fraction (HFpEF) who presented complaining of shortness of breath and diminished exercise capacity and was admitted for a COPD/HFpEF exacerbation. His admission echocardiogram (echo) showed normal systolic function with an increased pulmonary artery systolic with right-arterial and left-arterial dilation and right-ventricular hypokinesis. His chest x-ray showed interstitial edema with probable bilateral pleural effusion. He had a computed tomography angiogram that was negative for pulmonary embolism. His admission chemistry was notable for a HCO$_3$ of 48 mmol, which had been 29 mmol 4 months prior. His arterial blood gas (ABG) showed a chronic compensated respiratory acidosis with a P$_{CO_2}$ of 84 mm Hg, occurring subacutely over months, based on his last HCO$_3$ reading. His preadmission (baseline) pulmonary function tests showed severe obstruction with a low diffusing capacity of the lung for carbon monoxide. The patient was supported with oxygen, nocturnal BiPAP (though poorly compliant), daily diuresis (1–2 L), and a 5-day prednisone taper. After diuresis of ~14 L, he left the hospital 2 weeks later, with a dramatic improvement in his chronic respiratory acidosis. At presentation the patient was not taking narcotics, sedatives, or other centrally acting medications or drugs (urine toxicology screen negative). Although this individual has severe COPD, P$_{CO_2}$ elevations from COPD occur gradually (over years). Compensated (a.k.a. chronic) severe respiratory acidosis that develops subacutely, over weeks to months, often involves a combination of blunted ventilation and cardiogenic pulmonary edema.

2. Is this not just a heart failure presentation?
   Yes, but it has a very unique feature of profound central hypoventilation.
3. What causes pulmonary hypertension and right-sided heart failure, hypoxemia?
   Pulmonary hypertension (PH) and right-sided heart failure occur as part of the biventricular heart failure reflex. Resolution of hypoxemia happens quickly with oxygen supplementation, but resolution of the pulmonary hypertension, and the left sided heart failure that drives it, takes more time (weeks).

CHAPTER 9

LUNG CANCER

COMMON MISCONCEPTIONS AND MISTAKES

- Believing that IV contrast is required to screen for pathologic mediastinal adenopathy
- Being reassured about a lesion that has demonstrated growth over time because it is "cold on PET scan"
- Designing a therapeutic plan for advanced lung cancer without a multidisciplinary chest tumor board
- Comparing imaging reports rather than actual imaging
- Failing to ensure radiographic resolution of pneumonia
- Attributing enlarged mediastinal lymph nodes to acute bacterial pneumonia
- Performing a biopsy of a lung abscess

LUNG CANCER EPIDEMIOLOGY

- Lung cancer always grows, producing symptoms by occupying space and compressing/eroding into normal structures, ultimately killing the patient via a complication associated with the above process, or a systemic complication like venous thromboembolic disease or other paraneoplastic syndrome
- >95% of lung cancers are carcinomas (ie, epithelial cell origin)
- >85% of lung cancers are caused by cigarette smoking
  - Risk increases with the total number of cigarettes smoked
  - Precise quantification via "pack-years" = (average number of packs per day) × (number of years); useful in research, **not** clinically
  - Clinically, ~10 cigarettes a day for ≥ ~10 years equals a significant exposure, thereby increasing the risk of lung cancer (and chronic obstructive pulmonary disease [COPD])
  - Tobacco smoke contains tobacco-specific nitrosamines and polycyclic hydrocarbons, which are known carcinogens
  - Cigar and pipe smoking (less smoke inhalation) poses a significantly lower (but real) risk of lung cancer
- Other significant risk factors for lung cancer include:
  - Asbestos exposure, which dramatically increases the risk for lung carcinoma **and** is associated with the rare mesothelioma (pleural-based malignancy of mesothelial cell origin)
    - Risk of lung cancer is **very** high among smokers with asbestos exposure (synergy)
      - Asbestos alone confers a 2- to 5-fold increased risk
      - Cigarette smoking alone confers a 10-fold increased risk
      - Cigarette smoking and asbestos confer a 40-fold increased risk
  - Pulmonary fibrosis and other focal parenchymal scaring (eg, as seen after tuburculosis [TB])
  - Radon exposure (typically residential) which confers a definite risk of unclear magnitude
    - Radon (gas) decay product of radium-226 occurs naturally and is a known lung carcinogen
    - Exposure potentially occurs in homes (with basements built on soil/rock high in radium)

- Occupational exposures/risk factors other than asbestos
  - Heavy metals
  - Ionizing radiation in uranium miners
  - Halo ethers in chemical industry workers
  - Polycyclic aromatic hydrocarbons in petroleum and foundry workers
- Inherited genetic vulnerabilities
  - Individual genetic factors place some at higher risk after exposure to carcinogens than others
  - First-degree relatives of lung cancer patients have higher rates of lung cancer
  - Candidate genetic factors include:
    - Enzymes of the cytochrome P-450 system responsible for metabolizing cigarette smoke products to carcinogens
    - Role of the immune system in tumor surveillance and suppression
- Diets low in β-carotene and vitamin E
  - However, vitamin supplementation is not only ineffective, but it appears to cause more lung cancers
- Chronic exposure to wood smoke, via poorly ventilated indoor cooking, causes a significant amount of lung cancers (and COPD) worldwide, particularly among women

CONCERN FOR LUNG CANCER

- Concern for lung cancer usually arises because of abnormal thoracic imaging (most commonly a chest x-ray [CXR]) showing a focal, dominant opacity:
  - "Dominant," as opposed to "solitary" acknowledges that multiple unrelated small abnormalities are often present on thoracic imaging (eg, linear scaring)
- The most common cause of a focal CXR opacity is pneumonia
  - Pneumonia tends to:
    - **Be accompanied by symptoms of cough and fever**
    - Appear quickly (ie, clear CXR 2 months prior) (Fig. 9.1)
    - Have air bronchograms and vague borders (or complete lobar consolidation), suggestive of an alveolar filling process; much more common in pneumonia than cancer
- An opacity is concerning for lung cancer whenever the clinical radiographic presentation does **not** support pneumonia (in individuals over the age of 40 years)
  - Lung cancer tends to:
    - Appear slowly (ie, smaller opacity visible in the same location on prior imaging during the previous 1 to 2 years, often only in retrospect [Fig. 9.2])
    - Appear as a solid, often rounded opacity
    - Be asymptomatic, unless it is enormous and/or invading critical structures, causing pain and/or malfunction (eg, pathologic rib fracture or laryngeal nerve involvement)
- Concern for lung cancer increases with individual risk factors:
  - Personal history of lung cancer (single biggest risk factor)
  - Age >55 years
  - Total number of cigarettes smoked (cumulative)
  - Concomitant COPD
  - Family history of lung cancer
  - Other significant or synergistic exposures (eg, asbestos)
- Reviewing prior imaging (if available) is the first step in establishing concern or reassurance with regard to lung cancer (Fig. 9.3)
  - **A rapidly appearing opacity** (days to weeks) should be presumed infectious (eg, typical pneumonia or lung abscess), whereas a stable opacity (≥ 2 years) can be presumed to be benign (ie, scarring)
  - **Stability** of a solid lesion for ≥2 years or a ground glass lesion for ≥5 years provides reassurance that a lesion is nonmalignant and most likely represents scarring or a benign process (eg, hamartoma)

VERY RAPID GROWTH REASSURING WITH REGARDS TO LUNG CANCER

	Emergency Department,
• Chest x-ray obtained for cough and fever shows **5 cm rounded opacity** in the LLL	cc: cough
	HPI:
	60 y. o., past week he has had intermittant fevers, chills, and a cough.
• Portable Chest x-ray 2 mo. prior shows **NO nodule or mass**	Cough was initially dry but is now productive of brown sputum.
	lungs; Ill inspiratory crackles
• Doubling time 4-9 days (not lung cancer)	cxr: LLL pneumonia that looks rouned
	a/p;
• Fastest reported doubling time for lung cancer 25 days (small cell)	LLL pneumonia (patient last in hospital 2 months ago so will not need to treat for hospital acquired pneumonia)
• Patient ultimately diagnosed with oral anaerobic lung infection/ abscess	– will get sputum culture
	– moxifloxacin x 10 days
	– patient will need repeat cxr in 1 month since pneumonia is rounded and could be masking a mass

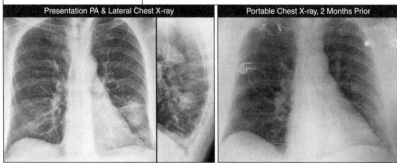

Presentation PA & Lateral Chest X-ray	Portable Chest X-ray, 2 Months Prior

Fig. 9.1 Encapsulated case showing the reassuring nature of **very** rapid growth with regard to lung cancer. Despite the opacities very concerning round, mass-like appearance, a doubling time of 4–9 days rules out lung cancer. Doubling time is estimated by assuming that a 0.1 cm to 1 cm opacity could have been missed on the initial film. Because of its concerning appearance, short-interval imaging follow-up is indicated (4–6 weeks) to ensure antibiotic response.

PROFOUND CENTRAL NECROSIS CLASSICALLY SEEN WITH SQUAMOUS CELL CARCINOMA

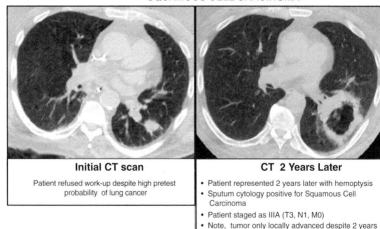

Initial CT scan	CT 2 Years Later
Patient refused work-up despite high pretest probability of lung cancer	• Patient represented 2 years later with hemoptysis
	• Sputum cytology positive for Squamous Cell Carcinoma
	• Patient staged as IIIA (T3, N1, M0)
	• Note, tumor only locally advanced despite 2 years of growth (classic squamous cell behavior)
	• The tumor appears to be more hole then wall

Fig. 9.2 Computed tomography (CT) scans (unfortunately) show the natural history of squamous cell carcinoma, highlighting the profound cavitation and the tendency to progress locally before metastasizing distantly.

DOMINANT OPACITY ON CHEST X-RAY, PATIENT HIGH RISK* FOR LUNG CANCER, NO Pneumonia Symptoms

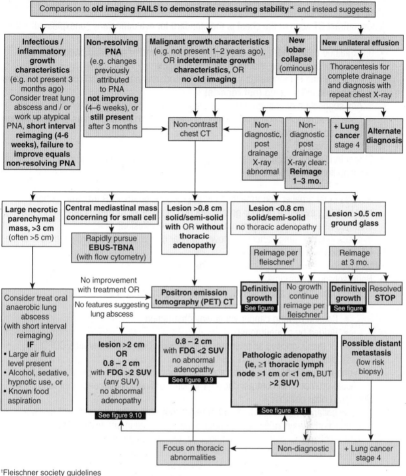

†Fleischner society guidelines
*Solid opacity present ≥2, ground glass ≥5 y
*High risk = former or current cigarette smoker, age >55

Fig. 9.3 Flow diagram outlining the evaluation of a dominant opacity seen on imaging that is concerning for lung cancer (because it is not associated with PNA symptoms). A noncontrast chest computed tomography (CT) scan and positron emission tomography (PET) scan provide most of the information required to decide whether a lesion should be reimaged, biopsied, or resected/definitively treated. Biopsy via endobronchial ultrasound transbronchial needle aspiration (EBUS-TBNA) is the preferred approach because it is low morbidity, high yield, and often provides diagnosis and stage in a single procedure. Additionally, if adenopathy is nondiagnostic, the primary lesion can often be approached by radial probe. Occasionally a lung abscess must be empirically treated before a diagnosis of lung cancer can be pursued. Biopsy of a lung abscess can lead to pleural seeding, empyema, and persistent bronchopleural (BP) fistula (see CH 11).

- **Pneumonia that fails to radiographically improve** in 3 to 6 weeks, and/or resolve in months, is **very** worrisome for lung cancer
- Steady growth of a lesion over several months to years makes it a cancer until proven otherwise
  - Growing from 1 cm to 2 cm in 3 months (doubling time of 30 days) is about as fast as lung cancer grows

- When growth characteristics are concerning for malignancy, indeterminate, or not known (ie, no prior imaging), a noncontrast chest computed tomography (CT) scan should be obtained
- A noncontrast CT scan of the chest is the standard for evaluating any "unexplained" CXR opacity
  - Unexplained means not easily attributable to acute and/or resolving pneumonia or known prior scarring (eg, stable from prior imaging)
    - Prior scarring is most reliably assessed by undertaking a detailed comparison of new imaging to old imaging **(not reports)**
    - Any suggestion of change over time should prompt consideration for CT scanning because adenocarcinoma of the lung is more likely to occur in areas of prior scarring (a.k.a. scar carcinoma)
- Noncontrast chest CT:
  - Characterizes the lesion as likely benign (eg, fat attenuation suggesting hamartoma) vs likely malignant (eg, necrosis)
  - Localizes the lesion
  - Reveals other smaller abnormalities not appreciated on the CXR that may either reassure (eg, evidence of prior granulomatous disease) or further increase concern (eg, enlarged hilar, mediastinal lymph nodes, or a small effusion)
  - In cases in which lung cancer is known (or near certain), chest CT provides 90% of the information required for staging
- Other common x-ray findings concerning for lung cancer:
  - Nonresolving pneumonia
    - Every pneumonia should be reimaged to complete resolution
      - Pneumonia can be:
        - Caused by lung cancer via airway obstruction
        - Hidden by a pneumonia
        - Or misdiagnosed as pneumonia (in an individual with bronchitis/COPD exacerbation)
    - A pneumonia that fails to radiographically improve in 6 weeks or persists for 3 months should prompt a noncontrast chest CT looking for findings concerning for lung cancer
  - Ominous Lobar collapse
    - Lung collapse not associated with foreign body aspiration or significant mucus production always raises concern for a (possibly malignant) airway lesion
    - Lobar collapse is particularly ominous (ie, worrisome for airway obstruction from lung cancer) when it occurs in the upper lobe (less likely to be aspirated foreign material or impacted secretion) in high-risk individuals
    - Additionally, collapse without the anticipated volume loss or collapse with volume gain are also very concerning for malignant airway obstruction (as the mass makes up for the lost volume of lung) (Fig. 9.4)
    - CT scan and bronchoscopy (with endobronchial ultrasound [EBUS] capability) is the preferred approach
  - Unilateral pleural effusion concerning for malignancy
    - Evaluation of a unilateral effusion begins with the fair presumption that it represents an exudative process
      - If the patient is obviously sick with pneumonia (eg, fever, cough, increased white blood cell count), a parapneumonic effusion is likely
    - If the patient has risk factors for lung cancer and does not have signs or symptoms of pneumonia, a malignant effusion should be high on the differential
- **Malignant pleural effusion** (Seen in lung cancer > metastatic cancer > lymphoma > mesothelioma)
  - Common presentation of stage IV lung cancer (often discovered by CXR imaging obtained to investigate gradual DOE)

RIGHT UPPER LOBE COLLAPSE, TYPICAL AND MALIGNANT

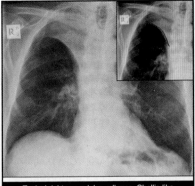

Typical right upper lobe collapse, Challis-like Appearance with volume loss (tracheal deviation)

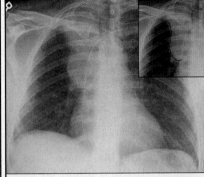

Malignant Right upper lobe collapse, showing the 'golden-S' sign of proximal mass causing RUL collapse without volume loss (trachea midline)

Fig. 9.4 Chest x-ray comparing typical right upper lobe collapse to ominous right upper lobe collapse. Ominous lung collapse has the concerning feature of volume gain, implying mass and collapse rather than airway obstruction from foreign body or mucus, which produces collapse with volume loss.

- Malignant effusions may occur from either:
  - Tumor-associated lymphatic obstruction, or
  - Tumor metastasis to the parietal pleural surface
- Malignant effusions are typically moderate to large at presentation
- Thoracentesis often reveals a macroscopically bloody pleural fluid appearance
- Pleural pressures should be measured during thoracentesis, because the likelihood of lung entrapment is high with malignant pleural disease (see CH 17)
- Diagnostic yield is maximized at 100 mL per thoracentesis
  - Overall diagnostic yield goes up with a second 100-mL sample during repeat thoracentesis and slightly again with a third 100-mL sample
- Management:
  - If the effusion is large enough to tap safely, a diagnosis should be attempted via thoracentesis
  - In general, a CT scan should be obtained **after** thoracentesis to maximize the ability to see underlying pathology
  - If CXR and ultrasound investigation reveal a complex pleural space (eg, adhesions or loculations), CT scan may be obtained before drainage (to help plan the procedure)
  - The initial thoracentesis should attempt complete drainage (possible when the total volume of fluid in the effusion is estimated to be $\leq$ ~2000 mL)
  - If the effusion is massive (ie, clearly >2–3 L) a small bore chest tube (placed via seldinger technique) should be considered (with overnight admission) to facilitate rapid, complete drainage
    - 1-2 L may be intermittently drained (q 4–6 hours) as tolerated by reexpansion symptoms
      - This aggressive approach aimed at timely, complete drainage is appropriate because it is indicated in the initial management of:
        - Parapneumonic effusion/empyema
        - Malignant effusion
        - Idiopathic exudative effusion
- Complete drainage may prevent recurrence up to 10% of the time in addition to maximizing the ability to visualize the lung and pleural surface on the subsequent postdrainage CT scan

- If the postdrainage CT scan shows a dominant parenchymal focus and pleural fluid is negative, consider repeat diagnostic thoracentesis (ie, 100 mL for cytology)
- If the repeat thoracentesis is nondiagnostic (or not technically feasible), attention should shift to any abnormal adenopathy or the parenchymal lesion itself
- If the CT scan reveals abnormal pleura without adenopathy or a dominant parenchymal focus, video-assisted thoracoscopic surgery (VATS) biopsy may be required to make the diagnosis
- VATS is a particularly attractive option if the fluid recurs and causes symptoms, because it may provide both diagnosis and definitive therapy (via pleurodesis)
- A persistent, unexplained, lymphocytic predominant exudate in a patient with advanced lung cancer (behaves statistically like, so) can be assumed to be malignant in origin, despite negative pleural cytology

EVALUATION AND MANAGEMENT OF THE WORRISOME PARENCHYMAL LESION(S) DURING A CHEST CT SCAN (NUMBER, SIZE, APPEARANCE, AND GROWTH)

- Evaluation and management of **multiple pulmonary nodules**:
  - Likelihood of lung cancer based on number of lesions:
    - The greater the number of nodules, **the lower** the likelihood of lung cancer
    - Multiple nodules occur most commonly in granulomatous infections (eg, nontuburculous mycobacteria [NTM] infection, miliary TB) or inflammation (eg, sarcoidosis)
      - Multiple small nodules (<0.8 cm) should be evaluated with sputum specimens for acid-fast bacillus (AFB), immunologic screening for TB, endemic fungal infection, and Aspergillus with serial imaging (initially at 3 months)
        - Steady growth of multiple nodules seen by serial imaging **strongly** suggests metastatic disease
        - Steady growth of a single nodule in a chest with multiple nodules is concerning for concomitant early stage lung cancer occurring in the setting of prior granulomatous disease
      - Three spiculated 1-cm lesions of the same size, in a patient with severe emphysema are more likely to represent atypical infection (eg, Aspergillus) rather then 3 synchronous primary lung cancers
  - Multiple malignant nodules are seen in cancer that is metastatic to the lung, from a primary lung cancer or an extrathoracic malignancy (eg, colon)
    - When multiple nodules represent metastatic lung cancer, a dominant lesion/mass is usually visible (Fig. 9.5)
    - Renal cell, melanoma, colon, and breast cancer can cause oligometastatic disease (ie, a single or handful of pulmonary metastases, typically round, smooth-edged, lower-lobe lesions of similar size)
      - ≤5 metastases may be definitively treated (external beam radiation therapy [XRT] or subanatomic/wedge resection) to slow disease progression (if systemic options are lacking or failing)
      - Multiple metastases (>5) must be treated systemically
    - Adenocarcinomas arising from the GI tract often metastasize widely to the lung
      - Colon typically involves the liver and lung, but rectal, pancreatic, small bowel, and gastric adenocarcinomas may "skip" the liver on their way to the lung
      - Bronchoscopy with blind transbronchial biopsies is a high-yield, low-morbidity approach to the diagnosis of metastatic adenocarcinoma to the lung when the pulmonary metastatic pattern is "too numerous to count (TNTC)" (Fig. 9.6)
      - Otherwise, needle aspiration of the most accessible metastatic lesion (often extrathoracic) provides diagnosis and staging

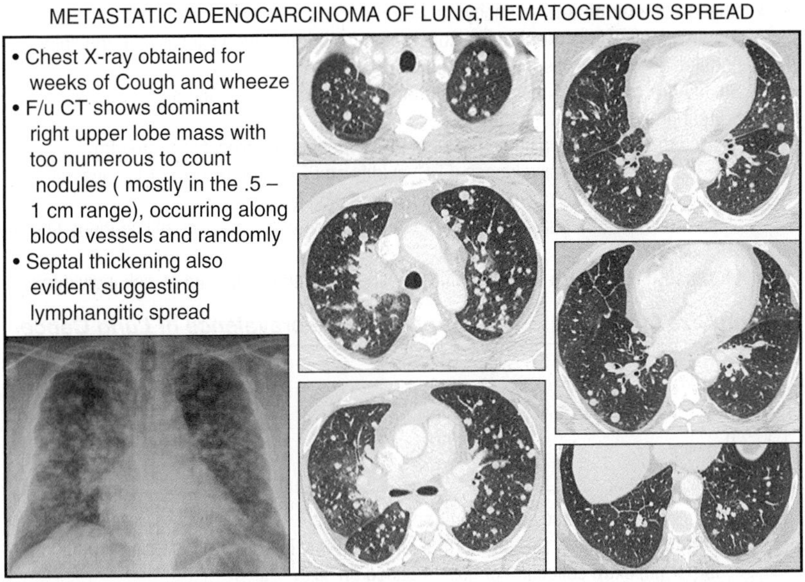

METASTATIC ADENOCARCINOMA OF LUNG, HEMATOGENOUS SPREAD

- Chest X-ray obtained for weeks of Cough and wheeze
- F/u CT shows dominant right upper lobe mass with too numerous to count nodules (mostly in the .5 – 1 cm range), occurring along blood vessels and randomly
- Septal thickening also evident suggesting lymphangitic spread

Fig. 9.5 Chest x-ray and computed tomography (CT) scan showing metastatic lung adenocarcinoma in a "too numerous to count pattern." The vessel associated and the random nature of nodules suggests that the majority of the metastasis was hematogenously spread.

METASTATIC ADENOCARCINOMA OF LUNG, LYMPHATIC SPREAD

- Chest X-ray Obtained for weeks of dry cough
- F/u CT shows dominant right lower lobe mass with too numerous to count nodules (mostly < the .5 cm) lining the perilymphatic structures
- At least two 1 cm sized blood vessel associated nodules appear hematogenously spread

Fig. 9.6 Chest x-ray and computed tomography (CT) scan showing metastatic lung adenocarcinoma in a "too numerous to count pattern." The perilymphatic, pleural, and fissure-based nodules suggest that the majority of the metastasis were lymphatically spread.

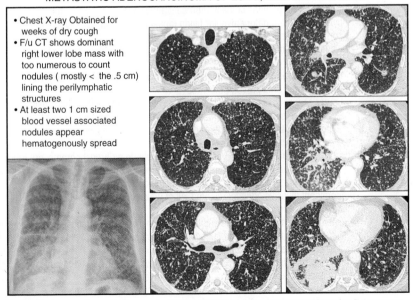

- Evaluation of a **dominant** parenchymal lesion:
  - A dominant lesion is **much** more concerning for primary lung cancer than multiple nodules of similar sizes
  - Steady growth of a lesion over time (months to years) creates the highest possible pretest probability for lung cancer
    - Growth trumps PET avidity (because PET avidity is a surrogate for growth)
      - Lack of fluorodeoxyglucose (FDG) avidity on PET scan (ie, cold PET) does not provide reassurance with regard to a growing lesion
      - It also is **not** a guarantee that the lesion is growing slowly, or will continue to grow slowly
  - **Increasing** lesion **size increases** the likelihood of lung cancer (in at-risk individuals):

Lesion Size (cm)	Approximate prevalence of Lung Cancer
<0.5	0.5%
<0.8	5%
0.5–1.0	20%
1.1–2.0	50%
>2.0	75%

- Likelihood of malignancy based on appearance:
  - **Solid lesions** imply that **no** normal lung anatomy is visible, suggesting granuloma or tumor (ie, extra collection of tissue) based on size
    - Principle differential diagnosis is granuloma vs hamartoma vs malignancy
      - Granulomas are typically <1 cm in size
      - Hamartomas are typically <3 in size
      - This is why solid lesions >3 cm are refereed to as a mass and presumed malignant until proven otherwise
  - **Semisolid lesions** raise the possibility of an infectious or inflammatory process where the nonsolid portions actually represent airways (appearing as a tubular lucency) and/or inflammatory alveolar filling (appearing as ground glass), and the solid portions represent consolidated lung
    - However, this constellation of findings may also be seen with invasive mucinous adenocarcinoma (Fig. 9.7)
    - Small semisolid lesions that persist or grow slowly are presumed to be invasive adenocarcinoma until proven otherwise
      - Larger semisolid lesions may represent tumor with obstructive atelectasis
        - Where the solid portion represents the malignancy and the more distal portion contains air bronchograms and ground glass consistent with a postobstructive process
  - **Ground glass lesions** alone, and/or lesions with definite air bronchograms, are more likely to represent an infectious or inflammatory process **but** may represent:
    - Adenocarcinoma in situ, minimally invasive adenocarcinoma or lepidic predominant invasive adenocarcinoma, all of which grow in a lepidic, alveolar filling, pattern mimicking pneumonia
      - Often starting as ground glass and then evolving more solid components over time
      - Differentiated from pneumonia because of is steady, slow growth over years; not compatible with infectious pneumonia
    - Small semisolid lesions (that persist or grow slowly) are presumed to be lepidic predominant invasive adenocarcinoma until proven otherwise
  - **Cavitation** (ie, a hole in a lesion that is not an airway or a preexisting emphysematous hole), implies **necrosis**
    - Pulmonary necrosis occurs in a limited number of disease sates, such that it is always a critical finding

INVASIVE MUCINOUS ADENOCARCINOMA
(THE TUMOR FORMERLY KNOWN AS MUCINOUS BAC)

Pulmonary diagnostic clinic reason for consult: abnormal chest CT
HPI: 51 yo M with h/o asthma, tobacco abuse, and asbestos exposure
who presents with an abnormal chest CT. He had a CXR performed for cough
that showed a questionable RUL nodule vs confluence of shadows. F/u chest CT
did not show a RUL nodule but did incidentally find a patchy opacity in the
RLL concerning for infection/inflammatory process. He had a f/u CT that
showed equivocal growth of the nodule. Recent repeat CT showed slight growth
Impression: 51 yo M with h/o tobacco abuse p/w irregular pleural based nodule in
the RLL with very slow growth over 1 year concerning for a BAC. Given the low
yield of needle biopsy for BAC, we favor consideration of a VATS

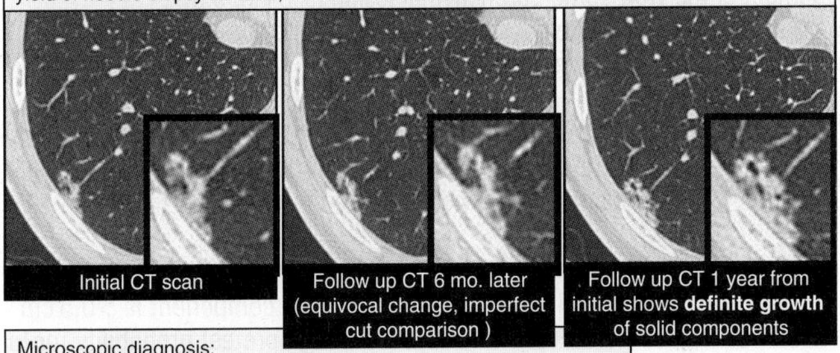

| Initial CT scan | Follow up CT 6 mo. later (equivocal change, imperfect cut comparison) | Follow up CT 1 year from initial shows **definite growth** of solid components |

Microscopic diagnosis:
A. lung, right lower lobe, wedge biopsy
    DX: BRONCHOALVEOLAR CARCINOMA, MUCINOUS TYPE
B. lung, right lower lobe
BRONCHIOALVEOLAR CARCINOMA, MUCINOUS TYPE
TUMOR SIZE: greatest dimension: 1.5 cm,
SYNOPTIC REPORT FOR RIGHT LUNG
HISTOLOGIC TYPE: bronchioalveolar carcinoma, mucinous type
HISTOLOGIC GRADE: G1; well-differentiated
PATHOLOGIC STAGING: pT2; tumor invades the visceral pleural
ADDITIONAL PATHOLOGIC FINDINGS: bronchio-alveolar dysplasia

Fig. 9.7 Serial computed tomography (CT) scans over a 12-month period show a semisolid lesion, subtly growing over a year. Note the very concerning growth in the solid components of the lesion. At 6 months, growth is equivocal because of imperfect cut comparisons. Positron emission tomography (PET) scan is of limited utility when evaluating these lesions (often they have no fluorodeoxyglucose [FDG] avidity) and biopsy may yield only broncho-alveolar dysplasia (missing the true carcinoma). Both of these findings may provide false reassurance. This lesion was empirically resected when it demonstrated definitive growth.

- Necrosis **either** implies rapidly growing tumor (outpacing its blood supply) or
- Infectious or inflammatory lung destruction
- Necrosis is commonly seen in lung cancer, especially **squamous cell**
  - Necrosis may also be seen in fast-growing tumors (eg, small cell, large cell) with neuroendocrine features and poorly differentiated adenocarcinomas
- Cavitary lesions where the wall thickness is >1 cm have >80% chance of being malignant
- Common nonmalignant conditions associated with cavitation include:
  - Lung abscess
    - Air fluid level is suggestive
  - Necrotizing pneumonia (staph or gram negative rods other than Haemophilus)
    - Clinical scenario of acute pneumonia
  - Endemic fungal infection, especially coccidiomycosis (thin-walled cavity)
  - Invasive fungal infection (eg, aspergillus)
  - Granulomatosis with polyangitis (GPA)
  - Necrotizing sarcoidosis
- Likelihood of malignancy based on the characteristics of the border:
  - Size is more predictive than border characteristics, so border characteristics are most helpful when assessing smaller nodules (ie, lesions <2 cm)

- **Spiculated** is more worrisome than **lobulated**, which is more worrisome than **smooth edge** (with regard to likelihood of primary lung cancer)
  - Spiculated lesions are the most concerning for primary lung cancer, but they may actually represent infections lesions in the setting of severe underlying emphysema (eg, aspergillus)
  - Lobulated lesions are also concerning for primary lung cancer, but they may actually represent a conglomerate mass of granuloma
  - Smooth-edged lesions suggest granuloma, hamartoma, **or** pulmonary metastasis
- Management of the worrisome parenchymal lesion (see Fig. 9.3)
  - Approach hinges on the pretest probability of malignancy
  - Pretest probability increases with:
    - Growth:
      - Lesions with potential malignant growth characteristics (steady growth over months to years) have the highest pretest probability for lung cancer and should be biopsied, resected, or empirically treated
    - Size:
      - Most lesions ≥2 cm should be biopsied, resected, or empirically treated
      - Note: small semisolid lesions, where the solid component is >0.5 cm and persists over time, have also have a high pretest probability for lung adenocarcinoma
    - Upper-lobe location
    - Spiculations
    - **Individual (additive) risk factors** (personal history of lung cancer, cigarette smoking, asbestos exposure)
  - Pretest probability decreases with benign features such as:
    - Central fat attenuation or calcification patterns specific for hamartomas (popcorn, central/target)
    - Signs of prior granulomatous disease:
      - Multiple other small nodules, calcified granuloma, calcified hilar adenopathy (normal sized), and splenic calcifications (suggesting histoplasmosis)
    - Young age (ie, <40 years)
- Pure ground glass lesions >0.5 cm should be reimaged at 3 months to check for resolution
  - Persistence requires reimaging per Fleischner Society guidelines
  - Growth of ground glass lesion over a 3-month period is concerning for adenocarcinoma, and a PET scan should be obtained looking for PET-avid adenopathy or distant metastasis, followed by definitive intervention (Fig. 9.8)
- Small solid/semisolid lesions <0.8 cm should be serial imaged per Fleischner Society guidelines
  - Growth over a 3 month period is very concerning, and a PET scan should be obtained looking for PET-avid adenopathy or distant metastasis, followed by definitive intervention (see Fig. 9.8)
- Lesions >0.8 cm should be initially evaluated by **PET scan** to assess the FDG avidity of both the primary lesion while screening for pathologic adenopathy or metastasis
  - Pathologically enlarged mediastinal lymph nodes, or FDG-avid mediastinal adenopathy of any size, should be evaluated by endobronchial ultrasound transbronchial needle aspiration (EBUS-TBNA) to rule out malignancy
  - Distant metastasis (eg, long bone, spine, or rib) may provide diagnosis and stage via a single low-morbidity biopsy
    - The liver is a common metastatic site for lung cancer, **but** liver biopsy has a high risk of hemorrhage (such that it should be avoided)
      - Liver metastasis from lung cancer should be diagnosed clinically/radiographically

DEFINITIVE GROWTH* OF ANY DOMINANT LESION (REGARDLESS OF SIZE OR FDG AVIDITY)

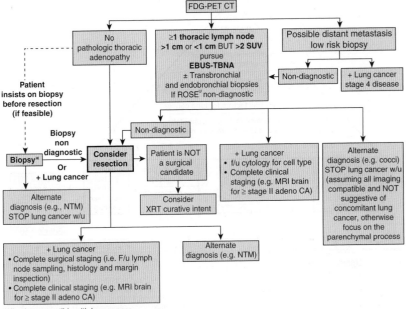

*Kinetics compatible with lung cancer

ᵂROSE (rapid on site evaluation) of cytology specimens

ˣBiopsy approach individualized based on location (e.g. peripheral vs. central / airway associated), endobronchial approach preferred to CT guided (less morbid)

Fig. 9.8 Flow diagram outlining the evaluation and management of a dominant pulmonary lesion that has demonstrated definitive growth over months to years, creating the highest pretest probability possible for lung cancer. In the absence of adenopathy or distant metastasis, resection should be considered. Patients who are not candidates for resection should consider empiric external beam radiation (XRT) with curative intent.

- Lesions measuring 0.8 to 2 cm with a standard uptake value (SUV) <2 pose the greatest challenge, because appropriate management ranges from **serial imaging** to **empiric resection** (based on the pretest probability of malignancy) (Fig. 9.9)
  - Pretest probability increases with size, concerning features, and individual risk factors
  - Pretest probability decreases with small size, evidence of prior granulomatous disease (eg, multiple smaller nodules, calcified granuloma, or calcified adenopathy), or imaging suggestive of hamartoma (eg, central fat attenuation and target or popcorn calcification)
  - Lesions with **high** pretest probability should be considered for empiric resection
    - An alternate diagnosis is required to "stand down" when pretest probability is high
    - Patients unable to tolerate resection should be considered for empiric XRT
  - Lesions with an **intermediate** pretest probability should be biopsied
    - Biopsy approach must be individualized based on location (eg, peripheral vs central/airway associated); endobronchial approach is preferred to CT-guided because its less morbid
    - If biopsy is not feasible (ie, unsafe based on underlying lung disease or lesion location), it may be serially imaged (to look for definitive growth) or empirically treated via resection or XRT
      - Patient preference and individual risk factors should be weighed heavily in this situation

0.8 – 2 CM SOLID / SEMI-SOLID DOMINANT LESION (WITH FDG <2 SUV, NO ABNORMAL ADENOPATHY)

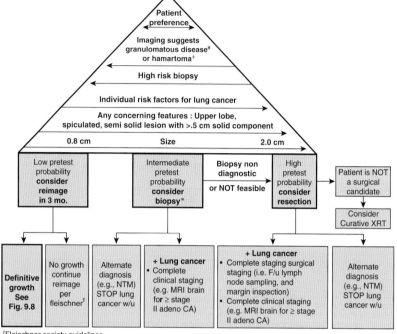

†Fleischner society guidelines
+ Central fat attenuation and target or popcorn calcification
¥Multiple smaller nodules, calcified granuloma or calcified adenopathy (<1 cm short axis)
*Biopsy approach individualized based on location (e.g. peripheral vs. central / airway associated), endobronchial approach preferred to CT guided (less morbid)

Fig. 9.9 Schematic diagram outlining the evaluation of smaller, non FDG avid positron emission tomography (PET). Low pretest probability lesions should be serially imaged, intermediate pretest probability lesions should be biopsied, and high pretest probability lesions should be empirically resected or treated with external beam radiation (XRT).

- Lesions with a low pretest probability of malignancy should be reimaged in 3 months
  - No growth at 3 months should prompt continued serial imaging per Fleischner Society guidelines
  - Growth of any lesion over a 3-month period is concerning for lung cancer, and a PET scan should be obtained (if not already done) looking for PET-avid adenopathy or distant metastasis, followed by definitive intervention (see figure 9.8)
- Larger lesions >2 cm (regardless of FDG avidity) or smaller lesions with an SUV >2 are likely malignant, such that they may be biopsied or definitively treated based on pretest probability (Fig. 9.10)
- Pathologic adenopathy occurring with a dominant lesion is concerning for advanced lung cancer, and lymph node aspiration via EBUS-TBNA should be pursued first (Fig. 9.11)
  - Endobronchial ultrasound transbronchial needle aspiration (EBUS-TBNA) is the preferred approach for sampling the mediastinum based on its high yield and low morbidity
  - EBUS should be paired with rapid onsite cytology examination, allowing for repeat sampling until diagnostic material is obtained
  - If EBUS is nondiagnostic, attention should then focus on the dominant parenchymal abnormality as previously outlined

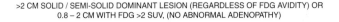

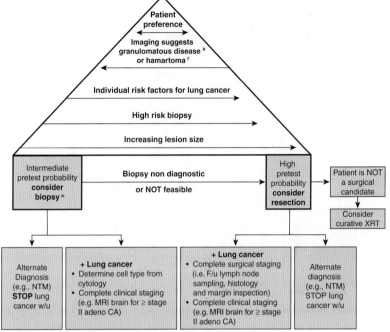

+Central fat attenuation and target or popcorn calcification
¥Multiple smaller nodules, calcified granuloma or calcified adenopathy (<1 cm short axis)
*Biopsy approach individualized based on location (e.g. peripheral vs. central / airway associated),
endobronchial approach preferred to CT guided (less morbid)

Fig. 9.10 Schematic diagram outlining the evaluation of larger lesions, or positron emission tomography (PET)–FDG avid smaller lesions. Pretest probability is intermediate to high in this group, such that serial imaging is **NOT** a satisfying option. These lesions should be biopsied, resected, or empirically treated with external beam radiation (XRT).

EVALUATION AND MANAGEMENT OF MEDIASTINAL ADENOPATHY AND CONCERN FOR N2 DISEASE

- Although intrapulmonary/hilar lymph nodes may enlarge reactively in the setting of a proximate, typical bacterial pneumonia, mediastinal lymph nodes should not, such that mediastinal adenopathy is **always** abnormal, requiring some degree of investigation (ie, serial imaging or biopsy)
- Pathologically enlarged or PET-avid mediastinal adenopathy occurring with an unexplained pulmonary lesion represents advanced lung cancer (ie, at least stage IIIA) until proven otherwise
- Thoracic lymph node definitions:
  - Hilar (intrapulmonary) lymph nodes are considered N1 and are signified by double-digit numbers (eg, stations 10 and 11)
  - Mediastinal lymph nodes are signified by single-digit numbers (eg, stations 4 and 7)
    - They are considered N2 nodes if they occur ipsilateral to the primary lung cancer, and N3 if they are contralateral

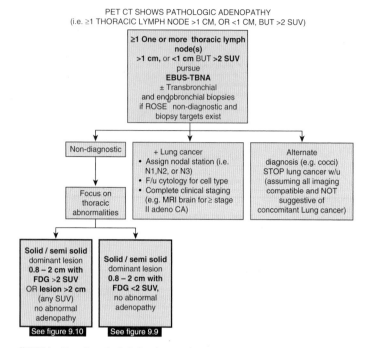

PET CT SHOWS PATHOLOGIC ADENOPATHY
(i.e. ≥1 THORACIC LYMPH NODE >1 CM, OR <1 CM, BUT >2 SUV)

≥1 One or more thoracic lymph node(s)
>1 cm, or <1 cm BUT >2 SUV
pursue
EBUS-TBNA
± Transbronchial
and endobronchial biopsies
if ROSE non-diagnostic and
biopsy targets exist

Non-diagnostic

+ Lung cancer
• Assign nodal station (i.e. N1,N2, or N3)
• F/u cytology for cell type
• Complete clinical staging (e.g. MRI brain for ≥ stage II adeno CA)

Alternate diagnosis (e.g. cocci) STOP lung cancer w/u (assuming all imaging compatible and NOT suggestive of concomitant Lung cancer)

Focus on thoracic abnormalities

Solid / semi solid dominant lesion **0.8 – 2 cm with FDG >2 SUV** OR **lesion >2 cm** (any SUV) no abnormal adenopathy
See figure 9.10

Solid / semi solid dominant lesion **0.8 – 2 cm with FDG <2 SUV,** no abnormal adenopathy
See figure 9.9

ωROSE (rapid on site evaluation) of cytology specimens

Fig. 9.11 Schematic diagram outlining the evaluation of abnormal thoracic adenopathy by endobronchial ultrasound transbronchial needle aspiration (EBUS-TBNA) with rapid onsite evaluation of specimens.

- N3 also refers to involved lymph nodes outside of the thorax (eg, supraclavicular or scalene)
- The most common mediastinal lymph node stations involved in the thoracic spread of lung cancer are stations 2, 4, 5, 6, and 7, which are found in predictable locations of the mediastinum and do **not** require contrast to visualize and/or precisely measure (Fig. 9.12)
  - In fact, poorly timed contrast in the superior vena cava (SVC) creates a streak artifact, making mediastinal nodal station examination more difficult
  - IV contrast is required to precisely screen for and define/measure hilar adenopathy
  - Lymph nodes should be measured in their **short** axis
    - Station 7 is often 2 cm in its long axis long (draped to the right side of thorax)
    - Classically, station 7 had to be >1.5 cm in the short axis to be considered pathologic, but current practice raises concern at 1 cm (as for all other thoracic nodes)

CENTRAL MEDIASTINAL MASS CONCERNING FOR SMALL CELL LUNG CANCER

- Small cell lung cancer grows so fast, and has such a propensity for distant metastasis (eg, brain), that its workup must be expedited (ie, biopsy within 2 weeks of presentation)
- Concern for small cell occurs when the primary thoracic abnormality is a contiguous conglomerate mass of mediastinal lymph nodes

THORACIC LYMPH NODE STATIONS

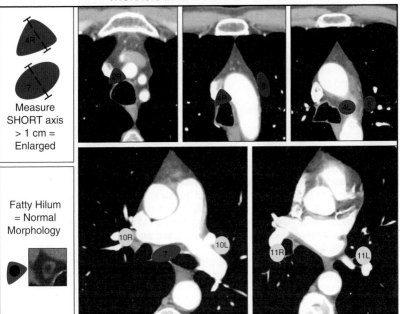

Fig. 9.12 Lymph node stations most commonly involved in lung cancer metastasis. Lymph nodes should be measured in their short axis. Normal mediastinal lymph nodes may have low attenuation centers. This is a benign finding implying normal lymph node architecture (ie, fatty lymph node hilum). IV contrast is required to precisely measure stations 10 and 11 (only).

- The differential diagnosis of this imaging has no benign entities and consists of aggressive lymphoma, large cell with neuroendocrine features, and poorly differentiated adenocarcinoma
- EBUS-TBNA with flow cytometry, looking for both a clonal population of lymphocytes (ie, lymphoma) and CD56 a small cell marker

Large Necrotic Parenchymal Mass (often >5 cm)

- The differential diagnosis for a large necrotic mass is the same as previously outlined for a cavitary lesion
- Consider treating with antibiotics aimed at oral anaerobes (ie, ampicillin/sulbactam) with short-interval reimaging (ie, 4–6 weeks) **if** the lesion:
  - Appeared quickly
  - Has a large air fluid level
  - Occurs in an individual with poor dentition, alcohol, sedative/hypnotic use, or known food aspiration
- If there are no features suggesting a lung abscess **or** no improvement with treatment, the mass should be worked up as a presumed cancer (see Fig. 9.3)

TYPICAL CLINICAL RADIOGRAPHIC AND HISTOPATHOLOGIC FEATURES OF LUNG CANCER (AND MESOTHELIOMA) BY CELL TYPE

- Almost all lung cancers fall within one of five histologic categories or cell types, with the majority being adeno, squamous, or small cell carcinoma:

Cell Type	Approximate Percentage of Lung Cancers
Adenocarcinoma	50%
Squamous cell carcinoma	20%
Large cell carcinoma	5%
Neuroendocrine spectrum tumors:	
Typical and atypical carcinoid	5%
Small cell carcinoma	15%
Large cell carcinoma with neuroendocrine features	5%

- The four cell types of lung cancer and mesothelioma (pleural cancer) have characteristic initial imaging, reflecting their underlying biological behavior
- This allows one to anticipate the cell type of grossly abnormal/obviously malignant imaging up to 85% of the time based on the thoracic pattern of disease (Fig. 9.13)
  - Adenocarcinoma makes up ~50% of lung cancers and is the most common cell type to affect young people (<50 years), nonsmokers, and women
  - Lung adenocarcinomas:
    - Display aggressive metastatic behavior, often involving a peripheral mass and N2 adenopathy during the initial examination, with intrathoracic and distant metastasis also common (Fig. 9.14)

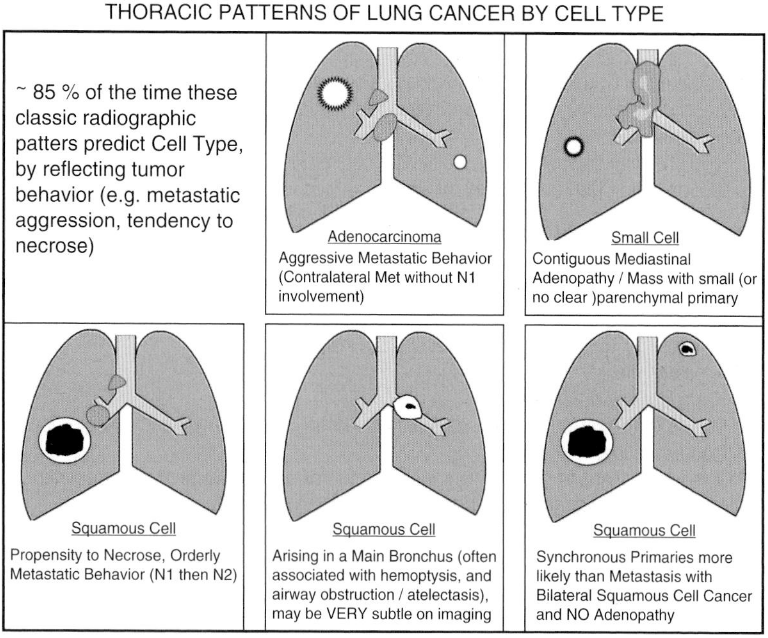

THORACIC PATTERNS OF LUNG CANCER BY CELL TYPE

~ 85 % of the time these classic radiographic patters predict Cell Type, by reflecting tumor behavior (e.g. metastatic aggression, tendency to necrose)

Adenocarcinoma Aggressive Metastatic Behavior (Contralateral Met without N1 involvement)

Small Cell Contiguous Mediastinal Adenopathy / Mass with small (or no clear)parenchymal primary

Squamous Cell Propensity to Necrose, Orderly Metastatic Behavior (N1 then N2)

Squamous Cell Arising in a Main Bronchus (often associated with hemoptysis, and airway obstruction / atelectasis), may be VERY subtle on imaging

Squamous Cell Synchronous Primaries more likely than Metastasis with Bilateral Squamous Cell Cancer and NO Adenopathy

Fig. 9.13 Cartoon images depicting the typical presenting computed tomography (CT) imaging pattern for the most common lung cancer cell types. When one of these classic patterns is seen, the cell type may be anticipated ~85% of the time.

ADENOCARCINOMA OF THE LUNG, TYPICAL IMAGING ON PRESENTATION

Chest x-ray obtained for chest pain (ultimately GI origin) shows a 5 cm, well circumscribed (round) mass sup. segment of the left lower lobe (Frontal Chest X-ray and Coronal and Sagittal CT scan Cuts). Axial CT and PET scan cuts show pathologically enlarged, PET Avid station 11L and 7 lymph nodes, as well as a contralateral nodule. Biopsy of station 7 by EBUS showed adenocarcinoma of lung, clinical stage IV (T2a,N2,M1a).

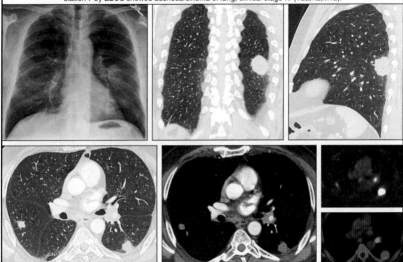

Fig. 9.14 Chest x-ray, computed tomography (CT) scan, and positron emission tomography (PET) imaging showing the classic radiographic presentation of lung adenocarcinoma, with a dominant peripheral mass, mediastinal adenopathy, and intrapulmonary metastasis.

- Are associated with paraneoplastic blood clots, specifically migratory superficial thrombophlebitis (a.k.a. Trousseau's syndrome) and hypertrophic osteoarthropathy (a.k.a. digital clubbing [often painful])
- Exist on a spectrum of histologic disease entities, each with unique radiographic appearances and growth characteristics (Fig. 9.15)
  - Adenocarcinoma in situ (a preinvasive lesion) is 100% curable if completely resected
  - Minimally invasive adenocarcinoma (mucinous, nonmucinous, mixed)
  - Invasive adenocarcinoma may be lepidic, acinar, papillary, micropapillary, predominantly solid, or characterized as invasive mucinous adenocarcinoma
- Have the propensity to grow in a lepidic fashion, giving them the potential to masquerade as infectious/inflammatory ground glass lesions
  - Small ground glass lesions with solid components are very concerning for adenocarcinoma because granulomas (the most common cause of small solid lesions) should not cause ground glass
  - These tumors are often not FDG avid and require empiric resection because biopsy may underestimate the lesion (by sampling hyperplasia only)
  - Tumors with a predominant lepidic pattern may grow very slowly such that pure ground glass lesions must demonstrate 5 years of stability before they can be deemed benign (unlike solid lesions, which only require 2 years of stability)
- Stain positive for TTF-1 and CK7, and negative for CK5/6
  - Metastatic adenocarcinomas of GI origin tend to be TTF-1 negative such that an adenocarcinoma that is CK7 and TTF-1 negative may actually represent metastatic disease to the lung from below the diaphragm
- Large cell carcinoma without neuroendocrine features behaves like, and is difficult or impossible to distinguish from, a very poorly differentiated adenocarcinoma

SPECTRUM OF LUNG ADENOCARCINOMA MORPHOLOGY

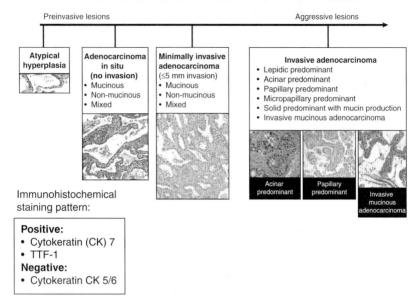

Fig. 9.15 Histologic and immunohistochemical staining pattern of lung adenocarcinoma.

- Squamous cell carcinoma makes up ~25% of lung cancers, is the most common lung cancer associated with smoking, **and**:
  - Is the least aggressive of the common lung cancers with regard to metastasis, tending to spread in an orderly fashion, growing (and often experiencing necrosis) locally for a time (years) before spreading to a hilar lymph node and then a mediastinal node (see Fig. 9.13)
    - Because of this, bilateral biopsy–proven squamous cell lung cancers presenting without adenopathy, are more likely to represent synchronous primaries
      - Unlike a poorly differentiated adenocarcinoma, which may metastasize to the contralateral lung (skipping the mediastinum)
  - Tends to form in the proximal airways and commonly presents with airway obstruction/lobar collapse, and/or hemoptysis
    - Lesions arising in the airway may have the majority of their mass intraluminal, making them hard to see by imaging before complete airway occlusion occurs (Fig. 9.16)
  - Is associated with parathyroid hormone-related protein (PTHrP) elaboration and hypercalcemia
  - Has two unique morphologic properties (Fig. 9.17):
    - Intercellular bridges (normally seen in skin) and
    - keratin pearls (often with an associated multinucleated giant cell reaction)
  - Stains positive for CK 5/6 and P63, and negative for TTF-1 and CK7
- Small cell carcinoma makes up ~15% of lung cancers, is strongly/uniformly associated with smoking, and exists as an aggressive member of the neuroendocrine spectrum lung cancers (Fig. 9.18)
  - Small cell:
    - Has the unique propensity to exist primarily as a central mediastinal mass, often with little or no obvious parenchymal component (Fig. 9.19)

SQUAMOUS CELL LUNG CANCER, TYPICAL IMAGING ON PRESENTATION

Follow up chest x-ray after PNA (not shown) suggested a persistent lingular nodule leading to a CT scan which INSTEAD revealed a 2 cm left mainstem nodule, difficult to see since it sits almost entirely inside the airway, blending with the air way wall. PET scan shows avid nodule without adenopathy or metastasis. Bronchoscopy with endobronchial biopsy revealed squamous cell carcinoma IIA (T2b,N0,M0)

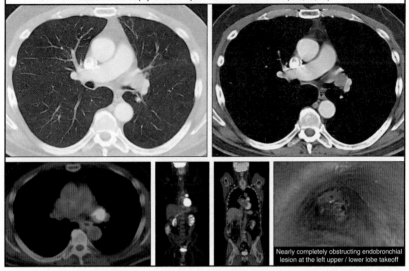

Nearly completely obstructing endobronchial lesion at the left upper / lower lobe takeoff

Fig. 9.16 Computed tomography (CT) scan, positron emission tomography (PET), and bronchoscopic images showing the classic radiographic presentation of squamous cell carcinoma arising in a mainstem bronchus. The lesion is difficult to see without PET imaging because it sits entirely in the airway. The tumor is a T2b, despite its small size, because it involves a main bronchus.

SQUAMOUS CELL CARCINOMA MORPHOLOGY

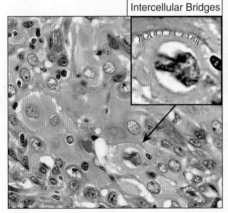

Intercellular Bridges

Keratinization in Squamous Cell Carcinoma, 'Keratin Pearl'

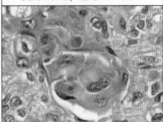

Immunohistochemical Staining Pattern:

Positive:
• Cytokeratin (CK) 5/6
• p63
Negative:
• TTF-1,
• CK7

Fig. 9.17 Histologic and immunohistochemical staining pattern of squamous cell carcinoma.

SPECTRUM OF NEUROENDOCRINE TUMORS

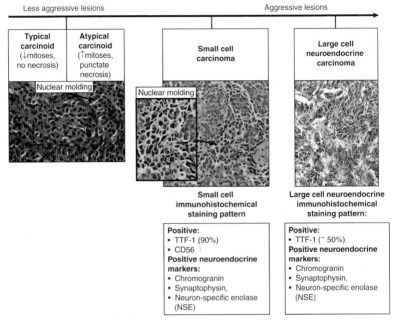

Fig. 9.18 Histologic and immunohistochemical staining pattern of neuroendocrine tumors of the lung.

SMALL CELL LUNG CANCER, TYPICAL IMAGING ON PRESENTATION

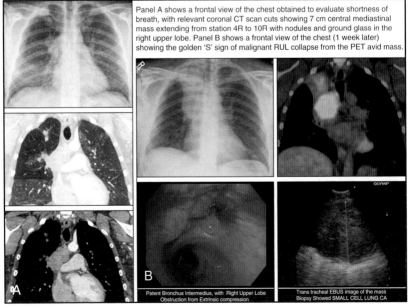

Fig. 9.19 A) Chest x-ray, computed tomography (CT) scan, and positron emission tomography (PET) imaging showing the classic radiographic presentation of small cell lung carcinoma. B) Bronchoscopic image showing submucosal disease and extrinsic compression of the RUL by tumor, with transtracheal EBUS image of the mass (just prior to biopsy).

- Is the most aggressive of the common lung cancer cell types, growing over months as opposed to years
  - Except for the very rare solitary pulmonary nodule presentation, small cell is uniformly metastatic during the initial examination and thus **not** amenable to (surgical) cure
- Typically responds very well to chemotherapy initially (often with no visible disease at the end of therapy)
- Unfortunately it almost always returns within 5 years (often 2), rapidly progressing after recurrence
- Is associated with paraneoplastic syndrome of inappropriate antidiuretic hormone secretion (SIADH), Lambert-Eaton myasthenic syndrome, and cerebellar degeneration
- Has the characteristic morphology of relatively small cells for cancer (ie, 2-3 times the size of a resting lymphocyte), nuclear molding, salt-and-pepper chromatin, scant cytoplasm, and a high mitotic rate
- Stains positive for TTF-1 and neuroendocrine markers (eg, chromogranin, synaptophysin, neuron-specific enolase)
- Carcinoid tumors represent the least aggressive of the neuroendocrine spectrum tumors, typically presenting as an SPN, often arising in the large airways (polypoid lesion), and rarely (if ever) associated with carcinoid syndrome
- Large cell with neuroendocrine features behaves clinically and radiographically like small cell
  - Morphologically, the cells are large and columnar
- Mesothelioma
  - Mesothelioma is a rare tumor of the pleura nearly uniformly associated with asbestos exposure, which tends to progress rapidly and cause pain and shortness of breath
  - Mesothelioma:
    - Is often associated with a pleural effusion (that may spontaneously resolve)
    - Has a propensity to cause medial pleural thickening and thus encasement of the lung
    - Often causes an intense inflammatory response in the adjacent pleura, making diagnosis difficult because biopsy may only show inflammation
    - VATS maybe required (Fig. 9.20)

LUNG CANCER STAGING

- Therapeutic approach and prognosis hinge on the clinical stage at diagnosis
- Stage is based on features of the primary tumor, nodal involvement, and the presence or absence of metastases (Table 9.1)
  - Tumor definitions : T1 = tumor ≤3 cm, T2 = tumor ≤7 cm, T3 = tumor >7 cm, T4 = tumor invading critical structures
    - T also increases with invasion and obstruction of critical structures and satellite nodules (see Table 9.1)
  - Thoracic lymph node definitions: N1 = hilar, N2 = ipsilateral mediastinal, N3 = contralateral mediastinal or extrathoracic
  - Metastasis definitions: M1a = thoracic metastasis, M1b = distant metastasis
- Metastasis and nodal involvement are more significant with regard to stage than tumor characteristics (see Table 9.2)
  - Metastatic disease is not curable
  - Metastatic disease is screened for by imaging:
    - Unexplained symptoms (eg, pain or neurologic complaints) in an individual with lung cancer should be pursued as possible metastatic disease with targeted imaging (ie, MRI of head or spine)

MESOTHELIOMA

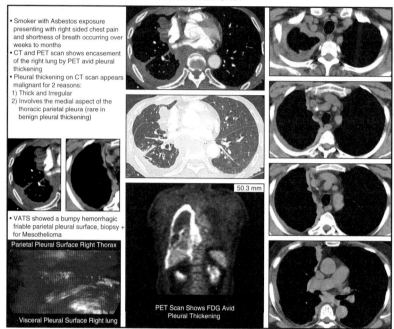

- Smoker with Asbestos exposure presenting with right sided chest pain and shortness of breath occurring over weeks to months
- CT and PET scan shows encasement of the right lung by PET avid pleural thickening
- Pleural thickening on CT scan appears malignant for 2 reasons:
  1) Thick and Irregular
  2) Involves the medial aspect of the thoracic parietal pleura (rare in benign pleural thickening)

50.3 mm

- VATS showed a bumpy hemorrhagic friable parietal pleural surface, biopsy + for Mesothelioma

Parietal Pleural Surface Right Thorax

Visceral Pleural Surface Right lung

PET Scan Shows FDG Avid Pleural Thickening

Fig. 9.20 Computed tomography (CT) scan, positron emission tomography (PET) imaging, and video-assisted thoracoscopic surgery (VATS) screen capture showing the classic radiographic and pleural appearance of mesothelioma; note the angry red intense inflammatory, pleural reaction (which can make diagnosis more challenging).

- Whole-body PET-CT (standard in the evaluation of all lung cancer) screens for other asymptomatic metastatic foci
- Individuals with adenocarcinoma stage IIA or greater or small cell should have a brain MRI looking for asymptotic brain metastasis
- N2 disease is a critical point in staging because it removes resection from the initial approach
  - N1 involvement has important prognostic implications but does **not** change initial approach
  - N3 disease removes surgery as an option (provides no clinical benefit)
- T4 describes tumors involving critical structures such that they are initially (and usually ultimately) unresectable

THERAPEUTIC APPROACH TO LUNG CANCER

- The therapeutic approach to lung cancer is based primarily on stage and, to a lesser extent, cell type
- The formulation of a therapeutic plan to treat lung cancer, especially for higher stage lesions (ie, III A), requires a wide variety of expertise (eg, surgeons, radiation oncologists, medical oncologists, radiologists, pathologists, pulmonologists) found in a multidisciplinary chest tumor board
  - Tumor boards are the standard of care for cancer centers and large health care systems
- Lung cancer is most reliably cured by anatomic resection (ie, entire lobe rather than wedge), such that this should be the goal for all resectable tumors, without N2 adenopathy, if lung function permits (ie, stage IA, IB, IIA, IIB, IIIA [T3, N1, M0])

Table 9.1 Lung Cancer Staging

TUMOR BY SIZE AND/OR LOCATION/INVASION	CLINICAL STAGE IF NO ADENOPATHY OR METASTASIS	OPTIMAL THERAPUTIC APPROACH	FIVE-YEAR SURVIVAL
T1a $\leq$2 cm **T1b** $\leq$3 cm	IA	▪ Lobar resection preferred to curative XRT	82%
T2a >3 ($\leq$5 cm) **or** **Any T** ($\leq$5 cm) involving: Main bronchus $\geq$2 cm from carina Lobar atelectasis/post obstructive lobar PNA Visceral pleural invasion (surgical stage)	IB	▪ Lobar resection preferred to curative XRT ▪ Consider adjuvant chemotherapy	66%
T2b >5 ($\leq$7 cm) **or** **Any T** ($\leq$7 cm) involving: Main bronchus $\geq$2 cm from carina Lobar atelectasis/post obstructive lobar PNA Visceral pleural invasion (surgical stage)	IIA	▪ Lobar resection preferred to curative XRT ▪ Adjuvant chemotherapy	52%
T3 > 7 cm or **Any T** involving: Main bronchus <2 cm from carina Whole lung atelectasis Chest wall Superior sulcus Phrenic nerve Diaphragm Parietal pleura (mediastinum, pericardium) Separate tumor nodules same lobe	IIB	▪ Lobar resection preferred to curative XRT ▪ Adjuvant chemotherapy	47%
T4 **Any T** ($\pm$ N1) involving: Carina (NOT in situ) Mediastinum, trachea, Esophagus, heart, or great vessels Recurrent laryngeal nerve Vertebral body Separate tumor nodules different lobe (ipsilateral)	IIIA	▪ Concurrent [†] vs sequential Chemotherapy and curative XRT ▪ Lobar resection if tumor shrinks to resectable (neoadjuvant approach)	36%

[†]Concurrent therapy has better efficacy than sequential therapy, BUT more toxicity, and is reserved for those with a good performance status. XRT = external beam radiation therapy (for unresectable tumors or those who cannot tolerate resection)

Table 9.2

Nodes:
Hilar (10 & 11 Right and Left)
Mediastinal (Right 2,4,7 and
  Left 4,5,6,7)
N1: Hilar
N2: Ipsilateral Mediastinal
N3: Contralateral Mediastinal
  or Extrathoracic
Metastasis:
M1a Thoracic
M1b Distant
	Clinical Stage
	IF
	Nodes
	or Metastasis
	Present
		Optimal Approach	Five Year
			Survival

N1 + T1 N1 + T2a	IIA	■ Lobar Resection preferred to Curative XRT ■ Adjuvant Chemotherapy	52%
N1 + T2b	IIB	■ Lobar Resection preferred to Curative XRT ■ Adjuvant Chemotherapy	47%
N1 + T3	IIIA	■ Lobar Resection preferred to Curative XRT ■ Adjuvant Chemotherapy	36%

N2 + T1-T3	IIIA	■ Concurrent † vs.
		  Sequential Chemotherapy
		  with Curative XRT
		■ Lobar Resection if N2
		  Disease Resolves
		  (Neoadjuvant Approach)	

N2 + T4	IIIB	■ Concurrent † vs.
		  Sequential Chemotherapy
		  and Curative XRT
			19%

N3 + any T	IIIB	■ Concurrent † vs.
		  Sequential Chemotherapy
		  and Curative XRT	

M1a
• Nodule(s) Contralateral
  Lung
• Malignant Pleural /
  Pericardial Effusion
M1b
• Distant Metastasis
	IV	■ Palliative Chemotherapy
		  for ECOG ≤ 2
		■ Palliative XRT for: Pain,
		  Hemoptysis, and or
		  Symptomatic Airway
		  Obstruction
		■ Targeted therapy for if
		  Driver Mutations Present
		  in Tumor
		■ Immunotherapy (e.g. PDL1
		  inhibitor)
			6%

† Concurrent therapy has better efficacy than sequential therapy, BUT more toxicity, and is reserved for those with a good performance status. XRT= External Beam Radiation Therapy (for Unresectable Tumors or those who cannot Tolerate Resection)

EMPIRIC CURATIVE RADIOTHERAPY

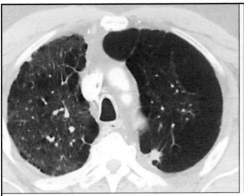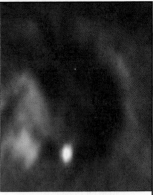

- Ct scan obtained to f/u an abnormal CXR in a former smoker with severe COPD, shows a 1.2 cm left upper lobe spiculated lesion. Pet scan shows that nodule is active (no adenopathy or other lesions identified)
- Given Location, and underlying lung disease Biopsy could cause a life threatening PTX (acutely) and or persistent BP fistula formation(sub acutely)
- Additionally pretest probability for Lung Cancer > 80% therefore alternate diagnosis required to stop Lung Cancer work up
- Patient not a candidate for resection therefore Empiric XRT was pursued

Fig. 9.21 Computed tomography (CT) scan and positron emission tomography (PET) imaging showing a classic example where underlying lung disease, the lesion location, and pretest probability make empiric external beam radiation (XRT) the only reasonable approach.

- Although XRT may also be curative for individuals who are not candidates for resection, it is most effective for small lesions and much less likely to cure large ones (Fig. 9.21)
- N2 involvement removes surgery as an initial approach (provides no clinical benefit)
  - Individuals with N2 involvement may become resectable if they respond well to chemotherapy and N2 lymph node disease disappears (by anatomic size criteria and FDG avidity)
    - This is known as a neoadjuvant approach
      - It may be considered in stage IIIA disease with N2 involvement
- T4 tumors involving critical structures (eg, carina, heart, great vessels, recurrent laryngeal nerve, vertebral body) are (at least initially) unresectable
  - If individuals have a great response to chemotherapy and radiation such that the primary tumor shrinks away from critical structures, resection can be considered
    - This is also a neoadjuvant approach
      - It is may be considered for patients with stage IIIA disease with T4 (especially in the case of superior sulcus tumors)
- **Ensuring an individual can tolerate lung resection:**
  - Individuals without lung disease can easily tolerate lobar, and even entire lung resection
  - Patients with lung cancer often have significant obstructive lung disease such that lobar resection might compromise them to a point of persistent postoperative respiratory failure (unacceptable outcome)
  - Traditional teaching states that a baseline forced expiratory volume in 1 second (FEV_1) >1.5 L should be able tolerate a lobectomy and an FEV_1 > 2.0 L should be able to tolerate a pneumonectomy

- In general, a calculation to predict postoperative FEV_1 should be done for everyone in whom resection is being contemplated
- Predicting postoperative FEV_1 and diffusing capacity of the lungs for carbon monoxide (DLCO):
  - Calculating the postoperative predicted FEV_1 and DLCO:
    - There are 19 total lung segments:
      - RUL = 3 segments, RML = 2 segments, RLL = 5 segments, LUL = 4 segments, LLL = 5 segments
    - (19) − (# of segments to be resected) = Postresection segment number (PRS#)
    - Postoperative predicted FEV_1 = (FEV_1) × (PRS#/19)
    - Postoperative predicted DLCO = (DLCO) x (PRS#/19)
    - Postoperative percent predicted = (percent predicted) x (PRS#/19)
    - If **both** the postoperative predicted FEV_1 and DLCO are >60%, the patient is at **low** risk for resection
    - If **either** the postoperative predicted FEV_1 and DLCO are <30%, the patient is at **high** risk for resection
    - If **either** the postoperative predicted FEV_1 and DLCO are between 30% and 60%, a functional study should be performed (eg, maximum cardiopulmonary exercise testing or stair climb assessment) to better assess risk
  - Alternatively, quantitative perfusion scanning can be done (most useful when lung function is borderline and the emphysema pattern is heterogeneous; eg, confined to the upper lobes)
    - Results are reported as the percent of blood flow to each lung zone, allowing for an estimated postoperative percent reduction in FEV_1 and DLCO
- Therapeutic considerations based on cell type:
  - **Small cell lung cancer** is staged like nonsmall cell lung cancer, but the therapeutic approach pragmatically takes into account its aggressive (metastatic at diagnosis) behavior
    - Aside from the **very** rare solitary pulmonary nodule presentation, small cell is **not** resected
      - The primary treatment modality is chemotherapy, which usually provides a dramatic initial response (eg, disease free imaging), before nearly uniformly recurring
      - Radiation therapy should be used (as an adjunct) if **all** visible disease is confined to the thorax and amenable to XRT
      - Prophylactic cranial irradiation should be considered in individuals who have a good response to chemotherapy
  - **Large cell carcinoma** with neuroendocrine features behaves, and is treated like, small cell
  - **Adenocarcinomas** (especially in nonsmoking Asians and females) have high rates of driver mutations (eg, EGFR/ALK), which can be specifically targeted with small molecule inhibitors
    - This targeted therapy approach may be used as a first line for stage IV disease (if mutation is present)
  - **Mesothelioma** has a very poor prognosis, and care is best delivered by a center of excellence (few and far between)
    - Centers of excellence offer aggressive surgical procedures on the spectrum from lung-sparing pleurectomy-decortication to the radical extrapleural pneumonectomy

STAGE IV DISEASE AND MANAGEMENT OF A PROVEN MALIGNANT PLEURAL EFFUSION

- Stage IV disease is not curable
  - Treatment is aimed primarily at alleviating symptoms:
    - Palliative chemotherapy has been shown to improve quality of life (and extend it by weeks) when given to individuals with a good performance status (ECOG ≤2)

- Palliative XRT is useful to treat pain, for airway obstruction, other critical structure impingement (eg, SVC), and/or hemoptysis
- Immunotherapy (eg, programmed death-ligand 1 inhibitor) is available for all stage IV nonsmall cell lung cancers
- Targeted therapy can be used for nonsquamous cell carcinomas demonstrating driver mutations (eg, EGFR mutation)
- Management of a malignant pleural effusion is based on symptom control such that if it is **not** responsible for symptoms (ie, dyspnea on exertion), it does not require intervention
  - Many individuals with end stage lung disease and advanced lung cancer suffer from severely limiting, multifactorial DOE, such that it is hard to tell whether or not symptoms are referable to the malignant effusion
  - This is best evaluated by the patient's subjective response to drainage
    - Individuals who respond to drainage may be offered serial thoracentesis (most reasonable when reaccumulation happens slowly, over weeks to months) vs a tunneled indwelling catheter, allowing for home drainage, which is most appropriate when reaccumulation is fast **or** when the patient has lung entrapment
      - Individuals with trapped lung (ie, failure of the lung to completely reexpand with fluid removal) may experience pain and are at risk for ex vacuo pneumothorax with recurrent, intermittent, larger-volume thoracentesis
        - Instead these individuals do better draining 200 to 300 mL at home on a daily basis ("taking the top off"' the effusion) to prevent collapse of remaining nontrapped lung
    - 10% of the time, systemic chemotherapy prevents recurrence of a malignant pleural effusion
    - Preventing and or treating volume overload dramatically reduces the reaccumulation rate of a malignant effusion (despite it being exudative)
      - Said differently, diuresis to euvolemia and maintenance of euvolemia may take an individual from requiring weekly taps to just once monthly
      - Exudates drain from the thorax (like transudates) via lymphatics in the parietal pleura/chest wall that drain into the IVC, such that high central venous pressure reduces and/or prevents thoracic lymphatic drainage, favoring effusion accumulation

QUESTIONS COMMONLY GENERATED BY THIS TEACHING

1. What is the difference between clinical stage and surgical stage?
   Every patient who undergoes surgery receives a surgical stage based on the additional information provided by the surgery—namely the exact tumor size and whether or not the visceral pleura is involved. If the surgical stage is higher than the clinical stage, patients should offered additional treatment based on the "new" stage (eg, chemotherapy).
2. When should I obtain a brain MRI to look for metastasis in patients with lung cancer, who don't have neurologic symptoms?
   Brain MRI should be obtained for all small cell carcinomas and adenocarcinomas that are stage II or higher. It should also be considered in large cell carcinomas with neuroendocrine features.

CHAPTER 10

ASPERGILLUS LUNG DISEASE

COMMON MISCONCEPTIONS AND MISTAKES

- Confusing an aspergilloma or fungus ball with chronic fibrosing pulmonary aspergillosis
- Failing to make the distinction between allergic bronchopulmonary aspergillosis (ABPA) and asthma with fungal sensitization
- Believing that invasive pulmonary aspergillosis only occurs in bone marrow transplant patients
- Not attempting antifungal therapy in a steroid-dependent asthmatic with mucus plugging and bronchiectasis, because of negative aspergillus serology
- Failing to diagnose and treat chronic fibrosing aspergillosis

ASPERGILLUS

- Aspergillus is:
  - The most common invasive mold
  - Ubiquitous—found in soil and decomposing organic matter (worldwide)
  - The most common contaminant seen in specimens exposed to unfiltered air (during processing)
  - A common colonizer seen in the sputum of ~3% of healthy individuals and ~10% of cigarette smokers, HIV-infected individuals, or those with chronic parenchymal lung disease
  - *Aspergillus fumigatus* causes ~90% of human diseases
    - Together, *Aspergillus flavus, Aspergillus terreus,* and *Aspergillus niger* are responsible for the rest
      - Serology is **not** available for these less common human-pathogen Aspergillus species
- Aspergillus disease begins with (the relatively common event of) accidental spore inhalation
  - In the normal host, inhaled spores are rapidly cleared by the immune system
  - In individuals with underlying lung disease or in those with immunologic sensitization to Aspergillus or immunosuppression, inhalation of spores may result in colonization, hypersensitivity, or invasive disease, respectively
  - Small clusters of invasive pulmonary aspergillosis have been reported when an environmental focus (eg, hospital construction) exposes a group of immunosuppressed patients (eg, bone marrow transplant ward)
    - Human-to-human transmission does not occur
- Aspergillus causes seven distinct pulmonary syndromes in allergic individuals and those with parenchymal lung disease or immunosuppression:
  - Atopic/allergic/asthmatic individuals are vulnerable to:
    1. **Severe asthma with fungal sensitization** (immunoglobulin E [IgE]-mediated asthma)
    2. **Allergic bronchopulmonary aspergillosis** (ABPA)
    3. **Hypersensitivity pneumonitis** (HP)

- Individuals with chronic parenchymal lung disease (especially chronic obstructive pulmonary disease [COPD]) are vulnerable to:
  4. **Aspergilloma**
  5. **Chronic pulmonary aspergillosis** (CPA)
     - Semiinvasive (noncavitary)
     - Chronic fibrosing (cavitary)
- Patients with any degree of immune suppression are at risk for:
  6. **Invasive pulmonary aspergillosis** (IPA) ranging from:
     - Atypical (nodular) bronchopneumonia to
     - Vessel-invasive disseminated disease
  7. **Tracheobronchial aspergillosis** (seen after lung transplant and in HIV infection)
- Significant overlap may be seen in these syndromes (eg, allergic disease may progress to invasive disease in the setting of high-dose prednisone therapy)

ALLERGIC ASPERGILLUS DISEASES

- **Severe asthma with fungal sensitization (IgE-mediated asthma):**
  - Patients with severe extrinsic IgE-mediated asthma triggered by environmental Aspergillus antigens (and many others) are different from individuals with ABPA
  - ~30% of individuals with asthma demonstrate fungal sensitization (immediate skin test reactivity to Aspergillus)
  - Asthma with fungal sensitization can be differentiated from ABPA by the **absence** of bronchiectasis, mucus plugging, and high IgE levels
    - IgE levels <1000 IU/mL (obtained off of prednisone) makes severe asthma with fungal sensitization more likely than ABPA
  - Avoidance of antigen (eg, moldy environments) is crucial for asthma control in these individuals
- **HP:**
  - Inhalation of organic matter contaminated with Aspergillus species has been associated with HP (eg, Malt-worker's lung)
  - Hypersensitivity pneumonitis is a clinical diagnosis such that specific allergen testing is not sensitive, specific, or helpful
- **ABPA:**
  - ABPA is a clinical syndrome involving a **hypersensitivity to A. fumigatus,** which occurs in predisposed individuals (ie, those with asthma or cystic fibrosis)
  - Age of onset is 30–50 years old
  - The clinical syndrome of ABPA is characterized by:
    - Episodic "or fleeting" chest radiograph infiltrates
    - Significant IgE elevations (>1000 IU/mL)
    - Poorly controlled asthma (~80% of the time)
  - Common symptoms of ABPA, aside from poorly controlled asthma, include:
    - Productive cough with mucus plugs
    - A history of recurrent pneumonia (diagnoses)
      - Often with a clinical radiographic discrepancy between a significant infiltrate on chest x-ray, and muted clinical findings
        - Fleeting ABPA infiltrates are often a result of mucus plugging and subsegmental atelectasis (rather than representing true infectious consolidations)
    - Intermittent fever (immune system activation)
    - Chest pain (often from mucus plugging and atelectasis)
    - Hemoptysis
      - Occurs on a spectrum from (nonmassive) blood-tinged sputum, secondary to mucosal irritation associated with coughing, to bronchiectatic bleeding (potentially massive)

- Radiographic findings seen in/suggestive of ABPA include:
  - The "finger in glove" sign describing branching tubular (vascular-looking) homogeneous opacities (actually representing mucus-impacted airways) (Fig. 10.1])
  - Fleeting upper lobe infiltrates and wedge-shaped infiltrates (subsegmental atelectasis) (Fig. 10.2)
  - Tramline and ring shadows (bronchial wall thickening)
  - Bronchiectasis, classically central (medial two-thirds of the chest), but may also be distal; often identified by computed tomography (CT) scan (see Fig. 10.2)
  - High-attenuation mucus (HAM) impaction seen on CT scan is nearly pathognomonic for ABPA and is predictive of relapsing, progressive disease
- The differential diagnosis of ABPA includes:
  - Allergic bronchopulmonary mycosis (same syndrome, different fungus, serology not available/helpful)
  - IgE-mediated asthma with fungal sensitization (as discussed previously)
  - pulmonary infiltration with eosinophilia syndromes, helminthic lung disease, and other types of hypersensitivity pneumonitis
- The diagnosis of ABPA can be confidently made when an individual has a compatible clinical syndrome and the following:
  - Asthma or cystic fibrosis (ie, predisposing condition)
  - Type I allergic response to Aspergillus (ie, positive serum IgE specific for Aspergillus or a positive skin test)

MUCUS IMPACTION IN ALLERGIC BRONCHOPULMONARY ASPERGILLOSIS THE 'FINGER IN GLOVE' SIGN

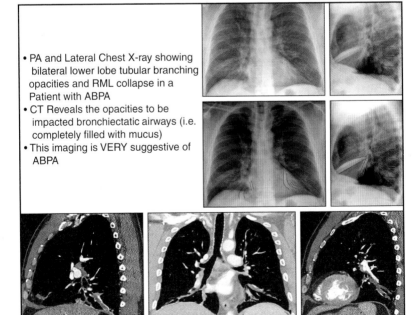

- PA and Lateral Chest X-ray showing bilateral lower lobe tubular branching opacities and RML collapse in a Patient with ABPA
- CT Reveals the opacities to be impacted bronchiectatic airways (i.e. completely filled with mucus)
- This imaging is VERY suggestive of ABPA

Fig. 10.1 Posterioranterior (PA) and lateral chest x-ray (with mark-up) showing the "finger in glove" sign of mucus impaction in allergic bronchopulmonary aspergillosis (ABPA). Computed tomography (CT) scan confirms that the tubular branching opacities are completely impacted airways.

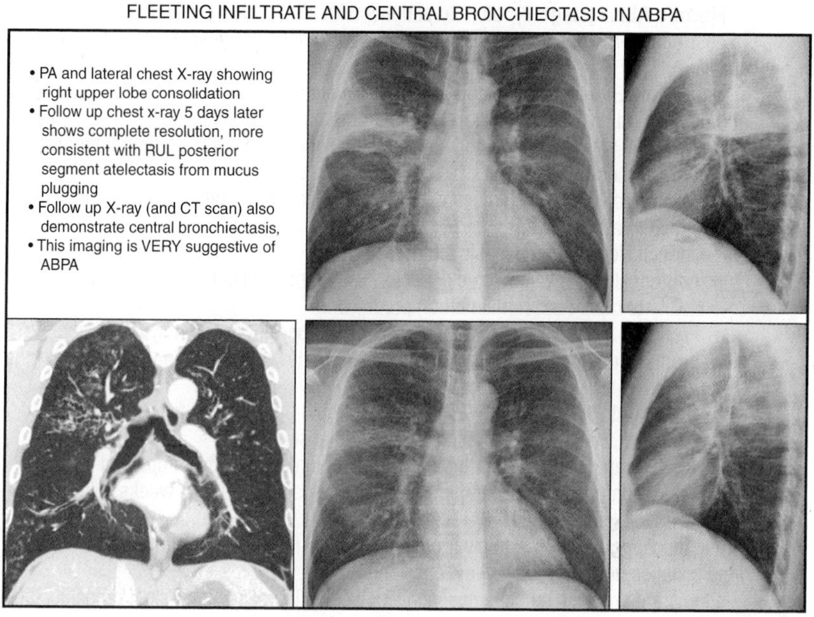

FLEETING INFILTRATE AND CENTRAL BRONCHIECTASIS IN ABPA

- PA and lateral chest X-ray showing right upper lobe consolidation
- Follow up chest x-ray 5 days later shows complete resolution, more consistent with RUL posterior segment atelectasis from mucus plugging
- Follow up X-ray (and CT scan) also demonstrate central bronchiectasis.
- This imaging is VERY suggestive of ABPA

Fig. 10.2 Posterioranterior (PA) and lateral chest x-ray (CXR) showing a "fleeting" or rapidly resolving consolidation (time course too fast for resolution of an infectious consolidation). Computed tomography (CT) scan shows central bronchiectasis occurring in the same region, supporting the diagnosis of subsegmental atelectasis from mucus impaction (rather than a pneumonic consolidation).

- Two of the following three:
  - Positive IgG specific to *A. fumigatus*
  - Imaging findings suggestive of ABPA (eg, fleeting infiltrates, bronchiectasis, or HAM plugs)
  - Total eosinophil count >500 cells/μL and/or IgE >1000 IU/mL (during a flare and while off prednisone)
- Patients with ABPA can be divided into five clinical stages:
  - **Acute ABPA (stage I)** describes the initial presentation of classic ABPA
  - **Remission (stage II)** is defined as no recurrence for at least 6 months after prednisone therapy is stopped
    - Remission is expected (and achieved in over 90% of all patients)
    - Relapse is common and may occur several years later
    - Patients in remission should be screened with serial IgE measurements every 3–6 months (for the first year)
  - **ABPA exacerbation (stage III)** occurs in nearly half of all patients and may be clinically silent, consisting only of asymptomatic infiltrates or an increase in IgE levels (2–10 times higher than baseline values)
    - Almost half of all patients with ABPA who experience exacerbations progress to steroid-dependent asthma
  - **ABPA with corticosteroid-dependent asthma (stage IV)** lacks the typical features of IgE elevation and fleeting infiltrates (because of prednisone)
    - Diagnosing ABPA at stage IV involves paring a clinically compatible history with imaging, demonstrating either:
      - Bronchiectasis, HAM impaction on chest CT, or previous fleeting upper lobe infiltrates

- **Fibrotic ABPA (stage V)** refers to patients with ABPA who develop mixed obstructive–restrictive lung disease with symptomatic bronchiectasis and respiratory failure
- Treatment of ABPA focuses on decreasing organism colonization and burden with antifungals and control of exaggerated inflammation with prednisone
  - Both the initial presentation and subsequent exacerbations should be treated with antifungal therapy
    - Itraconazole is first line (because of cost) but has poor oral absorption known to cause treatment failures
    - Voriconazole is a reasonable alternative
    - Antifungal therapy should be given for 3–6 months based on clinical improvement/ability to taper (and remain off of) prednisone
    - Prednisone should be initiated, dosed, and tapered based on symptomatic bronchospasm (as in asthma) rather than IgE levels in isolation (which take time to fall)
    - Once prednisone is stopped, individuals should be screened for recurrent infiltrates, clinical symptoms, or a rise in total serum IgE
  - ABPA should rapidly improve with therapy (resolution of infiltrates, improved asthma, reduced sputum, and decreased peripheral blood eosinophilia by 4 weeks, with decreased total serum IgE by 6 weeks)
  - Bronchoscopy can be used to clear proximal airway mucus impaction and segmental lung collapse not relieved by chest physiotherapy
    - Persistent proximal mucus impaction (>3 weeks) increases the risk of bronchiectasis
- **Allergic bronchopulmonary mycosis:**
  - Some individuals have the clinical syndrome of ABPA, involving to either a non-fumigatus species of Aspergillus or another environmental fungus, making serology and skin testing unhelpful
  - Because of this, most steroid-dependent asthmatics deserve an empiric trial of antifungal therapy before being condemned to lifelong prednisone

ASPERGILLOMA

- Aspergilloma (a.k.a. fungus ball) refers to a mobile, intracavitary mass of fungal mycelia, inflammatory cells, and tissue debris occurring in a **preexisting,** poorly communicating lung cavity, bullae, or cyst
- Aspergilloma commonly occurs in emphysematous bullae or in association with prior cavitary lung disease (eg, tuberculosis [TB], lung cancer treated with XRT, coccidioidomycosis, cysts)
- Most aspergillomas are discovered incidentally on chest imaging
  - Commonly appear as an intraluminal irregularity in an upper lobe cavity
  - Prone CT imaging and/or fluoroscopy should demonstrate mobility of the irregularity with positional changes (Fig. 10.3)
- Sputum culture for Aspergillus is positive ~50% of the time
- Aspergillus skin testing and serology are negative, unless there is a more invasive process (ie, CPA)
- Asymptomatic patients with stable chest imaging require no antifungal therapy
- 80% of aspergillomas remain stable and up to 10% demonstrate resolution of intraluminal material over time
- 10% are associated with recurrent (nonmassive) hemoptysis
  - Antifungal therapy can be given but will only be effective if there is a component of CPA (ie, a more invasive disease)
  - Embolization can be used for persistent hemoptysis (not relieved by antifungal therapy) or for massive hemoptysis
  - Resection can be considered in individuals with adequate lung function (rarely done)

ASPERGILLOMA

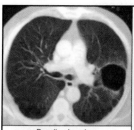 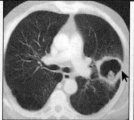 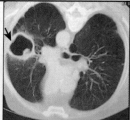

Baseline Imaging: Showing Bullous Emphysema	CT Obtained for COPD Exacerbation Showing Consolidation / Thickening around a preexisting bullae with intraluminal material / debris	Prone Imaging Shows Intraluminal Material is Freely Mobile: Imaging Pathognomonic for a Aspergilloma

Fig. 10.3 Computed tomography (CT) scans showing an aspergilloma (ie, preexisting cavity that has developed wall thickening and a freely mobile intraluminal debris). The wall thickening raises the concern for possible concomitant semi invasive aspergillosis.

CHRONIC PULMONARY ASPERGILLOSIS

- CPA encompasses a spectrum of indolent invasive Aspergillus infections
- Occurs in patients with underlying lung disease and often mild degrees of immunosuppression
  - Typically affects patients with COPD, but may complicate any underlying parenchymal lung disease (eg, sarcoidosis)
  - Mild immunosuppression (ie, diabetes mellitus, low-dose oral glucocorticoid therapy, alcoholism, poor nutrition, or connective tissue disease) is common but not required
- Aspergillus initially colonizes areas of abnormal parenchyma and then progresses via indolent, local invasion
- Although the diagnosis of CPA classically requires a tissue biopsy demonstrating branching hyphae in tissue, the contemporary approach involves correlating a compatible clinical and radiographic presentation with supportive evidence of invasive Aspergillus infection
- This change has occurred primarily because biopsy may be morbid and antifungal therapy is no longer toxic, such that a diagnostic/therapeutic trial is often the safest way to proceed
- CPA occurs in both **semiinvasive** and **chronic fibrosing** forms
- **Semiinvasive aspergillosis:**
  - Occurs when Aspergillus colonizes a preexisting cavity (eg, bullae) and then becomes locally invasive, causing areas of thickening and inflammation, often with a solid, nodular (pseudospiculated) component, mimicking an early (stage IA) lung cancer (Fig. 10.4)
  - May be asymptomatic or associated with worsening COPD symptoms (ie, cough, shortness of breath, and dyspnea on exertion)
  - Spontaneous improvement with resolution of nodules (and/or fleeting nodules) occurs commonly
  - Diagnosis is made primarily by correlating a compatible clinical and radiographic presentation with ancillary evidence—namely:
    - Demonstration of IgG-specific Aspergillus antibodies
    - Positive serum galactomannan
    - Growth of Aspergillus in sputum (least compelling)
  - Treatment with antifungal therapy is reserved for symptomatic individuals (a minority) or those who are being evaluated for a possible early-stage lung cancer (ie, a trial of antifungal therapy before reimaging/biopsy)

SEMI INVASIVE ASPERGILLOSIS WITHOUT CAVITATION
MIMICKING EARLY STAGE LUNG CANCER

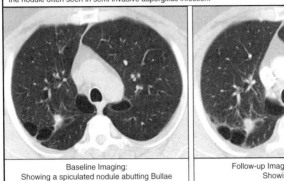

CT Scan obtained to evaluate a nodule seen on X-ray obtained for COPD exacerbation. Follow-up imaging 3 months later shows growth. Lesion resected via lobectomy based on high pretest probability for lung cancer. Lesion instead shows semi invasive aspergillosis. Note thickening around bullae walls in addition to growth of the nodule often seen in semi invasive aspergillus infection.

Baseline Imaging: Showing a spiculated nodule abutting Bullae	Follow-up Imaging 3 Months Later Showing growth

---- SURGICAL PATHOLOGY ----
Lung, right upper lobe, lobectomy
DX: FUNGAL HYPHAE WITH ACUTE AND NECROTIZING GRANULOMATOUS INFLAMMATTON, CORRELATION WITH MICROBIOLOGY RECOMMENDED

Fig. 10.4 Serial computed tomography (CT) scan showing a spiculated nodule abutting a bullae. Follow-up imaging 3 months later demonstrates growth of the nodule together with thickening around the bullae. Because of a high pretest probability for lung cancer, the lesion was resected and ultimately turned out to be semiinvasive aspergillosis. Note the lack of cavitation, fibrosis, and volume loss. Lesions like this often regress on their own.

- Oral itraconazole or voriconazole may be given for 2–3 months and stopped when clinical and radiographic improvement is noted
- Relapse is common
- Surveillance imaging is required both to ensure that fibrosis and cavitation do not occur (see chronic fibrosing aspergillosis below) and to rule out steady growth concerning for lung cancer
- **Chronic fibrosing aspergillosis:**
  - Occurs when Aspergillus colonizes abnormal lung parenchyma (eg, bullae, bronchiectatic airway) and then becomes locally invasive, causing areas of cavitation, fibrosis, and volume loss (Fig. 10.5)
  - Typical imaging involves multiple upper lobe, confluent thick-walled areas of cavitation with intraluminal irregularities, associated fibrosis, bronchiectasis, adjacent pleural thickening, retraction, and volume loss
    - Intraluminal material is often erroneously called a fungus ball, despite the fact that it represents lung necrosis (rather than debris collected in a preexisting bullae or cavity)
  - Despite dramatic progressive parenchymal destruction, symptoms may be muted or absent
    - Dry cough, recurrent hemoptysis, and/or dyspnea occur ~50% of the time
    - Weight loss is nearly universal (but is often attributed to pulmonary cachexia)
  - Fever and sputum production are not anticipated and instead suggest bacterial super infection and/or bronchiectasis exacerbation (which occur frequently)
    - During an episode of acute bacterial super infection, the parenchymal changes of chronic fibrosing aspergillosis may be erroneously attributed to (necrotizing) pneumonia, causing the diagnosis to be delayed or missed entirely (Fig. 10.6)

EARLY CHRONIC FIBROSING ASPERGILLOSIS

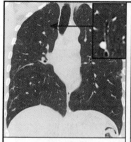

Baseline Imaging
History of Stage 2 sarcoidosis
Note Bronchiectatic Airway

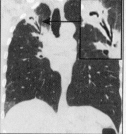

6 Years Later
CT Imaging for Fever and Cough
Treated for Lung Abscess

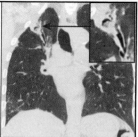

Follow-up Imaging 4 mo. Later Shows
Continued Necrosis Concerning for chronic
Fibrosing Aspergillus Infection (note upper
lobe volume loss)

- Serial imaging showing the development of fibrosing aspergillosis in the distal aspect of a bronchiectatic airway (note NO preexisting cavity)
- Initial cavitation attributed to traditional lung abscess (treated with antibiotics)
- Follow-up imaging 4 months later, to ensure resolution, instead shows continued cavitation, volume loss
- Note the development of intraluminal material consistent with necrotic lung tissue, NOT an aspergilloma, (since it is not occurring in a preexisting cavity)

Test	Result / Status
COCCI SEROLOGY IgG	NEGATIVE
COCCI SEROLOGY IgM	NEGATIVE

Test	Result / Status
Quantiferon Gold TB	Negative

Collection sample: SPUTUM
AFB CULTURE & SMEAR----------- completed
AFB SMEAR------------------------- completed
* MYCOBACTERIOLOGY FINAL REPORT
concentrate Acid Fast Stain: Negative
NO MYCOBACTERIUM ISOLATED AFTER 8 WEEKS

Site/Specimen: SPUTUM
GRAM STAIN: 2+ POLYMORPHONUCLEAR CELLS
4+ MIXED BACTERIA
CULTURE RESULTS: ASPERGILLUS FUMIGATUS 2+

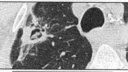

Test	Result / Status
ASPERGILLUS-CF	1:16
ASPERGILLUS-ID	POSITIVE

Fig. 10.5 Serial computed tomography (CT) scans show the development of chronic fibrosing aspergillosis occurring in an area of prior bronchiectasis. Note fibrosis and volume loss in addition to cavitation. The intraluminal debris should not be called a fungus ball or aspergilloma (benign condition occurring in a preexisting cavity that does not require treatment) because it actually represents lung necrosis, necessitating antifungal therapy to prevent further parenchymal destruction.

- Diagnosis involves exclusion of other conditions with similar presentations (eg, active TB, endemic fungal infection, lung cancer, nontuberculous mycobacterial [NTM]) infection by sputum examination, culture, and comparison with prior imaging
  - Differential diagnosis includes:
    - Lung abscess or infected bullae
      - The presence of a significant air fluid level within a cavity suggests bacterial superinfection
    - Lung cancer with necrosis (especially squamous cell)
    - Radiation fibrosis (in the appropriate setting)
    - TB and/or rapidly growing NTM
    - Endemic fungal infection (eg, coccidioidomycosis)
  - Biopsy is reserved for cases that are concerning for lung cancer (**not** to confirm invasive Aspergillus infection)
  - Bronchoscopy with bronchoalveolar lavage (BAL) may be helpful when sputum results are unrevealing, and the suspicion for TB or NTM are high
    - Additionally, bronchoscopy may support the diagnosis of CPA via BAL galactomannan and positive aspergillus culture results
  - Serum IgG Aspergillus–specific antibodies are present in >90%
    - May be falsely negative in patients taking systemic corticosteroids or in patients infected with non–*A. fumigatus* species
  - Weight loss is present in >90%
  - Sputum culture is positive for Aspergillus ~50% of the time
  - Serum or BAL galactomannan is also positive ~50% of the time

THE NATURAL HISTORY OF CHRONIC FIBROSING ASPERGILLOSIS

93 yo. with HTN, anemia, and COPD admitted with massive hemoptysis and shortness of breath. Admission chest x-ray showed a stable left apical bullae / cavity, with new dense consolidations and ground glass opacities in the left upper lobe. Comparison to an X-ray from 2 months prior showed preexisting left upper lobe fibrocavitary opacity with hilar retraction (appearance compatible with reactivation TB). The patient had left a upper lobe ectatic bronchial artery embolized with improvement in hemoptysis. Sputum and serologic tests were negative for bacteria, coccidioidomycosis, and AFB/TB. Sputum and serology did demonstrate exposure to aspergillus fumigatus, supportive of semi-invasive disease.

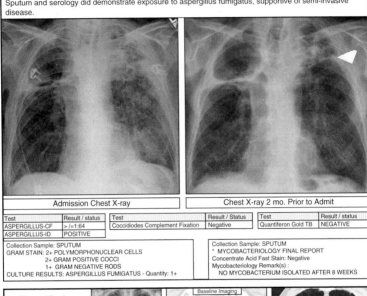

Admission Chest X-ray	Chest X-ray 2 mo. Prior to Admit

Test	Result / status	Test	Result / Status	Test	Result / status
ASPERGILLUS-CF	> /=1:64	Coccidiodes Complement Fixation	Negative	Quantiferon Gold TB	NEGATIVE
ASPERGILLUS-ID	POSITIVE				

Collection Sample: SPUTUM
GRAM STAIN: 2+ POLYMORPHONUCLEAR CELLS
2+ GRAM POSITIVE COCCI
1+ GRAM NEGATIVE RODS
CULTURE RESULTS: ASPERGILLUS FUMIGATUS - Quantity: 1+

Collection Sample: SPUTUM
* MYCOBACTERIOLOGY FINAL REPORT
Concentrate Acid Fast Stain: Negative
Mycobacteriology Remark(s) :
NO MYCOBACTERIUM ISOLATED AFTER 8 WEEKS

Record Review

• Review of chart and imaging reveals 7 years of progressive bilateral apical cavitation and fibrosis
• Pt admitted multiple times over the 7 years with complaints of dry cough, DOE and hemoptysis, treated for recurrent CAP
• Imaging shows worsening confluent thick walled cavities with intraluminal irregularities, associated fibrosis, adjacent pleural thickening, and volume loss
• Patient loses 40 lbs. over the course of the disease

Baseline 139 lbs.

Admission 7 years later → 100 lbs.

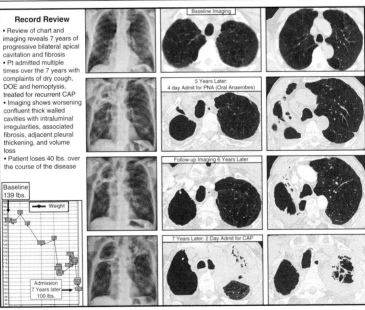

Fig. 10.6 Encapsulated case of an elderly gentleman with chronic obstructive pulmonary disease (COPD) who was treated for necrotizing upper lobe bacterial pneumonia twice. Both times the patient was discharged and prescribed oral antibiotics after clinical improvement. Importantly, his cavitary apical lesions did not resolve with antibiotic therapy and time (as is anticipated in bacterial necrotizing pneumonia). Instead his apices demonstrate progressive destruction over time, with cavitation, fibrosis, and volume loss, ultimately resulting in massive hemoptysis requiring embolization. This progressive apical fibrosis with cavitation is classic for long-standing chronic fibrosing aspergillosis. Note the dramatic (consumptive) weight loss over time.

- Massive hemoptysis is a significant cause of morbidity and mortality in individuals with chronic fibrosing aspergillosis
  - Bronchial artery embolization may be required
    - Recurrent bleeding from collateral blood vessels is common
  - Although surgical resection offers definitive treatment, severe underlying lung disease is usually prohibitive
    - Surgery is only considered for individuals with massive hemoptysis and adequate pulmonary reserve who fail embolization (or are unwilling to accept the small but real risk of paralysis via accidental spinal artery injury and spinal cord ischemia)
- Chronic fibrosing aspergillosis requires lifelong antifungal therapy
  - Because of this, posicianzole or isavuconazole is preferred to voriconazole (photosensitizing) and itraconazole (poor oral absorption)
- Radiographic improvement occurs gradually (eg, thinning cavity walls and resolving intraluminal irregularities)
- Treatment failures should prompt consideration for:
  - Inadequate absorption of oral medications (screened for by testing drug levels)
  - Mimics (eg, anaerobic bacterial superinfection or lung cancer)

INVASIVE PULMONARY ASPERGILLOSIS

- IPA represents a spectrum of acute invasive pulmonary Aspergillus infections that occur most commonly in patients with prolonged neutropenia, but also in patients with only modest degrees of immune suppression
  - ~90% of IPA cases occur in patients with hematologic malignancies and allogeneic hematopoietic stem-cell transplants
    - Acute and chronic graft versus host disease poses a greater risk for IPA than neutropenia in this group
  - ~10% of IPA occurs in patients with only modest degrees of immunosuppression (eg, solid organ transplant, AIDS, autologous hematopoietic stem cell transplantation)
  - ~1% of cases are reported in immunocompetent patients
    - Chronic granulomatous lung disease (eg, sarcoidosis) increases the risk of IPA
- ~70% of IPA presents as neutropenic fever with asymptomatic pulmonary radiographic changes (ie, halo sign), which if untreated progresses to symptomatic disease
- Common symptoms include fever, dry cough, pleurisy, and hemoptysis
- Patients with prolonged neutropenia are at risk for rapidly progressive, often fatal, IPA in which large-vessel pulmonary artery invasion causes massive hemoptysis and thrombosis, with death occurring from airway obstruction and/or acute right-sided heart failure
- Individuals with modest degrees of immunosuppression may have a more indolent IPA presentation, appearing like an atypical bacterial pneumonia (often round/nodular), which if not diagnosed and treated may progress to angioinvasive IPA
- The classic CT patterns of IPA are the halo and air crescent signs (Fig. 10.7):
  - The halo sign is seen in neutropenic patients and describes a circumferential rim of ground glass surrounding a more solid nodule (resulting from local vessel invasion and hemorrhage)
  - The air crescent sign is seen after the recovery of neutrophils and represents necrosis of the nodule (from neutrophil-mediated inflammation)
  - Initial serial CT imaging (first week) may demonstrate growth of IPA lesions despite adequate therapy as immune response and inflammation increase (should not diagnose therapeutic failure solely based on initial radiographic growth)
  - Other common CT findings in IPA include multiple small nodules, large nodules, and areas of dense/pneumonic consolidation
- The differential diagnosis includes pneumonia from other typical and atypical pathogens capable of causing nodular infiltrates with cavitation (eg, Pseudomonas, Staphylococcus,

INVASIVE PULMONARY ASPERGILLOSIS (IPA)
HALO AND AIR CRESCENT SIGNS (CT SCAN FINDINGS)

CT scan obtained to evaluate fever and neutropenia in a BMT patient revealed a 1 cm nodule with the 'halo sign' extremely suggestive of IPA. The patient was started on Voriconazole, defervesced and resolved his neutropenia. Follow-up imaging 3 weeks later showed growth and cavitation / necrosis, all of the anticipated findings as immune function returns. Despite what might be mobile intracavitary debris, it is NOT a fungus ball (since their was no pre existing cavity).

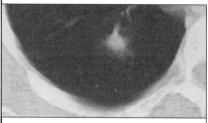

Chest CT in a BMT patient with Neutropenia and fever showing a ~ 1 cm nodule with surrounding ground glass 'halo'

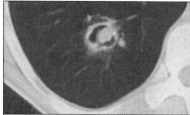

Follow-up Imaging 3 weeks later (after neutropenia resolved), showing that the lesion has increased in size and experienced necrosis, leading to the 'air crescent' sign

Fig. 10.7 Computed tomography (CT) imaging of the most sensitive and specific chest CT scan findings in invasive pulmonary aspergillosis—namely the halo and air crescent signs. These signs reflect the radiographic progression of invasive aspergillosis infection in an individual who is initially neutropenic (leading to a nodule with surrounding vessel invasion and hemorrhage) followed by necrosis as neutrophil function returns. This progression, in the right clinical setting, is pathognomonic for invasive pulmonary aspergillosis (IPA).

  Klebsiella, Nocardia, viruses, mycobacteria, and other fungi and noninfectious entities [eg, neoplasm, pneumonitis])
- Classically the diagnosis of IPA required a biopsy demonstrating tissue invasion (and culture growth)
  - However, transbronchial biopsy has a high false-negative rate and VATS lung biopsy carries a significant bleeding risk
- For most patients at risk for IPA, a presumptive diagnosis can be made by integrating chest CT imaging with BAL/sputum culture results and fungal antigen testing
  - Therapy is often started empirically, based on classical clinical and radiographic features
- Growing Aspergillus in sputum or BAL has a ~60% positive predictive value in at-risk patients
  - However, ~50% of patients with IPA have negative cultures
- Identifying branching hyphae on BAL cytology is strongly suggestive of invasive disease
- Aspergillus serology (IgG-Af) is unreliable, given the immunosuppressed status of at-risk patients
- Galactomannan is a polysaccharide produced by Aspergillus during hyphal growth, detected by an ELISA assay (≥ 0.5 [OD] equals a positive result)
  - False positives occur from dietary intake of galactomannan and poor bowel wall integrity
  - False negatives commonly occur when treatment has begun
- Voriconazole is first-line therapy for IPA, dosed at 6 mg/kg intravenously (IV) twice on the first day and then 4 mg/kg IV twice daily after that
  - Posaconazole or isavuconazole may be used for those intolerant to voriconazole
- Liposomal amphotericin B is second-line therapy, dosed at 3–5 mg/kg IV daily
  - Liposomal amphotericin B may be used as a first-line agent if mucormycosis is high on the differential

TRACHEOBRONCHIAL ASPERGILLOSIS

- Tracheobronchial aspergillosis (TBA) represents a unique situation in which Aspergillus invades the mucosa of the large airways, leading to thick, adherent, nodular plaques that cause endobronchial narrowing and sloughing, leading to life-threatening airway obstruction
    - TBA exists on a spectrum from mucosal ulceration to extensive pseudomembrane formation
- Symptoms include dyspnea, cough, and fixed wheeze, with chest x-ray evidence of lobar atelectasis
- Diagnosis is made by bronchoscopy with mucosal visualization, biopsy, and culture
    - Visually the mucosa may appear as a pale, devitalized pseudomembrane sloughing into the airway lumen
- TBA may cause respiratory failure and death from airway obstruction (or, more rarely, perforation of the trachea)
- Risk factors include hematologic malignancy, HIV infection, and lung transplant recipient status (at the anastomosis)
- TBA after lung transplant
    - Early (~1 month) after lung transplant, the bronchial anastomosis is uniquely vulnerable to Aspergillus colonization and subsequent invasion
        - Colonization occurs ~30% of the time
        - TBA occurs ~15% of the time
    - There is a ~80% response to antifungal therapy and bronchoscopic disimpaction
    - Despite therapy, stenosis at the bronchial anastomosis occurs ~20% of the time

COMMON QUESTIONS GENERATED BY THIS TEACHING

1. What is the difference between ABPA and severe asthma with fungal sensitization?
ABPA describes a syndrome in which asthmatics develop a hyperallergic response to Aspergillus airway colonization (typically with very high IgE levels). Severe asthma with fungal sensitization describes asthmatics with environmental Aspergillus antigen triggers. The latter may be controlled by avoiding moldy environments (and/or wearing a mask). Asthma with fungal sensitization should not cause mucus plugging and bronchiectasis. Antifungal therapy, which is critical against ABPA, does not help in cases of asthma with fungal sensitization.

2. I thought diagnosis of invasive aspergillosis required a biopsy showing histopathologic evidence of tissue invasion in addition to demonstrating growth of Aspergillus (from the surgical specimen).
Although the classic diagnostic criteria for invasive aspergillosis still exist, the practical, contemporary approach involves paring imaging, serology, culture, and fungal antigen testing with empiric treatment. This approach acknowledges the danger and false negative rate of biopsy together with the relatively safe nature of empiric antifungal therapy.

CHAPTER 11

ORAL ANAEROBIC LUNG INFECTION, ASPIRATION PNEUMONIA, LUNG ABSCESS, AND EMPYEMA

COMMON MISCONCEPTIONS AND MISTAKES

- Using the term "aspiration" without clearly defining the clinical aspiration syndrome you are concerned with

- Believing that aspiration pneumonia is solely a disease of swallowing difficulty and food aspiration

- Believing that aspiration pneumonia is a disease of gastroesophageal reflux disease

- Pursuing drainage of a lung abscess

- Treating a drained empyema with prolonged antibiotics (>14 days)

- Failing to treat a lung abscess with prolonged antibiotics until (often >30 days) radiographic improvement and/or resolution of necrosis

- Narrowing antibiotic coverage of an empyema based on the growth of a dominant pathogen (eg, MRSA) when commensurate infection with oral anaerobes is routine (oral anaerobes should always remain covered)

- Believing aspiration only occurs in dependent lung zones

ASPIRATION DEFINED

- Aspiration is defined as the inhalation of **anything** (besides a gas) past the vocal cords into the lower airway

- The reflexes of the oropharynx, glottis, and epiglottis are designed to prevent aspiration; therefore aspiration often occurs at times of central sedation when these reflexes are blunted (eg, sleep, sedation)

- There are six major types of aspiration events (Table 11.1)

- Microaspiration of oral contents occurs nightly in individuals, followed by cough and little else

- All typical pneumonias occur when individuals experience a microaspiration event (oral contents) at a time when they are also asymptomatically carrying a pathogenic organism in their oral pharynx (eg, *Streptococcus pneumoniae*)
  - Often occurs in the setting of impaired host defenses (eg, postviral period, sleep deprivation, stress)
  - This is unlike many **atypical pneumonias**, which are **inhaled** (eg, tuberculosis [TB], legionella, fungal)

Table 11.1 Major Types of Aspiration Events

TYPE OF ASPIRATION EVENT	TYPE OF INDIVIDUAL	ASSOCIATED CLINICAL SYNDROMES	REMEDY
Microaspiration (− pathogen)	Everybody	None	None
Microaspiration (+ pathogen)	Everybody	Typical pneumonia (predisposed)	Antibiotics
Macroaspiration (oral secretions)	Alcohol and/or sedative use; often with poor dentition (increases oral bacteria load)	Oral anaerobic lung infection Spillage of oral secretions into preexisting parenchymal cavity Pneumonia Lung abscess Empyema	Antibiotics vs observation Antibiotics Prolonged antibiotics Drainage and antibiotics
Food aspiration	Impaired swallowing as seen: After stroke After therapy for head and neck cancer Bulbar presentations of neuromuscular disease	Atelectasis and/or airway impaction with food Oral anaerobic lung infection Pneumonia Lung abscess Empyema	Bronchoscopy followed by speech and swallow evaluation and a modified diet Antibiotics Prolonged antibiotics Drainage and antibiotics
Gastric aspiration (large volume, aspiration of emesis)	Obtunded (often from general anesthesia or narcotics)	Aspiration pneumonitis Pneumonia/ARDS	Observation Antibiotics Lung protective ventilation
Gastroesophageal reflux (recurrent reflux and aspiration of gastric contents while sleeping)	Individuals with GERD	Basilar fibrotic changes	Gastroesophageal reflux treatment

ARDS, adult respiratory distress syndrome; *GERD*, gastroesophageal reflux disease

- Food aspiration occurs in patients with impaired swallowing and leads to food impaction with associated postobstructive pneumonia, lung abscess, and/or empyema
  - Impacted food may have to be mechanically removed via bronchoscopy, in addition to treatment with antibiotics covering oral anaerobes

- Gastric aspiration occurs when patients are sedated and experience a large volume emesis of gastric contents/secretions
  - Causes instantaneous chemical injury (pneumonitis) with varying degrees of food-particle impaction, depending on how recently the patient ate
    - Bronchoscopy is only useful for removing large particulate matter
      - Lavage right after gastric aspiration does not mitigate the instantaneous alveolar chemical injury seen with gastric aspiration
  - may progress to ARDS
  - To minimize risk, patients are made nil per os (NPO) for several hours before sedation

- Gastroesophageal reflux disease with recurrent nocturnal aspiration may lead to basilar fibrotic changes (misconstrued or concerning for pulmonary fibrosis)
  - Gastric aspiration is often clinically silent and may need a pH probe study to confirm
  - Interventions include acid suppression, elevation of the head of the bed, and promotility agents (ie, metoclopramide)

ORAL ANAEROBIC LUNG INFECTION

- Spectrum of lung infections caused by **macro**aspiration of bacteria-rich oral secretions, often occurring during sedated sleep
- Causes four distinct clinical/radiographic syndromes (existing on a spectrum)
  1. **Aspiration pneumonia** (Fig. 11.1)
     - Subacute presentation (eg, days of coughing with low-grade fevers), nontoxic appearing, and an often normal or only slight elevated white blood cell (WBC) count
     - Chest x-ray film typically shows patchy, basilar, nodular, and round opacities, often with an effusion
       - May have small areas of necrosis
     - Sputum Gram stain and culture typically show polymorphonuclear leukocytes (PMNs) and "normal oral flora" only (eg, culture negative)
  2. **Lung abscess** (cavitary [necrotizing] parenchymal lung lesion with an air-fluid level)
  3. **Empyema** (complicated parapneumonic effusion)
     - Often with air and pus in the pleural space (ie, hydropneumothorax)
     - May only have small areas of parenchymal consolidation/pneumonia (dominant feature/process is the effusion)
  4. **Accumulation/spillage** into areas of **preexisting parenchymal abnormality** appearing as **"pseudonecrosis"**

Aspiration Pneumonia

Subacute presentation with low grade fever, productive cough, and a normal WBC count
Chest x-ray shows left lower lobe patchy, nodular, round, opacities, and a small effusion

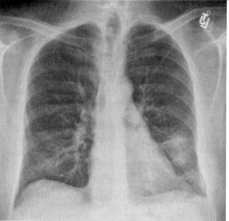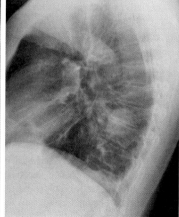

Fig. 11.1 Posterioranterior (PA) and lateral chest x-ray films of a patient who was recently started on narcotics because of a wrist fracture and presented with a week of low-grade fevers and productive coughing. The frontal view shows nodular, patchy opacities in the left lower lobe. The lateral film shows a dominant round lesion and a blunted costophrenic angle (CPA) suggesting effusion.

- Associated with **poor oral hygiene, central sedation** (alcohol or sedatives), and sleep
- Fever and productive cough are **not** typical presenting features of **lung abscess** and **empyema**
  - Spectrum of chief complaints associated with radiographic presentation (Fig. 11.2):
    - **Asymptomatic**: seen with spillage of oral contents into areas of preexisting parenchymal abnormality
    - **Malaise**: weight loss, fatigue, and night sweats are seen with lung abscess
    - **Chest pain**: seen with early empyema presentation (as the infection penetrates the pleural cavity)
    - **Shortness of breath**: seen with late empyema presentation (as the effusion causes whole lung atelectasis)

Chief Complaint Based on Presentation

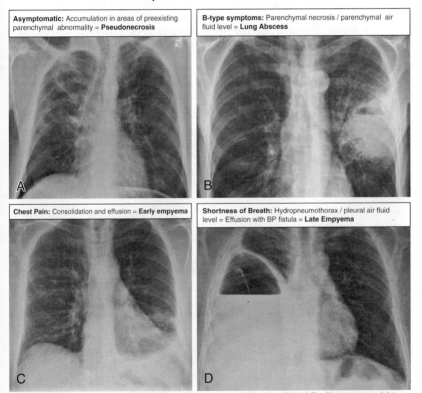

Asymptomatic: Accumulation in areas of preexisting parenchymal abnormality = **Pseudonecrosis**

B-type symptoms: Parenchymal necrosis / parenchymal air fluid level = **Lung Abscess**

Chest Pain: Consolidation and effusion = **Early empyema**

Shortness of Breath: Hydropneumothorax / pleural air fluid level = Effusion with BP fistula = **Late Empyema**

Fig. 11.2 (A)Chest x-ray obtained for preoperative clearance in an asymptomatic individual. The film suggests a right apical nodular cavitary process. This opacity actually represents a preexisting emphysematous area with superimposed oral aspiration (a.k.a. pseudonecrosis). (B) Chest x-ray with a large, dense, well-circumscribed, round opacity with necrosis evidenced by an air-fluid level (straight line in the cavity) demonstrating the classic appearance of a lung abscess. The patient presented with a chief complaint of weight loss (no pulmonary complaints and normal white blood cell count) and was admitted with the diagnosis of "failure to thrive" before the chest x-ray resulted. (C) Chest x-ray of a patient who presented with sudden onset severe left-sided chest pain (woke him from sleep). He denied cough or fevers. The film shows a patchy left lower lobe consolidation with an effusion; constellation most commonly representing pneumonia and parapneumonic effusion. Chest pain in this scenario (pleural in origin) likely represents pleural spread of infection. (D) Chest x-ray of an individual presenting with shortness of breath, demonstrating a large right-sided hydropneumothorax. This constellation of findings occurring spontaneously (ie, **not** after a thoracentesis) is seen when both a pleural effusion and a BF fistula are present (the amount of air is too much to be attributed to gas-forming organisms) and is most commonly seen in empyema. The patient required urgent chest tube placement to prevent "tension physiology"

- Clinical radiographic disconnect is common, often with a muted clinical presentation:
  - Imaging looks terrible patient looks good
  - Normal or slightly elevated WBC count and afebrile
    - Late empyema (as in Fig. 11.1) typically has abscess-level WBC count (eg, 20,000–30,000)
- Differential diagnosis (things that cause necrotic pulmonary masses):
  - **Lung cancer**, especially squamous cell carcinoma, given its proclivity for necrosis
    - Establishing growth characteristics with previous imaging is invaluable for distinguishing oral anaerobic lung infection (disease of weeks to months) from non-small-cell lung cancer (disease of years) (Fig. 11.3)
  - **Typical necrotizing pneumonia** (eg, staph or aerobic GNR) (Fig. 11.4)
    - Has classic pneumonia presentation (acute onset fever, high WBC count, and dramatic productive cough), **unlike** oral anaerobic lung infection
  - Reactivation tuberculosis (TB)
    - TB always needs to be considered with cavitary nodular lung disease especially in individuals with sub-acute cough, wt loss and or night sweats
      - History (TB exposure/purified protein derivative [PPD]) and imaging (fibronodular opacity in the apical posterior segments) may significantly heighten or lessen the concern for TB
      - Low threshold for respiratory isolation, sputum examination for acid-fast bacilli (AFB), and quantiferon testing

Growth Characteristics Differentiate Lung Abscess from Lung Cancer

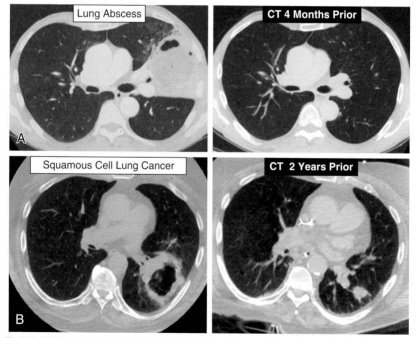

Fig. 11.3 (A) A chest computed tomography (CT) scan with a large left upper lobe lung abscess. A baseline CT scan of the patient's chest obtained 4 months prior is without abnormality. These growth characteristics are *almost* incompatible with malignancy. (B) A chest CT scan with a large left lower lobe cavitary mass. A CT scan of the chest 2 years prior shows a spiculated lung nodule. A thick-walled cavity evolving from a spiculated nodule over 2 years represents the natural history of squamous cell carcinoma. Given that lung abscess and lung cancer may have identical clinical radiographic presentations, growth characteristics (if previous imaging is available) are critical.

Typical Necrotizing or Cavitary Pneumonia

> X-ray shows left mid lung zone opacity with central lucency, suggesting necrosis
> "Typical" pneumonia presentation, suggests infection with typical organisms associated with
> necrotizing pneumonia (eg, Staph, Klebsiella). Patient diagnosed with
> Staph Pneumonia (post influenza).

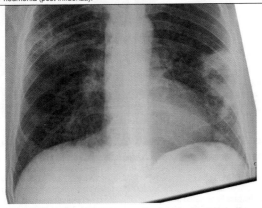

Fig. 11.4 Lung cavitation occurring with acute fever, cough, and leukocytosis suggests typical necrotizing bacterial pneumonia and should prompt empiric antibiotic coverage aimed at Staphylococcus and Klebsiella (and other Gram-negative rods [GNRs]). Acute presentations with high fever and dramatic cough are not common with oral anaerobic lung infection.

- Pseudonecrosis
  - Occurs when aspirated oral contents and subsequent anaerobic infected material accumulate in areas of preexisting parenchymal abnormality (eg, emphysema), leading to the appearance of a necrotic pneumonia (ie, a consolidation with lots of holes and small air-fluid levels)
    - Actually preexisting emphysematous holes
    - Typically asymptomatic
  - Diagnosis hinges on the presence of old imaging demonstrating that the areas appearing as necrosis on the current film actually represent preexisting holes
  - Differential diagnosis (DDx): Includes entities that cause asymptomatic, dense consolidations in patients with parenchymal lung disease:
    - Chronic necrotizing aspergillosis, reactivation TB, lung cancer, and cryptogenic organizing pneumonia (COP)
  - Treatment is he same as it is for lung abscess (ie, oral anaerobic coverage until radiographic resolution)
- c–ANCA vasculitis (rare)
  - Associated pathology (eg, sinus disease, glomerulonephritis, mononeuritis multiplex) raises suspicion
- Necrotizing sarcoidosis (rare)
  - Multiple lesions, no response to antibiotics

INFECTED BULLAE (A.K.A. "BULLAETIS"): A LUNG ABSCESS MIMIC

- Similar to pseudonecrosis (previously described), occurs when a preexisting cavity or bullae fills with oral secretions and/or phlegm; much less morbid than a lung abscess
  - Indolent and less responsive to antibiotics; do not treat in the absence of symptoms
  - Diagnosis made by old imaging, demonstrating the preexisting cavity (Fig. 11.5)

Infected Bullae a.k.a BULLAETIS

| CT Scan showing R basilar air fluid level | CT Scan 4 m prior showing preexisting bullae |

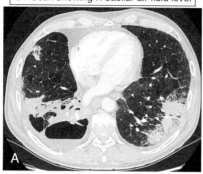 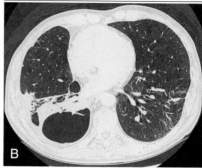

Fig. 11.5 Presenting computed tomography (CT) scan showing large, right base air-fluid level with adjacent consolidation, demonstrating bronchiectasis and possible cavitation. The fluid collection appears to be pleural based (a.k.a. hydropneumothorax [ie, exudative effusion with BP fistula]), which would require drainage. Additionally, the left base has a dense, peripheral consolidation with the appearance of multiple small cavities (peripheral holes). A CT scan 4 months prior clarifies the case by revealing that the fluid collection is **not** pleural based but rather occurring inside a preexisting basilar bullae (a.k.a. bullaetis). This process must **not** be drained. Drainage is unnecessary and risks the creation of a persistent/infected BP fistula. The left base cavitary consolidation, suggested on the presenting CT scan, is actually a dense consolidation occurring in an area of preexisting small holes (pseudonecrosis).

DISTINGUISHING A LUNG ABSCESS (DO NOT DRAIN) FROM AN EMPYEMA (MUST DRAIN)

- If the infected collection/air-fluid level is located in the **parenchyma**, it is a **lung abscess**
  - **Lung abscesses** require prolonged antibiotics until necrosis (air-fluid level) resolves (often >6 weeks)
  - Must **not** drain a lung abscess, given the risk of creating an empyema (via spillage) and/or an infected bronchopleural (BP) fistula (given that the needle tract passes through infected lung)

- If the infected collection/air-fluid level is located in the **pleura**, it is an **empyema**
  - **Empyemas** require drainage to obtain source control and to ensure that the effusion does not progress, leading to rapid lung collapse and ultimately impaired venous return (ie, tension physiology)

- A CT scan, ideally with IV contrast for pleural enhancement (though **not** required), is helpful in separating parenchymal collection from pleural collection, and is better for defining the space in preparation for chest tube placement (Fig. 11.6)

LUNG ABSCESSES

- Present indolently with night sweats and weight loss

- Cough and fever may be minimal or absent
  - Acute presentation suggests "typical" necrotizing pneumonia (eg, staph or aerobic Gram-negative rods [GNR])

- Signs and symptoms:
  - WBC count may be normal or only slightly elevated
  - Patients occasionally report, and demonstrate, halitosis
  - Classically (but infrequently) patients recall nocturnal episodes of sudden awakening with dramatic coughing

- DDx: non-small-cell lung cancer (especially squamous cell carcinoma), reactivation TB, infected bullae, c-ANCA vasculitis, and necrotizing sarcoidosis

Differentiating lung abscess from Empyema

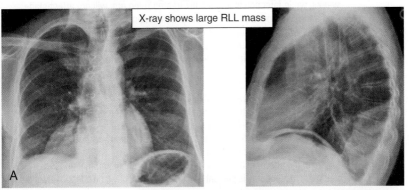

X-ray shows large RLL mass

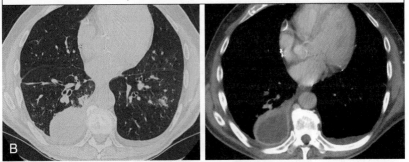

CT shows fluid collection is pleural based (effusion), and likely exudative (spilt pleura sign)

Fig. 11.6 (A) Posteroanterior and lateral chest x-ray films. The frontal view shows a large, well-circumscribed right lower lobe mass with effusion (blunting of the right costophrenic angle [CPA]). The lateral view also suggests mass and loculated effusion. (B) Simultaneous chest computed tomography (CT) scan with contrast, revealing that the opacity is actually entirely pleural based (ie, an exudative pleural effusion). The appearance is exudative because of the bowing "under pressure look" of the visceral pleura together with the "split pleura sign" (visceral and parietal pleural enhancement). The CT scan fails to show any associated parenchymal abnormality (eg, pneumonia or mass). A paucity of parenchymal findings is common in oral anaerobic empyemas, unlike malignancy or an empyema associated with a typical pneumonia. This collection (like most exudative effusions) required complete drainage, with a chest tube.

- Workup involves **ruling out infectious tuberculosis** and **worrying about malignancy**
  - Ruling out infectious (reactivation) tuberculosis:
    - Patients with a productive cough (not typical in lung abscess) should have TB ruled out by having three sputum specimens screened for AFB
    - Negative quantiferon testing is also very reassuring
    - Patients with significant TB risk factors and/or concerning imaging (eg, apical/ posterior upper lobe lesions) or a positive quantiferon, who do not produce adequate sputum specimens for AFB inspection, should have bronchoscopy considered as part of the initial evaluation (obtaining a bronchoalveolar lavage [BAL] with polymerase chain reaction [PCR] testing for TB)
  - Worrying about malignancy:
    - A lung abscess and lung cancer may have nearly identical clinical radiographic presentations
      - The diagnosis of lung cancer should **not** be pursued while active infection is (or might be) present, because it is:
        - **Confounding**: infection causes "atypical cells" and FDG avid opacities
        - **Potentially morbid**: BAL during active (untreated) bacterial infection may lead to endobronchial spread of infection

- **Unnecessary**: delaying the diagnosis of non-small-cell lung cancer by a few weeks, while infection is empirically treated/ruled out, will not affect stage
- Early diagnostic procedures aimed at ruling out cancer should be reserved for patients with very ominous imaging (eg, mass-like malignant adenopathy suggestive of small-cell lung cancer)
- Patients should be empirically treated with antibiotics and followed closely for a response
  - PA and lateral chest x-rays should be obtained, and patients should be evaluated every 1–2 weeks (initially)
- Failure of empiric antibiotics to shrink the lesion should prompt further workup:
  - Fungal serology and c-ANCA should be checked
  - Bronchoscopy (with BAL) looking for nocardia, actinomyces, coccidioides, and tuberculosis should be pursued
  - Failure of the above measures to yield a diagnosis should prompt an EBUS if pathologic adenopathy is present or a lung/lesion biopsy if no adenopathy is present

- Drainage/aspiration contraindicated
  - Lung abscesses should **not** be drained
    - Needle aspiration is often complicated by the development of an infected bronchopleural fistula with empyema (Fig. 11.7)
  - Lung abscesses need not be drained
    - The compliance of the lung is so great that the accumulation of puss does not increase local tissue pressure significantly, such that blood flow and antibiotic penetration continue despite the collection (not true of soft tissue collections)

Do Not Aspirate a Lung Abscess

IR guided biopsy of a cavitary LUL lesion, (thought to be malignant), yields inflammatory cells and debris.

Lesion was actually a focus of cavitary pseudomonas pneumonia.

A

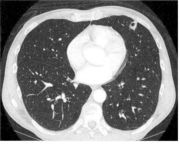
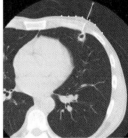

Patient Admitted 2 days later with pseudomonal empyema and BP fistula

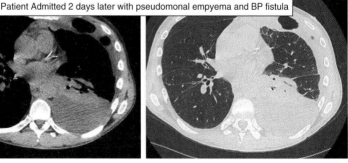

B

Fig. 11.7 (A) A chest computed tomography scan of an immunosuppressed patient, demonstrating a left upper lobe cavitary nodular consolidation. The leading diagnosis was cavitary intrapulmonary lymphoma, prompting a biopsy. Unfortunately the lesion actually represented a small focus of cavitary pseudomonal pneumonia and the inadvertent aspiration was complicated by spillage of infected material into the pleural space, resulting in an empyema. The significant amount of pleural air (seen anteriorly) was not present immediately after the biopsy and implies the presence of a BP fistula (B). Though not truly a lung abscess, this case illustrates the dangers of aspirating infected parenchymal lung collections.

- Additionally, airways may assist in puss drainage
- **Treat with ampicillin combined with sulbactam, start IV, and transition to PO (eg, unasyn to augmentin)**
  - Treat for a prolonged course until radiographic resolution of air-fluid level, 3 weeks to 3 months (Fig. 11.8)
- **Always cover oral anaerobes in addition to other dominant pathogens recovered (eg, *S. Pneumoniae* or MRSA)**
  - Second-line agents include clindamycin, respiratory quinolones, metronidazole (in combination with an additional antistrep pneumonia agent), or macrolides
- **<1% of lung abscess fail antibiotic therapy and require surgical intervention**

Lung Abscess at the Onset and End of Antibiotic Therapy

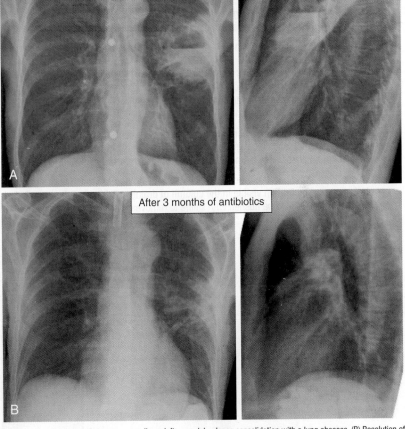

Hospital Discharge

After 3 months of antibiotics

Fig. 11.8 (A) A discharge chest x-ray revealing a left upper lobe dense consolidation with a lung abscess. (B) Resolution of the air-fluid level/cavity after 3 months of antibiotics. The remaining opacity likely represents pleural-based scarring and resolving infiltrate. Imaging to resolution should be pursued. If a residual opacity remains, a CT scan should be obtained for better characterization (to rule out underlying lung cancer). This is true of all pneumonias.

EMPYEMA AND COMPLICATED PARAPNEUMONIC EFFUSIONS

- Empyemas and complicated parapneumonic effusions must be drained to achieve sterility of the pleural space, ensuring that:
  - The patient will defervesce
  - The pleural space is stabilized (ie, the effusion will not progress and cause lung collapse and tension physiology)
  - Optimal healing and aeration will occur, avoiding significant trapped lung and restriction after the infection resolves

- Spectrum of acute presentations:
  - **Early: chest pain** (with pleural invasion of infection)
    - WBC often normal or mildly elevated
  - **Late: shortness of breath** from complete lung atelectasis
    - Often with mediastinal shift and decreased venous return physiology
    - WBC count may be at abscess level (ie, 20,000–30,000)

- If the parapneumonic effusion is too small to drain safely on initial evaluation, observe closely (ie, repeat chest x-ray in 12 to 24 hours)
  - If it is an empyema or a complicated parapneumonic effusion, it will grow, often quickly (Fig. 11.9)

- Hydropneumothorax common (Fig. 11.10):
  - DDx being bronchopleural fistula (lots of air) vs gas-forming organism (few bubbles)

- Preferred method of drainage is a Seldinger technique placed chest tube (12–14 F) via ultrasound guidance
  - Preferred location for insertion is in the "trial angle of safety", midaxillary line at the level of the nipple (5th intercostal space) between the latissimus dorsi and the pectoralis major
  - CT scanning is helpful in defining complex pleural anatomy (eg, adherent lung)
  - May require IR help for difficult locations

- Small-bore chest tubes are vulnerable to occlusion with thick fibrinous material
  - Continuous suction should be applied when initial drainage slows (assuming the postplacement chest x-ray did not reveal a hydropneumothorax; CH 17)

- When drainage stops **and** the tube fails to tidal (ie, fails to demonstrate respiratory-cycle pleural pressure fluctuation visible in the column of draining fluid), the tube is occluded
  - Occluded tubes should be flushed with saline to remove obstructing material via the inline three-way stopcock

Empyema Progresses from Too Small to Tap to Moderate Sized in Hours

Admission chest x-ray: Left lower lobe PNA and a small pleural effusion.	Follow up chest x-ray the next morning showing dramatic increase in the size of the pleural effusion.
Ultrasound exam: Effusion too small to tap	Effusion now drainable.

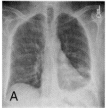 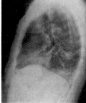 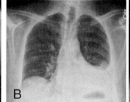 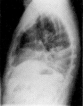

Fig. 11.9 (A) Admission chest x-ray of a patient presenting with left lower lobe pneumonia and a small parapneumonic effusion. Ultrasound examination revealed a small amount of fluid (too small to tap safely). (B) Follow-up chest x-ray ~15 hours later showing a dramatic increase in the size of the effusion, now amenable to safe drainage.

Empyema with Hydropneumothorax

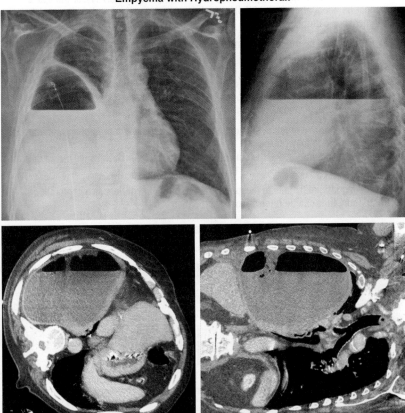

Fig. 11.10 Posteroanterior and lateral chest x-ray films show a large hydropneumothorax in a patient presenting with shortness of breath and a white blood cell count of ~25,000. A computed tomography scan (and ultrasound) reveals adherent lung near the inferior border of the triangle of safety. Lacerating or tearing adherent lung during chest tube placement may create an even larger BP fistula. Atelectatic lung can be seen as a dense, band-like consolidation medially and laterally.

- First the drainage portion of the system (stopcock to pleurovac) should be flushed with saline
- Then a syringe should be placed in line with the chest tube, and aspiration should be attempted
- Finally, sterile saline may be flushed into the thorax in an attempt to open occluded drainage holes
- Tube occlusion should prompt more frequent tissue plasminogen activator (tPA) use or more frequent tube flushing

- Intermittent tPA is very helpful after initial drainage stops **and** residual fluid remains
  - **Even** if it appears to be loculated far away from the chest tube (ie, apical collection/basilar tube)
  - Some advocate standing tPA orders:
    - tPA 7–10 mg (±DNase), dwell × 1 hour, BID for 3 days
  - tPA should be used more cautiously in patients requiring anticoagulation, because there is an incidence of hemothorax in this group

- If the pleura fail to oppose (ie, the lung fails to reexpand; see CH 17), or the space cannot be adequately drained (failure to defervesce), consider early video-assisted thoracoscopic surgery (VATS)

- Patients should be treated with antibiotics active against oral anaerobes (first line is ampicillin or sulbactam)
  - Patients should receive 14 days of antibiotics, starting from the point that their pleural space is completely drained (ie, **after** the chest tube is removed)
  - Pleural fluid culture results are often negative
    - *S. Milleri* is the most commonly recovered organism

- After all the fluid is drained, the lung will often suffer some degree of entrapment, requiring time to fully reexpand
  - Persistent volume loss at the time of discharge is common as inflamed pleura takes time to fully reexpand (Fig. 11.11)

- If the lung ultimately fails to reexpand **and** the patient experiences symptomatic restriction, they can be referred for decortication

Empyema Requiring Early Decortication

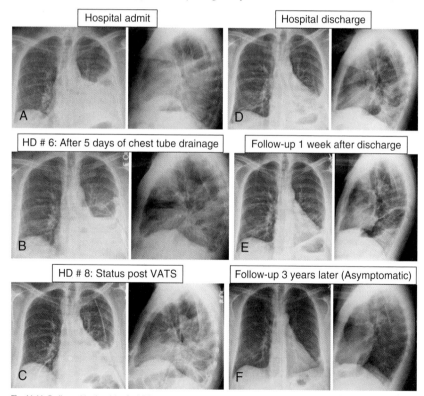

Fig. 11.11 Radiographic chronicle of a left lung empyema, culture negative, presumed secondary to oral anaerobes. (A) Large, left-sided pleural effusion. (B) Chest x-ray despite 5 days of chest tube drainage demonstrates failure, evident by the persistent air-fluid level without an air leak (failure of the lung to reexpand, ie, entrapped lung) and failure to defervesce, prompting video-assisted thoracoscopic surgery (VATS). (C) Post-VATS chest x-ray film showing two new chest tubes (apical and basilar). The lung is better expanded (no air-fluid level) but still demonstrates significant left lower lobe (LLL) consolidation with volume loss. The patient defervesces. (D) Discharge imaging with persistent but improved LLL consolidation and volume loss. (E) Imaging at 1 week after discharge. The patient complains of improving but persistent intermittent pleuritic chest pain. (F) Imaging 3 years later (patient asymptotic) shows, LLL pleural-based scarring causing lateral tenting and elevation of the left hemidiaphragm.

COMMON QUESTIONS GENERATED BY THIS TEACHING

1. How can I be sure that a necrotic pulmonary mass is really an abscess and not lung cancer?
   If growth characteristics are not definitive, you cannot be sure on presentation. Failure to respond to antibiotic therapy should prompt aggressive workup, including biopsy.

2. What should I do when the chest tube stops draining, despite tPA and flushing, and the CT scan suggests lung entrapment with a small residual collection?
   Most of the time, at this point, the chest tube should be removed and the patient should be followed closely with PA and lateral chest x-ray (at 2–3 days initially) to screen for reaccumulation.

CHAPTER 12

COUGH

COMMON MISCONCEPTIONS AND MISTAKES

- Evaluating and treating a chronic purulent cough in the same fashion as a chronic dry cough
- Failing to obtain chest imaging in individuals complaining of a subacute and/or chronic cough
- Abandoning a diagnosis of the upper airway cough syndrome before maximally and simultaneously treating all of its components
- Prematurely diagnosing a chronic chough as psychogenic
- Believing that bronchoscopy is an important, early part of the evaluation of chronic cough

THE COUGH REFLEX ARC

- A cough starts with the stimulation of irritant receptors located in the mucosa of the posterior oral pharynx, vocal cords, trachea, and airways
- Irritant receptors are activated by mechanical, thermal, chemical, and pH stress disturbance, such that the presence of any foreign material or fluid triggers a cough
- Afferent nerve impulses travel to the medulla, where efferent impulses are generated, producing a stereotyped sequence of events collectively known as a cough
  - Inspiration, glottic closure, diaphragmatic relaxation, and forceful expiratory muscle contraction (raising intrapleural pressure transiently to 300 mm Hg) is followed by sudden glottic opening
  - The explosive release of this high transpulmonary pressure gradient leads to high-velocity airflow, which is designed to expel foreign material from the airways

Acute Cough (<3 weeks) in Individuals with No Significant Comorbidities (Fig. 12.1)

- Most commonly from bronchitis (viral more so than bacterial)
  - Should be self-limited
- Cough may be dry **or** purulent
  - Purulent cough is more common in bacterial bronchitis
- **Chest pain, shortness of breath, frank hemoptysis** (blood without sputum), and/or high fever are **not** anticipated with bronchitis and should prompt a **chest x-ray** looking for typical or atypical pneumonia (eg, tuberculosis [TB]) and/or other pathology (eg, lung cancer, effusion, pneumothorax)
  - If chest imaging is normal and a workup fails to reveal an alternate explanation, these individuals typically deserve antibiotics, given the chance that early pneumonia may explain their additional symptoms (despite a clear chest x-ray)
- Cough may be associated with significant morbidity by causing:
  - Disturbed sleep
  - Work absence
  - Persistent blood-tinged sputum (from upper airway/large airway mucosal inflammation)
  - Posttussive emesis

ACUTE COUGH LASTING LESS THAN 3 WEEKS
NO SIGNIFICANT LUNG DISEASE OR IMMUNOSUPPRESSION

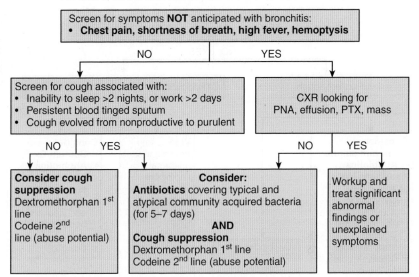

Fig. 12.1 Flow diagram outlining the evaluation and treatment of acute cough occurring in individuals without underlying lung disease or immunosuppression. The majority of healthy individuals with acute cough do not need antibiotics. Antibiotics should only be considered in those who have symptoms concerning for early pneumonia or those whose cough has persisted/worsened, leading to days of missed sleep or work.

- Incontinence
- Rib fracture
- Syncope
- Cough suppression should be offered to those whose cough is bothersome (most individuals who seek medical attention)
  - Dextromethorphan is first line because of its safety profile
  - Codeine has better efficacy and should be used for dextromethorphan failures
- Antibiotics typically are **not** indicated for healthy individuals with acute cough **but** should be considered in individuals whose cough has:
  - Caused persistent blood-tinged sputum
  - Prevented sleep or work for more than 2 days
  - Evolved from being nonproductive to purulent after several days (concerning for postviral bacterial superinfection)
- If antibiotics are used, they should cover atypical and typical community-acquired bacterial pathogens (eg, doxycycline, azithromycin)
- Individuals with recurrent posttussive emesis deserve consideration for pertussis infection and a course of macrolide antibiotics

Acute Cough (<3 weeks) in Individuals with Lung Disease or Immunosuppression (Fig. 12.2)

- Individuals with lung disease or immunosuppression are at increased risk for:
  - Pneumonia caused by typical bacteria, atypical bacteria, and fungal organisms
  - Pneumonia with muted clinical signs (eg, dry cough, afebrile)
  - Progression from bronchitis to pneumonia
  - Rapid clinical deterioration, given little pulmonary and/or immunologic reserve

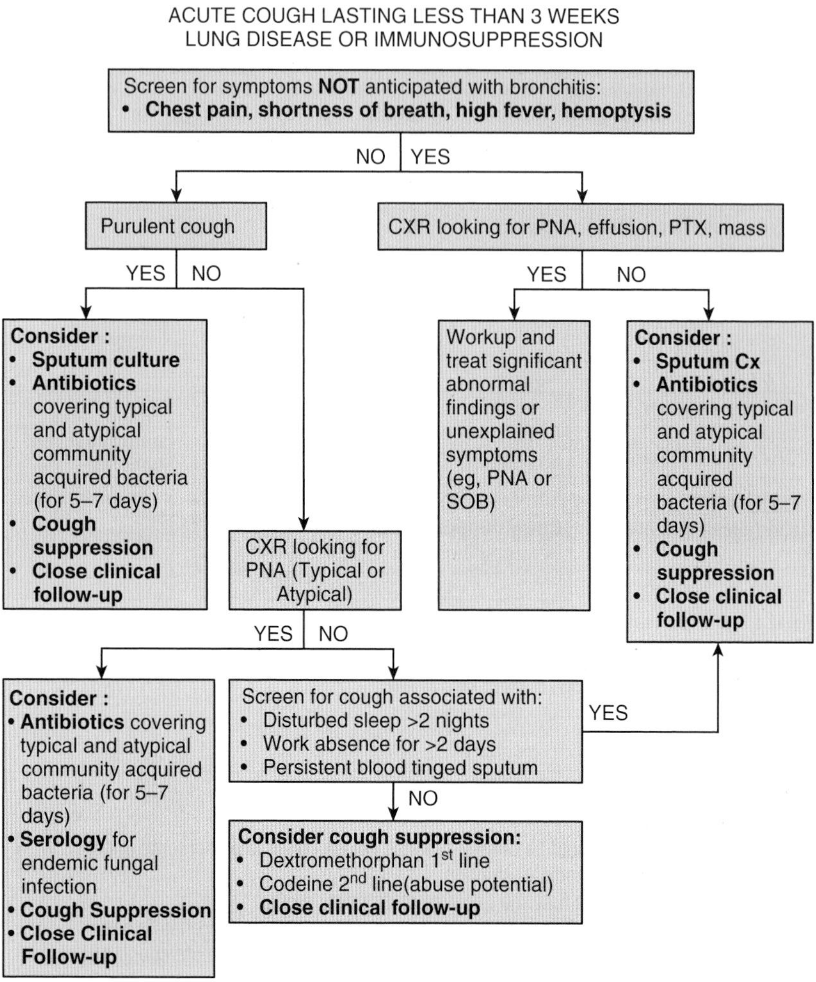

ACUTE COUGH LASTING LESS THAN 3 WEEKS
LUNG DISEASE OR IMMUNOSUPPRESSION

Fig. 12.2 Flow diagram outlining the evaluation and treatment of an acute cough occurring in individuals with underlying lung disease or immunosuppression. These individuals are much more vulnerable to bacterial infection and often require empiric antibiotics for a purulent cough. A dry cough occurring as part of an upper respiratory viral syndrome (or a resolving cough) may be observed as long as a chest x-ray is obtained and fails to show a new infiltrate.

- Chest pain, shortness of breath, significant hemoptysis, and/or high fever are **not** anticipated with bronchitis and should prompt a **chest x-ray** looking for typical or atypical pneumonia (eg, TB) and/or other pathology (eg, lung cancer, effusion, pneumothorax)
  - If chest imaging is normal and a workup fails to reveal an alternate explanation, these individuals typically deserve antibiotics, given a concern for early pneumonia
- There is a low threshold to obtain a sputum culture and prescribe empiric antibiotic therapy in individuals with lung disease or immunosuppression who have a purulent cough
  - An x-ray may be unnecessary if the decision to give antibiotics has been made
  - Empiric antibiotics should cover typical and atypical community-acquired bacteria (eg, respiratory quinolones or azithromycin)

- Antibiotics should also be considered in individuals whose dry cough has caused persistent blood-tinged sputum or prevented sleep or work for more than 2 days
- Cough suppression should be offered to all individuals whose cough has been disruptive
- Patients with lung disease or immunosuppression who do not appear to need empiric antibiotic therapy (eg, those with a short-duration, dry cough associated with a viral syndrome or a resolving cough) should have an x-ray obtained to ensure they do not have pneumonia (with a muted clinical presentation)
  - These individuals may be managed conservatively (ie, without antibiotics) if their chest x-ray fails to show a new infiltrate
- Close clinical follow-up is warranted in all individuals with immunosuppression or lung disease who are evaluated for acute cough

Subacute Dry Cough (Lasting 3–8 Weeks in the Absence of Radiographic Abnormality) (Fig. 12.3)

- A cough lasting more than 3 weeks should be evaluated with a chest x-ray
  - An opacity discovered in this context should prompt a workup for atypical pneumonia and its mimics (eg, lung cancer, diffuse parenchymal lung disease [DPLD])

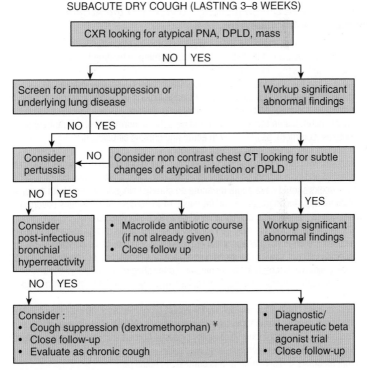

Fig. 12.3 Flow diagram outlining the evaluation and treatment of a subacute dry cough (lasting 3–8 weeks), starting with a chest x-ray looking for atypical pneumonia (eg, mycoplasma, chlamydia, endemic fungus) and its mimics (eg, diffuse parenchymal lung disease [DPLD], lung cancer). Individuals with immunosuppression or underlying lung disease may require a chest computed tomography (CT) scan to rule out more subtle parenchymal changes. Empiric treatment for pertussis and/or postinfectious bronchial hyperreactivity may also be warranted. In the absence of pertussis and postinfectious bronchial hyperreactivity, a subacute dry cough may be observed for several weeks or evaluated as chronic cough.

- There is a low threshold to obtain a noncontrast chest computed tomography (CT) scan in individuals with immunosuppression or underlying lung disease looking for subtle changes related to atypical pneumonia or diffuse parenchymal lung disease
- Subacute cough is typically dry (or occasionally productive of white sputum)
- Most commonly postinfectious, occurring after upper or lower respiratory tract infections
  - Often secondary to viral, mycoplasma, chlamydia, or pertussis infection
- A course of macrolide antibiotics is typically warranted for a subacute cough (despite little data supporting pertussis treatment after 2 weeks)
- Cough suppression with dextromethorphan should also be considered
  - Codeine should not be used for a subacute or chronic cough, given its potential for addiction and abuse
- May represent postinfectious bronchial hyperreactivity (formerly known as postinfectious reactive airway disease)
  - Consider diagnostic/therapeutic β-agonist trial (works faster than inhaled corticosteroid)
- Ultimately, a subacute cough should be self-limited
  - Patients without relief from this approach may be observed for weeks **or** evaluated as having a chronic cough (see next section)

Subacute Purulent Cough (Lasting >3 Weeks in the Absence of Radiographic Abnormality) (Fig. 12.4)

- A purulent cough lasting more than 3 weeks should be evaluated with a chest x-ray
  - An opacity discovered in this context should prompt a workup for atypical pneumonia and its mimics (eg, lung cancer, DPLD)
- There is a low threshold to obtain a noncontrast chest CT scan in individuals with immunosuppression or underlying lung disease looking for subtle changes related to atypical pneumonia or diffuse parenchymal lung disease
- Purulent secretions (in the absence of radiographic abnormality) originate in either the:
  - Sinuses (common), as occurs with acute and chronic sinusitis, or
  - Bronchiectatic lower airways (less common)
- Individuals with sinus symptoms (nasal congestion, nasal discharge, sinus tenderness, headache) and/or a history of chronic sinusitis who have a productive cough lasting more than 3 weeks should have acute (or acute on chronic) sinusitis treated with nasal steroids, antihistamines, decongestants, and (at least) 14 to 30 days of antibiotics covering oral anaerobes (eg, amoxicillin/clavulanic acid or a respiratory quinolone)
  - Six weeks of antibiotics may be required in severe cases and/or in cases in which the sinuses are anatomically abnormal (eg, deviated septum, nasal polyps)
- Individuals without sinus disease who complain of a productive cough lasting more than 3 weeks deserve a screen for bronchiectasis consisting of a:
  - Sputum culture looking for nontuberculous mycobacteria (NTM) and gram negative rods (GNRs)
  - Noncontrast chest CT scan looking for occult bronchiectasis, as may occur in NTM infection; allergic bronchopulmonary aspergillosis (ABPA); chronic aspiration; or, less commonly, immunoglobulin deficiency or cystic fibrosis transmembrane conductance regulator (CFTR) mutation
- If bronchiectasis is discovered in this context, it should be:
  - Worked up by screening for NTM infection, ABPA, chronic aspiration, immunoglobulin deficiency, or CFTR mutations
  - Treated with pulmonary hygiene (postural drainage/airway clearance devices) and a 14-day course of a respiratory quinolone or amoxicillin/clavulanic acid
    - Ciprofloxacin should be considered if a sensitive pseudomonas is recovered
- In the absence of sinus disease or bronchiectasis (ie, negative sputum cultures and a normal chest CT scan), a productive cough lasting more than 3 weeks may be evaluated and treated as chronic chough (see next section)

SUBACUTE PURULENT COUGH LASTING >3 WEEKS

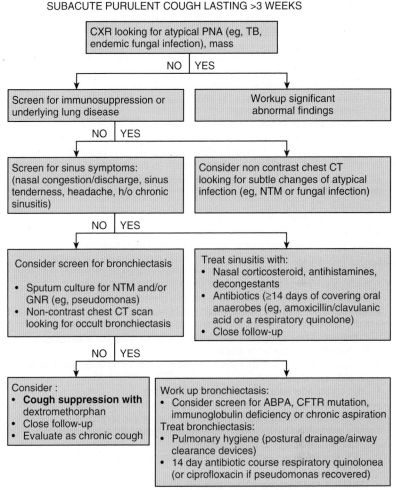

Fig. 12.4 Flow diagram outlining the evaluation and treatment of a subacute purulent cough (lasting >3 weeks), starting with a chest x-ray looking for atypical pneumonia (eg, tuberculosis, endemic fungus) and its mimics (eg, lung cancer). Individuals with underlying lung disease or immunosuppression typically deserve a noncontrast chest computed tomography (CT) scan to rule out subtle parenchymal findings associated with atypical lung infection. In the absence of parenchymal pathology, purulence commonly originates in the sinuses (ie, sinusitis). In the absence of sinus disease, parenchymal abnormality, and/or pathogen recovery (sputum culture), a subacute purulent cough may be observed for several weeks or evaluated as a chronic cough.

Chronic Cough (ie, Nonproductive Cough Lasting More Than 8 Weeks in the Absence of Radiographic Abnormality) (Fig. 12.5)

- Screen for angiotensin-converting-enzyme (ACE) inhibitor therapy or active tobacco use:
  - ACE inhibitor therapy:
    - Approximately 15% of patients taking ACE inhibitors experience an irritant-mediated cough
    - Typically within the first 6 months (but may occur after years of therapy)

- Likely secondary to bradykinin accumulation (also broken down by ACE)
- Patients taking ACE inhibitors complaining of a chronic dry cough should change to an angiotensin receptor blocker (ARB)
- Active smokers:
  - Chronic cough is common among active cigarette smokers; however, the majority do not seek treatment
  - Those who do are typically worried about lung cancer
  - Work up with PFTs, a chest x-ray, and consideration for lung cancer screening in individuals who meet criteria
  - Treat COPD if PFTs show obstruction or mixed disease (ie start inhalers)
  - Smokers also must be repeatedly counseled about smoking cessation, especially during the evaluation of potential COPD and or lung cancer (teachable moment)
- More than 95% of chronic nonproductive chough (in the absence of a radiographic abnormality) is caused by the upper airway cough syndrome (UACS), attributable to (one or more):
- Postnasal drip (PND)
- Cough-variant bronchial hyperreactivity
- Gastroesophageal reflux disease (GERD)
- History and physical screens for obvious GERD and/or PND symptoms
  - Individuals with GERD and chronic cough should receive counseling regarding lifestyle changes (weight loss, head of bed elevation, smoking cessation, and dietary modification) in addition to twice daily proton pump inhibitor therapy
  - A GERD-related cough may take up to 8 weeks to resolve
  - Individuals with PND and chronic cough should receive a diagnostic/therapeutic trial of twice daily nasal steroid (first line) or first-generation antihistamine (second line)
    - Oral leukotriene antagonists and nasal cromolyn are third-line alternatives
    - Cough may take weeks to resolve
- In the absence of GERD or PND, consider cough-variant bronchial hyperreactivity and/or eosinophilic bronchitis
  - Often occurs after an upper respiratory tract infection
  - More likely to occur in individuals with atopy and/or childhood asthma
  - A diagnostic and therapeutic medication trial of an inhaled corticosteroid (ICS) and a short-acting beat agonist (SABA) should be conducted either sequentially or simultaneously (weighing patient preference)
    - ICS: first line, given better efficacy with eosinophilic bronchitis
    - SABA: second line
  - The cough may disappear immediately with a SABA (suggestive of cough-variant postinfectious bronchial hyperreactivity), or it may take days to weeks to resolve with an ICS (suggestive of eosinophilic bronchitis)
- When this approach fails to resolve the cough, consider treating **all** three entities (GERD, PND, and bronchial hyperreactivity) simultaneously
  - Often all three diseases require maximal therapy in order for the chronic cough to resolve
- When combined therapy for PND, GERD, and bronchial hyperreactivity fails, consider:
  - Cough hypersensitivity syndrome (a.k.a. chronic idiopathic cough):
    - Thought to be secondary to an increased sensitivity of mucosal irritant receptors (and their coupled ion channels)
    - No specific therapy exists
    - Individuals may experience relief with:
      - Oral benzonatate pearls
      - Nebulized lidocaine (eg, 3 mL of a 2% solution)
      - Gabapentin (at doses from 300 to 1800 mg daily)

CHRONIC DRY COUGH (LASTING >8 WEEKS) NON-SMOKER, NOT ON
ACE INHIBITOR, NO RADIOGRAPHIC ABNORMALITY ¥

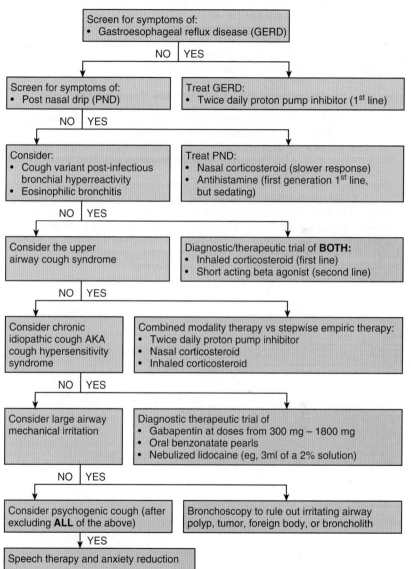

¥ Chest x-ray should have been obtained after 3 weeks of cough

Fig. 12.5 Flow diagram outlining the evaluation and treatment of a chronic dry cough (lasting >8 weeks) in nonsmokers who are not taking an angiotensin converting enzyme (ACE) inhibitor and who have no acute radiographic abnormality seen by chest imaging. Most chronic cough is a result of gastroesophageal reflux disease (GERD), paroxysmal nocturnal dyspnea (PND), bronchial hyperreactivity, or a combination of all three, collectively known as the upper airway cough syndrome (UACS). The diagnosis of UACS is based on medication response and should not be abandoned until an adequate trial (2–3 months) of simultaneous maximal therapy is completed.

- Large airway mechanical irritation from endobronchial pathology (eg, tumor, foreign body, broncholith)
  - Will usually be visible by CT scan (if obtained)
  - Evaluate with bronchoscopy
- After excluding all other causes, consider psychogenic cough
  - The cough behaves like a tic
  - Emotional stress is the predominant cough trigger
  - Speech therapy and anxiety reduction may be of benefit

COMMON QUESTIONS GENERATED BY THIS TEACHING

1. When patients describe a cough as occasionally productive of white sputum, should this be considered a purulent cough from the standpoint of evaluation?
   Patients with a purulent cough produce thick, colored sputum most of the time. A cough, occasionally productive of white sputum, should be considered "dry" from the standpoint of workup and management.
2. When should I perform a bronchoscopy as part of the evaluation of a chronic cough?
   Individuals with chronic cough and normal chest imaging who have failed a combined trial of therapy for GERD, PND, and bronchial hyperreactivity are unlikely to have an irritating airway abnormality as the etiology. However, individuals who associate the onset of their cough with an aspiration event, or those focused on the cough coming from a large airway punctate focus, may obtain reassurance (and subsequent cough relief) after a bronchoscopy is preformed and no abnormality/foreign object is discovered.

COUGH SYNCOPE

CHAPTER 13

COMMON MISCONCEPTIONS AND MISTAKES

- Believing that cough syncope is caused by coughing-induced vagal tone and bradycardia, leading to systemic hypotension and syncope (ie, vasovagal syncope as a result of cough)
- Believing that cough syncope is caused by decreased venous return secondary to the high intrathoracic pressure of forceful coughing, leading to systemic hypotension and syncope

COUGH SYNCOPE

- The most common cause of syncope is cerebral hypoperfusion associated with transient systemic hypotension
- Forceful coughing may transiently decrease blood pressure by either:
  - Causing increased vagal tone with subsequent symptomatic bradycardia, hypotension, and syncope (ie, vasovagal syncope as a result of cough) or
  - Causing increased intrathoracic pressure, with subsequent decreased venous return, reflex tachycardia, hypotension, and syncope
    - Patients with pulmonary hypertension and preexisting right-sided heart failure may be more vulnerable to a sudden decrease in preload, predisposing them to this physiology
- Cough syncope (originally known as laryngeal vertigo) describes a syndrome of syncope occurring with forceful coughing that is **not** associated with systemic hypotension
  - Responsible for approximately 2% of all syncope cases
- **Classic phenotype and presentation**
  - Most commonly affects stocky men (muscular and overweight) with abdominal obesity and chronic obstructive pulmonary disease (COPD)
  - Episodes start with a forceful crescendo of coughing, leading to a transient loss of consciousness (seconds)
  - Syncope occurs **without** systemic hypotension (and/or bradycardia)
    - Often syncope occurs in the setting of tachycardia and hypertension driven by the adrenergic nature of forceful coughing
  - Patients uniformly recall coughing before losing consciousness
    - Often they report prior episodes and/or endorse frequent episodes of presyncope with coughing
  - Over half of individuals experience jerking or rhythmic movements of the limbs with syncope (often erroneously interpreted as seizure activity)

PATHOPHYSIOLOGY OF COUGH SYNCOPE

- Coughing increases intrathoracic pressure, which increases central venous pressure, which increases intracranial venous pressure
- The intracranial veins cannot absorb this pressure with distension (as occurs in other tissues in the body), because the brain is enclosed in the skull and surrounded by a noncompressible fluid

- Therefore a sudden increase in central venous pressure can cause a sudden increase in intracranial pressure (ICP)
- When ICP rises, cerebral perfusion pressure (CPP) drops, decreasing cerebral blood flow (CBF)
  - CPP = mean arterial pressure (MAP) – intracranial pressure (ICP)
  - In normal individuals, CBF flow decreases with forceful coughing, but **never** reaches zero
  - In individuals with cough syncope, forceful coughing leads to transient cessation of cerebral blood flow
    - As ICP exceeds diastolic blood pressure (BP), diastolic flow reversal occurs in the intracranial arteries
      - CBF drops close to zero, and syncope ensues
      - With syncope, coughing stops, intrathoracic pressure falls, ICP falls, perfusion returns, and consciousness is restored

CONDITIONS TO BE EXCLUDED WHEN COUGHING IS ASSOCIATED WITH SYNCOPE

- A standard syncope workup should be pursued because coughing may provoke other causes of syncope
  - Forceful coughing decreases venous return, potentially unmasking preload-dependent states:
    - Pulmonary hypertension and isolated right-sided heart failure (ie, acute and chronic venous thromboembolism)
    - Outflow tract obstruction (eg, hypertrophic obstructive cardiomyopathy [HOCM])
    - Pericardial effusion with tamponade physiology
  - Coughing may precipitate arrhythmia:
    - Coughing (and its active suppression) may increase vagal tone, acting as a Valsalva maneuver and triggering bradycardia and/or heart block
    - Alternatively, coughing paroxysms may be hyperadrenergic, triggering atrial tachyarrhythmias
  - Coughing may increase ICP, unmasking:
    - Baseline elevations of ICP from an intracranial/brainstem mass
    - Significant intracranial arterial stenosis (manifesting as an inability to maintain CPP in the face of a rising ICP)
- Echocardiogram, cardiac monitoring, intracranial imaging, and carotid and vertebral artery Doppler assessments are typically indicated

DIAGNOSIS OF COUGH SYNCOPE

- Diagnosis hinges on demonstrating that the cough-induced loss of consciousness occurs without systemic hypotension
  - Reliable noninvasive BP measurements can be difficult to make during a forceful coughing paroxysm
  - Invasive BP monitoring (eg, an arterial line) may be used in hospitalized patients
- Vasovagal syncope associated with coughing-induced bradycardia (and subsequent hypotension) may be screened for by heart rate monitoring using telemetry for inpatients and event/Holter monitors for outpatients
- Transcranial Doppler studies are not widely available, making the demonstration of diastolic flow reversal during coughing an impractical approach
- Electroencephalogram monitoring is capable of detecting decreased cerebral blood flow by demonstrating characteristic hypoxia-generated wave forms (Fig. 13.1)
- Ruling out hypotension and arrhythmia, together with exclusion of other causes (as previously outlined), may suffice

77 yo male with severe COPD and HTN, presented with 2 days of increased cough and multiple episodes of witnessed syncope (>10), all occurring after coughing paroxysms. LOC lasted seconds and was followed immediately by normal mentation.

- Physical exam notable for bruising, scattered wheezes, and the absence of murmurs, and edema
- CXR hyperinflated / flattened diaphragms
- EKG with P-pulmonale (RA enlargement)
- CTA negative for pulmonary embolism
- Echocardiogram suggested isolated right heart failure (ie, cor pulmonale)
- While on monitor, with an A-line, the pateint had multiple episodes of transient loss of consciousness, **ALL** occurring during forceful coughing
- Episodes were preceded by sinus **tachycardia** and **hypertension**, and were followed by varying degrees of twitching and gaze deviation
  - Raising the concern for seizure
- EEG was obtained during an episode (ruling out seizure), instead suggesting transient hypoxia
- Patient diagnosed with **Cough syncope**
- Cough increases ICP which reduces cerebral perfusion pressure (CPP) and cerebral blood flow (CBF)
- Transient cessation of cerebral blood flow, during forceful coughing causes syncope

COUGH SYNCOPE

Chest x-ray

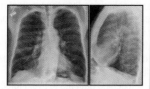

PFTs

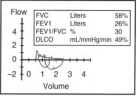

FVC	Liters	58%
FEV1	Liters	26%
FEV1/FVC	%	30
DLCO	mL/mmHg/min	49%

CT angiogram (main PAs)

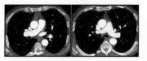

EKG

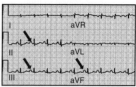

Cardiac echocardiogram

The left ventricular chamber size is normal. There is no left ventricular hypertrophy.
There is normal left ventricular systolic function with no wall motion abnormalities.
The left atrial chamber size is normal.
The right ventricle is mildly dilated. The right ventricular function is hypodynamic.
The right atrium is mildly dilated.
The inferior vena cava appears normal in size. There is a greater than 50% respiratory change in the inferior vena cava dimension. *Poorly defined TR jet. Difficult to accurately assess degree of pulmonary hypertension.*

Neurology consult

During the episodes, there were EEG changes strongly consistent w/hypoxia. Episodic seizure-like events are most likely due to increased ICP causing hypoxia.

Fig. 13.1 Encapsulated case of an individual with severe chronic obstructive pulmonary disease (COPD) presenting with worsening cough and abrupt onset of cough syncope. The patient had evidence of cor pulmonale (isolated right ventricular [RV] failure) based on his severe COPD and an echocardiogram suggesting high right- and low left-sided pressures. Typically, as in this case, the carbon monoxide diffusing capacity (DLCO) lung function test must be reduced to less than 50% predicted (ie, over half of the vasculature lost) to cause pulmonary hypertension at rest. Additionally, his electrocardiogram (ECG) showed the classic P-pulmonale pattern (peaked p waves in II, III, and F) of right atrial enlargement. Because of this, the initial impression was that the patient's cough was increasing intrathoracic pressure high enough to impair venous return, aggravated by preload-dependent physiology from his preexisting right-sided heart failure. Because the patient's lung disease was long-standing and his presentation was acute, a concomitant pulmonary embolism was ruled out. The patient was then admitted to the intensive care unit (ICU) and proceeded to have multiple syncopal events while lying in bed, all occurring after coughing paroxysms, with no evidence of bradycardia or hypotension (by noninvasive blood pressure [BP] measurements obtained as close to loss of consciousness [LOC] as possible). This led to the insertion of an A-line for invasive BP monitoring, which instead revealed mild hypertension at the point of LOC, raising concern for seizure activity instead of syncope. This led to an electroencephalogram (EEG), which instead revealed cerebral hypoxia without systemic hypotension or arterial hypoxemia, only explained by isolated cerebral hypoperfusion occurring in the setting of cough (ie, cough syncope). With treatment of COPD exacerbation, allergic rhinitis, and cough suppression, the patient's cough syncope resolved.

TREATMENT OF COUGH SYNCOPE

- Treatment is aimed at cough reduction and behavior modification
- Reducing cough can be done by optimizing the management of COPD, allergic rhinitis, gastroesophageal reflux disease, and bronchiectasis (when applicable)
  - Cough suppressants may also be used
    - Dextromethorphan (DM) is first line because of its safety profile
    - Codeine has better efficacy, but its abuse potential makes it second line
    - Sedation may be a limiting side effect of both
- Behavior modification involves teaching patients to avoid forceful coughing spells
  - Patients are often able to develop personal strategies to avoid coughing themselves to the point of collapse, and to avoid injury should they start coughing, once the syndrome is explained to them

COMMON QUESTION GENERATED BY THIS TEACHING

1. I had a patient who got a pacemaker placed for cough syncope (question implied by tone). The patient either had vasovagal syncope triggered by coughing or inappropriately received a pacemaker. Many cough syncope patients are offered or receive pacemakers based on the belief that bradycardia must be the culprit.

SARCOIDOSIS

CHAPTER 14

COMMON MISCONCEPTIONS AND MISTAKES

- The stages of sarcoid reflect disease progression (stage 1, early disease; stage 4, late disease)
- Pulmonary sarcoidosis is a steroid-responsive disease
- Believing that most individuals experience sarcoidosis as a chronic disease

PATHOPHYSIOLOGY OF SARCOIDOSIS

- Sarcoidosis is an idiopathic, systemic disease in which granuloma formation is pathologically triggered in a susceptible individual, presumably by inhalation of various environmental antigens (eg, mycobacteria, tree pollen, mold, inorganic particles)
- Symptoms are caused by organ dysfunction secondary to granuloma accumulation, which impinge on normal structures (eg, airways) or by cytokine elaboration (eg, TNF-α) and vitamin D metabolism
- Granuloma formation is designed to surround and contain organisms that cannot be opsonized:
  - Antigen-presenting cells stimulate an oligoclonal population of CD4+ T cells
  - Activated CD4+ T cells secrete IL-2, interferon-γ, and TNF-α, stimulating macrophages to differentiate to epithelioid cells
    - Epithelioid cells gain secretory antibacterial activity (in lieu of phagocytic ability)
  - Epithelioid cells fuse to form multinucleated giant cells
  - Granulomas covert vitamin D, leading to hypercalciuria and occasionally hypercalcemia
- Epidemiology of sarcoidosis:
  - Typically affects the young (20–40 years old)
  - Females more than males
  - African Americans are afflicted three times more than Caucasian Americans
    - Often older onset (40–50 years old)
    - Worse prognosis
  - Low income and poor socioeconomic status correlate with more severe sarcoidosis
  - Individuals with an affected family member/siblings are at higher risk
  - Patterns of organ involvement (eg, ocular, hepatic) track with families
- Natural history:
  - 50% experience remission within 3 years of diagnosis, and 66% experience remission within 10 years of diagnosis
  - Recurrence after a year of remission is rare (<5%)
  - 33% experience unrelenting disease and organ injury
  - Mortality is <5% and is most often associated with pulmonary fibrosis, followed by cardiac and neurologic involvement
  - Pulmonary fibrosis occurs in 20%–25% of individuals presenting with stage 2–3 disease
    - May occur despite resolution of granulomas
  - The stages of sarcoidosis are not progressive, but rather represent presentations

- Individuals typically maintain the same stage throughout the course of their disease
  - The exception being the occasional progression form stage 2 to stage 3
- Diagnosis:
  - Sarcoidosis is a diagnosis of exclusion because adenopathy, nodules, and granulomas occur commonly in many infectious, inflammatory, and malignant diseases
  - Requires a compatible clinical radiographic scenario with a tissue biopsy showing well-circumscribed noncaseating granulomas (with negative stains and cultures for acid-fast bacilli, fungi, and foreign matter)
    - Biopsy may not be required for acute sarcoidosis presentations (Löfgren's and Heerfordt's)
  - The easiest biopsy target should be pursued first (eg, skin, conspicuous peripheral lymph node)
  - Bronchoscopy is **often** required:
    - Endobronchial ultrasound-guided transbronchial needle aspiration (EBUS-TBNA) of thoracic lymph nodes, followed by transbronchial biopsy if aspirate is nondiagnostic (or if rapid on-site evaluation [ROSE]) is not available
    - This approach has a high sensitivity and specificity for both ruling out other entities (eg, malignancy) and making the diagnosis (>90% yield)
  - In the absence of adenopathy (stage 3), performing random transbronchial biopsies (eight samples, multiple segments, one side) also has a high diagnostic yield (~85%)
  - Angiotensin-converting enzyme (ACE) is produced by granulomas, and levels are elevated in 60% of patients with sarcoidosis
    - Limited diagnostic utility, given that the positive and negative predictive values are 84% and 74%, respectively

SARCOIDOSIS CLINICAL PRESENTATIONS (ACUTE, STAGES 1–3, STAGE 4, AND UNIQUE)

- **Acute sarcoidosis** (Löfgren's and Heerfordt's syndromes) represents ~20% of clinical presentations (Fig. 14.1)
  - **All have bilateral hilar adenopathy** and **fever** with extrapulmonary manifestations
    - Löfgren's syndrome
      - Bilateral, symmetric ankle or knee arthritis
        - Lasts for weeks; treat pain with nonsteroidal antiinflammatory drugs (NSAIDs)
        - More common in men
      - Erythema nodosum
        - More common in women
        - Occurs in ~10% of acute sarcoid presentations
        - Nonspecific, painful raised nodules on the lower extremities (shins)
          - Caused by a nonspecific septal panniculitis such that biopsy is **not** useful for diagnosis of sarcoid
        - Lasts for weeks; treat pain with NSAIDs
    - 90% spontaneous resolution of adenopathy (within 2 years)
    - No biopsy or treatment required
  - **Heerfordt's syndrome** (a.k.a. uveoparotid fever)
    - Uveitis and parotid gland swelling
    - Unilateral facial nerve palsy
    - Diagnosis confirmed by lacrimal gland biopsy **or** gallium scan showing the lambda panda sign
      - Characteristic, symmetric uptake in the lacrimal, parotid, submandibular glands and thoracic lymph nodes
    - Treat with prednisone
- **Stage 1 sarcoidosis presentation: hilar and mediastinal adenopathy without parenchymal involvement on chest computed tomography (CT) scan** (Fig. 14.2)
  - Majority of cases are incidentally discovered by a chest x-ray obtained for another reason (eg, preoperatively)

Acute Sarcoidosis Presentations
(Bilateral Hilar Adenopathy, Fever, Extrapulmonary Symptoms)

Löfgren´s Syndrome:
- Symmetric Knee / Ankle Arthritis, male predominance

and or
- Erythema Nodosum, female predominance

Evaluation and Treatment:

- No Biopsy
- No Primary Treatment
- NSAIDs for Arthritis (resolves in weeks)
- 90% resolve adenopathy within 2 years

Erythema Nodosum

Bilateral Hilar Adenopathy

Heerfordt's Syndrome
(Uveoparotid Fever):

- Uveitis
- Parotid, Lacrimal and Submandibular gland swelling
- Unilateral facial nerve palsy

Right CN VII Paralysis

Evaluation and Treatment:
- Lambda Panda Gallium Scan
- Lacrimal Gland Biopsy (vs. empiric therapy)
- Prednisone Indicated

Gallium Scan
Lambda Panda Sign

Nasopharynx (normal uptake)
Lacrimal Glands
Parotid Glands
Submandibular Glands
Right Paratracheal Adenopathy
Left Hilar Adenopathy
Right Hilar and Subcarinal Adenopathy

Fig. 14.1 Clinical radiographic aspects of the two most common acute sarcoid presentations, Löfgren's and Heerfordt's. Both share the features of hilar adenopathy and fever. Löfgren's features the extrapulmonary manifestations of symmetric knee/ankle arthritis and/or Erythema nodosum. Heerfordt's (a.k.a. uveoparotid fever) is more serious, given that the cranial nerve VII (facial nerve) is commonly involved. Because of this, prednisone is indicated. Although the clinical syndrome of uveitis, parotitis coupled with the lambda panda sign, is sensitive and specific, lacrimal gland biopsy is a low-morbidity, high-yield procedure for the diagnosis of Heerfordt's.

Chest Imaging in Stage 1 Sarcoidosis

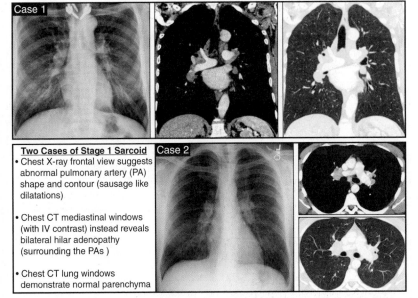

Case 1

Two Cases of Stage 1 Sarcoid Case 2
- Chest X-ray frontal view suggests abnormal pulmonary artery (PA) shape and contour (sausage like dilatations)

- Chest CT mediastinal windows (with IV contrast) instead reveals bilateral hilar adenopathy (surrounding the PAs)

- Chest CT lung windows demonstrate normal parenchyma

Fig. 14.2 Two examples of the chest imaging of stage 1 sarcoidosis (ie, hilar and mediastinal adenopathy alone). On a frontal radiograph, hilar adenopathy often appears as large, abnormally contoured pulmonary arteries. Chest computed tomography (CT) lung windows show no significant parenchymal involvement.

- May have mild pulmonary symptoms (eg, dry cough, dyspnea, chest pain/tightness, wheezing)
- Systemic symptoms (eg, fatigue, night sweats, and weight loss) occur less commonly
- The differential diagnosis of stage 1 sarcoid is the same as the differential for **isolated hilar and mediastinal adenopathy:**
  - Primary tuberculosis (TB), endemic fungal infection, lymphoma, small cell lung cancer, and metastatic adenocarcinoma (eg, breast, colon)
- **Evaluation** (Fig. 14.3)
  - Immunologic workup:
    - Quantiferon testing
      - A positive quantiferon should prompt sputum sampling for mycobacterium tuberculosis (MTB)
    - Complement fixation test for coccidioidomycosis and serum cryptococcal antigen (CrAg) in endemic areas or exposed individuals (sensitive and specific for active disease)
      - A positive complement fixation titer (may take 6 weeks to occur) implies active disease and should prompt consideration for treatment
        - One should **not** attempt to biopsy or process tissue specimens containing cocci because it is a hazard to laboratory workers (and diagnosis can be made serologically)

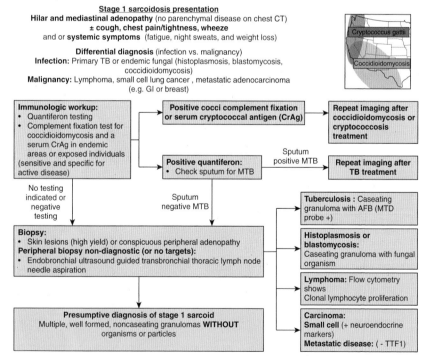

Fig. 14.3 Flow diagram outlining the workup of possible stage 1 sarcoidosis. Evaluation hinges on excluding infectious and/or malignant causes of hilar and mediastinal adenopathy. Tuberculosis (TB), coccidioidomycosis, and cryptococcosis can (and should) be screened for immunologically. The remainder of diseases are ruled out by lymph node aspirate/biopsy.

- Significant peripheral eosinophilia or the presence of a pleural effusion in the right patient (ie, young, no cancer risk factors) may increase the suspicion for cocci enough to warrant waiting 4–6 weeks to repeat complement fixation titer before lymph node biopsy
- A negative workup for active TB or coccidioidomycosis necessitates tissue sampling/biopsy:
  - Any new raised or nodular skin lesions should be evaluated for biopsy (except erythema nodosum)
  - Peripheral adenopathy is less helpful unless it is conspicuously pathologic
  - If skin/peripheral targets are nonexistent, or nondiagnostic, a mediastinal/hilar lymph node biopsy is indicated
    - The highest yield approach involves EBUS-TBNA of thoracic lymph nodes with flow cytometry to rule out lymphoma
    - If cytology specimens are nondiagnostic (or not available in real time), additional endobronchial and transbronchial specimens should be considered when clinical suspicion is high (even in the absence of visualized disease)
- **Stage 2 sarcoidosis presentation: Hilar and mediastinal adenopathy with parenchymal involvement on chest CT (reticulonodular pattern or diffuse parenchymal lung disease [DPLD] pattern)**
  - More likely to be symptomatic (eg, dry cough, dyspnea, chest pain/tightness, wheezing, and systemic symptoms)
  - Differential diagnosis based on CT pattern of parenchymal lung disease:
    - Nodular/reticular nodular (TB, nontuberculous mycobacteria [NTM], endemic fungal infection, metastatic carcinoma, lymphangitic spread of tumor, pneumoconiosis) (Fig. 14.4)

Chest Imaging in Stage 2 Sarcoidosis: Nodular Pattern

- Chest X-ray frontal view suggests abnormal pulmonary artery (PA) shape and contour with a diffuse reticulonodular parenchymal pattern
- Chest CT mediastinal windows (with IV contrast) reveals bilateral hilar and subcarinal adenopathy (surrounding the PAs)
- Chest CT lung windows demonstrate multiple pulmonary nodules (.3 mm to 1 cm) in a bronchovascular and perilymphatic distribution, with thickening of fissures and some interlobular septae

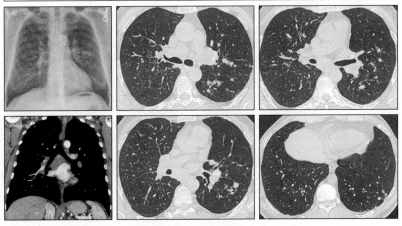

Fig. 14.4 Typical chest imaging of **stage 2 sarcoidosis, *nodular* pattern**.

Chest Imaging in Stage 2 Sarcoidosis: DPLD Pattern

- Chest X-ray frontal view suggests a widened mediastinum with a DPLD pattern including multifocal ground glass opacities (GGO), reticular markings and areas of more dense consolidation
- Chest CT mediastinal windows (with IV contrast) reveals bilateral paratracheal (and less conspicuous but present) hilar and subcarinal adenopathy (Red Rings)
- Chest CT lung windows demonstrate upper lobe reticulonodular pattern with GGO, middle and lower lobes GGO, pleural thickening and peripheral areas of dense consolidation (with multiple small nodules throughout)

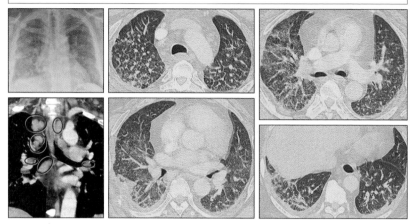

Fig. 14.5 Example of chest imaging of **stage 2 sarcoidosis, *diffuse parenchymal lung disease (DPLD)* pattern**.

- All other diffuse parenchymal lung disease patterns usual interstitial pneumonia (UIP), nonspecific interstitial pneumonia (NSIP), cryptogenic organizing pneumonia (COP), hypersensitivity, chronic eosinophilic pneumonia (CEP) (Fig. 14.5)
- **Evaluation** (Fig. 14.6):
  - Exclude active tuberculosis and coccidioidomycosis/cryptococcosis with quantiferon testing/sputum samples, complement fixation, and serum antigen testing, respectively
  - Biopsy should be pursued when TB and cocci/crypto have been excluded
    - New plaques or nodular skin lesions should be evaluated by biopsy
    - If skin/peripheral targets are nonexistent or nondiagnostic, a thoracic lymph node biopsy by EBUS-TBNA should be pursued
    - If lymph node aspirates are nondiagnostic or rapid on-site cytology evaluation is not possible, additional endobronchial and transbronchial specimens should be considered (high yield for the diagnosis of sarcoid)
    - If bronchoscopy with EBUS-TBNA and transbronchial biopsies are nondiagnostic, metastatic carcinoma and sarcoidosis become **much** less likely and DPLD much more likely
    - Consider video-assisted thoracoscopic surgery (VATS) lung biopsy (in attempts to make a definitive diagnosis, if possible) vs empiric steroids (for possibly steroid-responsive DPLD)
- **Stage 3 sarcoidosis presentation: Nodular/reticulonodular pattern withoutthoracic adenopathy and a clinical scenario suggesting sarcoid (eg, individual susceptibility/family history, mixed obstructive-restrictive pattern on pulmonary function tests [PFTs])**
  - Because stage 3 disease has much less (if any) conspicuous adenopathy, individuals present for evaluation of DPLD

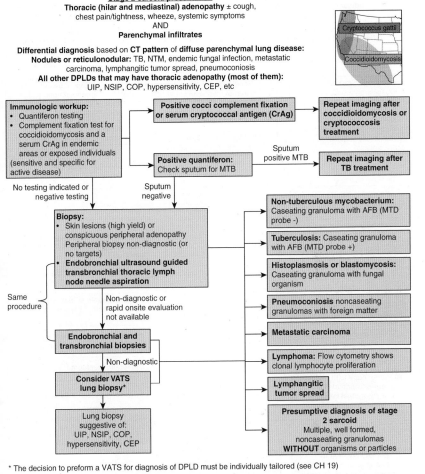

Fig. 14.6 Flow diagram outlining the workup of possible stage 2 sarcoidosis. Evaluation begins by excluding infectious and/or malignant causes of multiple pulmonary nodules (and/or diffuse parenchymal lung disease [DPLD]) with hilar and mediastinal adenopathy. Tuberculosis (TB), coccidioidomycosis, and cryptococcosis should be screened for immunologically. The remainder of diseases are ruled out by lymph node aspirate/lung biopsy. If aspirates and biopsies are nondiagnostic, the likelihood of granulomatous disease and/or malignancy drops significantly, and the focus should change to a workup of DPLD (see CH19).

- Suspicion for sarcoid occurs when a nodular pattern is seen on the a chest CT scan of a susceptible individual (eg, 45-year-old African American female with two affected siblings) or an individual with mixed obstructive-restrictive pattern on PFTs
- The differential diagnosis is the same as the differential diagnosis of nodular DPLD (ie, TB, NTM, endemic fungal infection, metastatic carcinoma, lymphangitic tumor spread, pneumoconiosis)
- **Evaluation (**Fig. 14.7**):**
  - Exclude active tuberculosis, NTM infection, and coccidioidomycosis/cryptococcosis with quantiferon testing, sputum samples, coccidioidomycosis complement fixation, and serum CrAg antibody testing

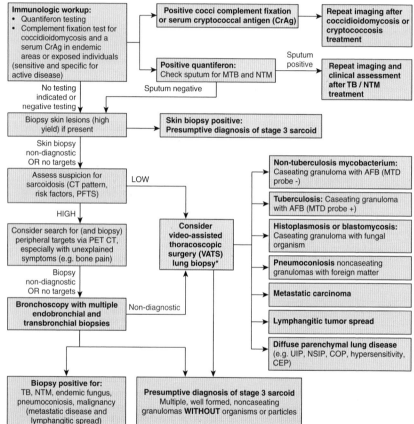

Fig. 14.7 Flow diagram outlining the workup of possible stage 3 sarcoidosis. Evaluation begins by excluding infectious and/or malignant causes of multiple pulmonary nodules and/or diffuse parenchymal lung disease (DPLD) mimics (eg, nontuberculous mycobacteria [NTM]). Tuberculosis (TB), coccidioidomycosis, and cryptococcosis should always be screened for immunologically. The remainder of the diseases are ruled out by lung biopsy. The decision to perform a bronchoscopy for the purpose of a random/blind transbronchial biopsy hinges on the pretest probability for sarcoidosis **or** other diseases in which transbronchial biopsy is high yield (eg, TB, NTM, endemic fungus, pneumoconiosis, metastatic disease, lymphangitic spread of tumor). If suspicion for granulomatous disease is **low**, the focus changes to the workup of DPLD (see CH19).

- Evaluate new nodular skin lesions for biopsy
- If **suspicion** for sarcoid is high and the patient has additional unexplained symptoms (eg, bone pain), consider a positron emission tomography–computed tomography scan looking for other peripheral biopsy targets (Fig. 14.8)
- If additional biopsy targets are nondiagnostic or nonexistent, consider bronchoscopy with multiple endobronchial and transbronchial biopsies (and bronchoalveolar lavage for acid-fast bacilli culture)

Chest CT and whole Body FDG PET Imaging in Stage 2 Sarcoidosis: Nodular Pattern, with Diffuse Bony Involvement

- Pt with sarcoidosis and diffuse bony pain
- Chest CT shows multiple nodules in a bronchovascular and perilymphatic distribution (along fissures and pleura)
- Chest CT mediastinal windows (with IV contrast) reveals bilateral hilar and subcarinal adenopathy
- Whole Body FDG – PET scan shows PET avid mediastinal adenopathy, hepatic and spleen lesions, with diffuse bony involvement of the spine and femurs bilaterally (mimicking metastatic disease)

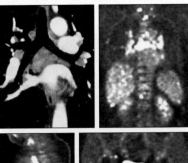
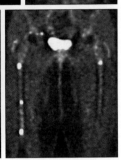
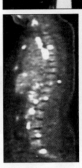
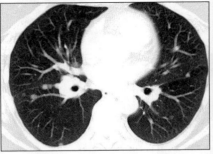

Fig. 14.8 Chest computed tomography (CT) scan and whole body fluorodeoxyglucose-positron emission tomography (FDG-PET) imaging of stage 2 sarcoidosis; **nodular** pattern reveals diffuse bony involvement (as well as liver and spleen) in a woman complaining of diffuse bony pain in her spine and legs.

- Consider VATS if bronchoscopy fails to yield a diagnosis, or before bronchoscopy if suspicion for sarcoid is low
- **Stage 4 sarcoidosis presentation: bilateral perihilar fibrosis with traction bronchiectasis and diffuse fibrotic bands in an individual with a history of biopsy-proven sarcoidosis or in a susceptible individual reporting a clinical history compatible with previously active sarcoidosis (despite no definitive diagnosis)** (Fig. 14.9)
  - Patients complain of exercise limitation and symptomatic bronchiectasis (not symptoms referable to active granulomatous inflammation)
  - During stage 4 disease, granulomatous inflammation has transitioned to fibrosis, causing traction bronchiectasis and limiting exercise via restrictive physiology
  - Patients may also experience symptomatic bronchiectasis (eg, chronic purulence, recurrent infections, and hemoptysis)
  - Stage 4 sarcoidosis should be considered in individuals with DPLD and a history of biopsy-proven sarcoidosis, or individuals with **very** suggestive imaging, such as bilateral perihilar fibrosis with traction bronchiectasis and diffuse fibrotic bands (fibrosis in a bronchovascular bundle distribution)
  - No specific workup is required for stage 4 sarcoid
  - The differential diagnosis includes diseases known to cause bronchiectasis (eg, NTM, aspiration, prior endemic fungal infection, chronic fibrosing aspergillosis, rounded atelectasis [as seen with asbestos exposure], cryptogenic organizing pneumonia)
  - PFTs are more likely to demonstrate restriction (rather than mixed disease)
  - Risk factors for progressive fibrosis, despite resolution of granulomatous inflammation, include:
    - African American
    - male gender

Stage 4 Sarcoid Presentation

Bilateral Perihilar Fibrosis with Traction Bronchiectasis and diffuse Fibrotic Bands
AND a **History of Biopsy Proven Sarcoidosis** or a **Susceptible individual** reporting a clinical
history compatible with previously active sarcoidosis

Differential Diagnosis e.g. NTM, Aspiration, Prior Endemic Fungal Infection, Chronic fibrosing
aspergillosis, Rounded atelectasis, COP

Stage 4 Sarcoid

- Non-progressive (burned out) fibrotic disease
- Biopsy no longer indicated or expected to yield granulomas (fibrosis only)
- Normal size thoracic lymph nodes (may be calcified)
- Risk Factors For Progression to Fibrosis in Sarcoid:
  - African American, male, onset > age 50, poor socioeconomic status
- Differential Diagnosis: NTM, Aspiration, Prior Endemic Fungal Infection,Chronic fibrosing aspergillosis, Rounded atelectasis, cryptogenic organizing pneumonia
- Presents with exercise limitation and symptomatic bronchiectasis (e.g. recurrent sputum production, lung infections, and hemoptysis)
- Pulmonary Function Testing shows restriction (much more commonly then mixed obstructive restrictive disease)

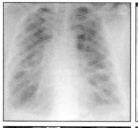
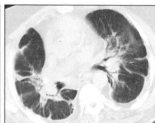
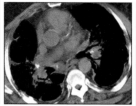
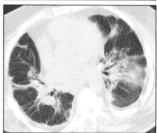

Fig. 14.9 Stage 4 sarcoid includes symptoms of pulmonary fibrosis (nonprogressive/"burned out") and has a restrictive physiology with traction bronchiectasis and linear scarring. The diagnosis is made, historically, in individuals with biopsy-proven sarcoidosis. The diagnosis can be considered in susceptible individuals with a compatible history and no alternate explanation for their pulmonary fibrosis. The differential diagnosis involves entities that cause traction bronchiectasis and fibrosis along bronchovascular structures (eg, nontuberculous mycobacteria [NTM], aspiration, prior endemic fungal infection, chronic fibrosing aspergillosis, rounded atelectasis). Frontal view of the chest shows multiple bilateral linear scars and diaphragm tenting. Chest computed tomography (CT) mediastinal windows show small (nonpathologic), calcified hilar lymph nodes bilaterally.

- age of onset >50 years
- poor socioeconomic status
- Unique, rare sarcoid presentations:
  - Sarcoid has the ability to injure any organ (eg, renal failure from granulomatous interstitial nephritis)
  - Additionally, a correctly placed granulomas may cause anything from pancreatitis to focal neurologic dysfunction/mononeuritis multiplex
  - ~13% of patients with neurosarcoidosis have isolated central nervous system (CNS) disease, mimicking intracranial tumors
  - These cases are ultimately diagnosed by biopsy

EVALUATION AND TREATMENT AFTER A DIAGNOSIS OF SARCOID IS MADE (TABLE 14.1)

- Sarcoidosis is a systemic disease in which the visualized abnormalities during the initial examination represent "the tip of the iceberg" with regard to the extent of granuloma formation
  - Because of this, a thorough review of systems and a complete physical examination are crucial

Table 14.1 Symptoms, Evaluation and Treatment by Organ

PRESENTING SYMPTOMS BY ORGAN SYSTEM	EVALUATION BY ORGAN SYSTEM (DESCENDING ORDER OF FREQUENCY)	TREATMENT BY ORGAN SYSTEM
Ocular • Eye pain and irritation • Decreased visual acuity	**Abnormal Slit Lamp and/or Fundoscopic Examination ~80%** • Anterior uveitis (65%) • Posterior uveitis (30%) • Optic neuritis (5%)	**Anterior Uveitis:** • Topical Corticosteroid **Posterior uveitis/optic neuritis:** • Prednisone 20–40 mg every day
Pulmonary • Dyspnea on exertion • Cough, wheeze, and chest tightness	**Abnormal PFT ~65%** • Restriction • Mixed obstructive-restrictive	**Mild Symptoms or PFT Abnormalities** • Inhaled corticosteroid **Moderate-Severe Symptoms or PFT Abnormalities** • Prednisone 20–40 mg every day
Calcium Homeostasis • Fatigue • Kidney stones (~10%)	**Abnormally elevated Urinary Calcium ~40%; Serum Calcium ~10%** • Hypercalciuria with kidney stones • Hypercalcemia	**Hypercalcemia or Hypercalciuria with Kidney Stones** • Hydroxychloroquine 400 mg every day • Prednisone 20–40 mg every day
Skin • Cosmetically significant lesions on face, nape of neck, upper back, extremities, and trunk	**Abnormal Skin Examination ~30%** **Macules, Papules, and Plaques in Single Lesions or Crops** **Lupus Pernio** • Indurated, lumpy, facial lesions (nose, cheeks, lips, and ears) with granulomas eroding into cartilage and bone	**Cosmetically Significant Plaques and Nodules** • Prednisone 20–40 mg every day • Hydroxychloroquine 400 mg every day **Lupus Pernio** • Prednisone 20–40 mg every day • Hydroxychloroquine 400 mg every day • Thalidomide 100–150 mg every day • Methotrexate 10–15 mg every week
Central Nervous System • Cranial nerve palsy • Headache • Ataxia • Cognitive dysfunction • Seizures • Focal neurologic deficits	**Abnormal Neurologic/Cranial Nerve Examination ± MRI Scan and/or Lumbar Puncture ~10%** • CSF shows oligoclonal immunoglobulin bands (mimicking MS) ~33% • MRI with gadolinium sensitive for CNS disease • mimics intracranial tumors (eg, meningiomas, optic nerve gliomas)	**Cranial Nerve Palsy** • Prednisone 40 mg every day **Intracerebral Involvement or Spinal Cord Involvement** • Prednisone 40 mg every day • Azathioprine 150 mg every day • Hydroxychloroquine 400 mg every day

Continued

Table 14.1 Symptoms, Evaluation and Treatment by Organ—cont'd

PRESENTING SYMPTOMS BY ORGAN SYSTEM	EVALUATION BY ORGAN SYSTEM (DESCENDING ORDER OF FREQUENCY)	TREATMENT BY ORGAN SYSTEM
Systemic • Fever • Night sweats • Weight loss • Symptomatic cholestasis	**Abnormal Liver Function Tests ~10%** • 99% asymptomatic hepatitis • <1% cholestatic granulomatous hepatitis	**Cholestatic Granulomatous Hepatitis** • Prednisone 20–40 mg every day • Ursodiol (15 mg/kg) every day
Cardiac • Palpitations • Arrhythmia • Syncope • Systolic dysfunction • Sudden death	**Abnormal Electrocardiogram, Echocardiogram, Cardiac MRI, or Electrophysiology Study ~5%** • Heart block/conduction delay • Systolic dysfunction • Extensive myocardial sarcoidosis • Ventricular tachycardia	**Heart Block** • Pacemaker • Prednisone 20–40 mg every day **Extensive Myocardial Sarcoid** • Echocardiogram ± EP study **Systolic Dysfunction** • AICD • Prednisone 20–40 mg every day **EP Study Shows VT/VF** • AICD • Prednisone 20–40 mg every day
Musculoskeletal • Asymptomatic (or painful) bone, joint, and muscle lesions • Mimic metastatic cancer (eg, prostate)	**Abnormal Whole Body** • FDG-PET scan • Bone, joint, and muscle involvement	**Symptomatic** • Granulomatous bone, joint, and muscle involvement • Prednisone 20–40 mg every day

AICD, Automatic implantable cardioverter-defibrillator; CNS, central nervous system; EP, electrophysiology; FDG-PET, fluorodeoxyglucose-positron emission tomography; MRI, magnetic resonance imaging; PFT, pulmonary function tests; VF, ventricular fibrillation; VT, ventricular tachycardia.

- **All** individuals diagnosed with sarcoidosis should have:
  - **Ophthalmologic evaluation** with a slit lamp and fundoscopic examination to rule out ocular involvement (very common)
  - **Electrocardiogram** (ECG) to rule out evidence of conduction system disease (eg, heart block)
  - **Serum calcium measurement**
- Specific attention should be given to screening for cardiac symptoms (ie, heart failure, palpitations, presyncope/syncope)
  - Low threshold for ECG and cardiac magnetic resonance imaging (MRI) (because cardiac sarcoid may cause sudden death)
    - Cardiac sarcoid is diagnosed by MRI, **not** biopsy (which is high risk, low yield)
    - Consider an electrophysiology (EP) study screening for ventricular tachycardia when extensive cardiac sarcoid is seen by MRI or when the patient reports presyncope/syncope
- Bone pain, musculoskeletal symptoms, or other unexplained symptoms may be investigated with a whole body PET scan
- Neurologic symptoms should be investigated with MRI

Treatment

- Most individuals with stage 1 sarcoidosis (vast majority) do not require treatment
- Prednisone is the mainstay of therapy in the following situations:
  - All cases with neurologic or cardiac involvement
  - Pulmonary involvement with abnormal PFT and symptoms (eg, cough, wheeze, dyspnea on exertion)
- Prednisone response in pulmonary sarcoid is typically underwhelming (unlike steroid-responsive nonspecific interstitial pneumonia [NSIP] or eosinophilic lung disease)
  - However, complete lack of a response suggests:
    - Inadequate prednisone dose
    - Medication noncompliance
    - Irreversible fibrotic disease
- Prednisone dosing (per expert opinion) involves 20–40 mg daily for 3 months, followed by attempted taper to 10–15 mg daily for a total of 9–12 months
  - Methotrexate may be used as a steroid-sparing agent, for those who respond, but cannot be tapered
- Hydroxychloroquine may be used for hypercalcemia, CNS, and skin diseases
- Azathioprine and TNF-α blockers (infliximab and etanercept) can be considered as second- and third-line agents, respectively

QUESTIONS COMMONLY GENERATED BY THIS TEACHING

1. Is progression from granulomatous inflammation to fibrosis synonymous with stage 4 sarcoidosis?
   No. Patients with stage 2 and stage 3 sarcoidosis may experience focal areas that progress to fibrosis without changing their imaging stage (ie, despite the persistence of adenopathy).
2. Why can't blastomycosis and histoplasmosis be diagnosed serologically?
   Unfortunately, available tests lack the required sensitivity and specificity for active disease.

CHAPTER 15

ACUTE VENOUS THROMBOEMBOLIC DISEASE

COMMON MISCONCEPTIONS AND MISTAKES

- Believing that the target of heparin is the already embolized clot (preventing its extension in the pulmonary vasculature)
- Missing the most common **abnormal** chest x-ray (CXR) finding in pulmonary embolism (PE) (subsegmental atelectasis and a small effusion)
- Assuming a VQ scan will be useless in an individual with underlying lung disease
- Failing to realize that thrombosis in the superficial femoral vein **is** a deep vein thrombosis (**DVT**)
- Undertreating an upper extremity DVT occurring in the outpatient setting

OVERVIEW OF ACUTE VENOUS THROMBOEMBOLIC DISEASE

- Represents a spectrum from DVT to symptomatic PE
- Every acute DVT will have caused tiny, subclinical (asymptomatic and/or undetectable) pulmonary emboli based on the unstable nature of a newly formed clot in the deep veins
- **Therefore**, when DVT is found in the absence of pulmonary symptoms, **presume asymptomatic PE**
  - **Treat DVT** and **asymptomatic PE** the same way
  - No need to perform thoracic imaging to attempt to prove asymptomatic PE once DVT is diagnosed
- Every acute PE that is diagnosed is a "**heralding event"**
  - If survived, the individual's intrinsic fibrinolytic system will lyse the embolized clot (often quickly)
  - Therefore the already embolized clot is **not** the focus of acute management
  - The primary goal of acute management is to prevent the next PE (ie, recurrent embolism) with anticoagulation
    - Each recurrent embolism carries a mortality risk of approximately 25%
- Although the CXR is normal the majority of the time in acute PE:
  - The most common **abnormality** seen by CXR is a small effusion with subsegmental atelectasis reflecting focal inflammatory mediator release (eg, histamine) and bronchoconstriction
- CT angiography (CTA) is useful in the initial diagnosis of PE, often providing an alternate explanation for symptoms when PE is not discovered
- A VQ scan is a reasonable alternative if the patient has a contraindication to IV contrast or an individual desire to minimize CT-related radiation exposure
- Once a symptomatic PE is diagnosed, patients should be risk stratified with an echocardiogram ECG, BNP, and troponin, looking for RV strain
- IV heparin is the anticoagulant of choice for individuals at risk of clinical deterioration, given its ability to be reversed and resumed quickly
- Urgent inferior vena cava (IVC) filter placement should be pursued in individuals who have a contraindication to anticoagulation

- Individuals with an unprovoked venous thromboembolism (VTE) (and a normal bleeding risk) should be offered indefinite anticoagulation
- Patients with VTE disease should be screened for persistent perfusion defects by VQ scan after 6 months of anticoagulation, or at the time anticoagulation is to be stopped (eg, 3 months for small provoked VTE)
- Individuals with persistent perfusion defects should be screened for chronic thromboembolic pulmonary hypertension (CTEPH) via an echocardiogram looking for an elevated pulmonary artery systolic pressure (PAS) and isolated right-sided heart failure

PATHOPHYSIOLOGY OF PULMONARY EMBOLISM

- A DVT (typically in the leg or pelvis) has both of the following:
  - A **stable**, organized edge that is attached to the vessel wall
  - And an **unstable** leading edge, extending into the lumen of the vessel
    - Fresh clot extends from this leading edge until shear forces cause it to break off and embolize to the lung
    - This process repeats until death (from obstructive, right ventricular [RV]-mediated cardiogenic shock), anticoagulation, or IVC filter placement
    - Symptomatic PE occurs when clot extension and breakage creates a large enough fragment to cause significant pulmonary artery (PA) occlusion
    - Heparin (anticoagulation) stops this extension and embolism cycle, stabilizing the leading edge and dramatically reducing the risk of significant recurrent PE
    - Contraindication to anticoagulation mandates urgent IVC filter placement to prevent death from recurrent PE
- PE symptoms and causes:
  - **Pleuritic chest** pain is caused by either:
    - Atelectasis causing pleural traction (common)
    - Pulmonary infarct (less common)
      - Pulmonary infarction occurs when PE is accompanied by shock (systemic hypotension)
        - Compromising both the pulmonary artery and bronchial artery circulation
  - **A-a gradient and hypoxemia** are caused by VQ mismatch related to:
    - Atelectasis from local inflammatory mediator release (eg, histamine) and bronchoconstriction
    - Alveolar edema occurring in the **unobstructed** regions of the lung from the increased blood flow
      - Unobstructed pulmonary arteries receive the entire cardiac output
  - **Tachypnea** and **dyspnea** occur with:
    - **Respiratory alkalosis (low Pco_2)**, which may be caused by pain, anxiety, and/or hypoxemic mediated hyperventilation
    - **Normal or high Pco_2** from the increased dead space created by the **obstructed** regions of the lung
  - **Tachycardia** and **hypotension** represent the spectrum of right-sided cardiogenic shock
    - Tachycardia is compensatory, attempting to maintain cardiac output (CO) in the face of a falling stroke volume
    - Hypotension reflects the failure to maintain CO (despite compensatory tachycardia and increased systemic vascular resistance [SVR])
- Acute respiratory failure from PE:
  - PE is an **uncommon** cause of respiratory failure in individuals **without** underlying lung disease
    - Patients with obstructive lung disease and PE are prone to hypercapnic failure from an inability to compensate for the increased dead space caused by the PA obstruction
    - Hypoxemia (from VQ mismatch) is typically easy to support with $\leq 6\,L$ of O_2 by NC

- Shunt physiology (ie, marginal oxygenation despite a 100% FiO_2) is **uncommon** but may be seen with:
  - Right-to-left shunting through an intracardiac shunt (eg, patent foramen ovale [PFO])
    - Increased PA and right-sided intracardiac pressure occur with low left-sided intracardiac pressure, promoting right-to-left shunting
      - Screen for this with a contrast echocardiogram (ie, immediate left-sided bubbles with IV agitated saline infusion)
    - PE with refractory hypoxemia from shunting though a PFO is a reason to consider thrombolysis (in hopes of rapidly dropping right-sided pressure)
  - Massive saddle emboli that fragment diffusely may cause shunt physiology (Fig. 15.1) from the combination of:
    - Atelectasis, adjacent to obstructed segments, via local inflammatory mediator release with bronchoconstriction
    - Alveolar edema occurring in the unobstructed segments, as they receive the entire cardiac output
      - This causes mechanical pulmonary capillary injury and alveolar edema, clinically similar to cardiogenic edema (ie, pink, frothy fluid that responds quickly to PEEP)

VTE DIAGNOSIS AND RISK STRATIFICATION (FIG. 15.2)

- Diagnostic approach hinges on presenting signs and symptoms
- DVT (extremity) signs and symptoms occurring alone should be evaluated by ultrasound
  - Unilateral lower extremity edema should be evaluated with bilateral lower extremity ultrasound
    - May identify undetected clot burden by identifying a contralateral DVT that was not appreciated during the physical examination
  - Demonstration of a DVT ends the VTE workup
    - Patients with a DVT and **no** cardiopulmonary signs or symptoms can be presumed to have suffered small, asymptomatic pulmonary emboli (based on the pathophysiology of VTE disease)
      - Because of this, DVT and asymptomatic pulmonary embolism are treated the **same**
- PE (cardiopulmonary) signs and symptoms occurring alone should be evaluated by CTA (ie, 1.25-mm chest CT with contrast timed for PA opacification)
  - CTA is the preferred mode for PE evaluation because of its ability to provide an alternate diagnosis for the cardiopulmonary symptoms (eg, tumor, pneumonia)
    - Major limitations to CTA for the diagnosis of PE (timing and artifact):
      - Poorly timed contrast, which inadequately opacifies the pulmonary arteries, can lead to a *false* negative study
      - Motion artifact with volume averaging (especially at the bases) and streak artifact can decrease intraluminal contrast opacification, leading to a *false* **positive** study
    - An equivocal CTA should be followed up with a VQ scan (to minimize the risk of radiation exposure from repeating the CTA)
      - Normal perfusion in an area that was equivocally opacified during CTA is **very** reassuring
  - In those in whom CTA is contraindicated, or "relatively" contraindicated (eg, poor renal function), the VQ scan is the second-line modality for PE diagnosis:
    - Made by identifying regions of the lung that demonstrate ventilation **without** perfusion (ie, unmatched perfusion defect)
      - This separates PE from parenchymal disease that affects **both** ventilation and perfusion (ie, matched perfusion defect) via hypoxemic vasoconstriction

Massive Pulmonary Embolism Mechanically Dislodged and Fragmented by Chest Compressions Leading to Transient Lung Failure (shunt **AND** extreme dead space physiology)

- 59 year old, POD # 30 after c-spine fusion, suffered a syncopal episode while ambulating with physical therapy on inpatient rehab
- Physical exam revealed the patient to be in moderate distress, asking for help, expressing a sense of doom (angoranimi)
- HR 112, RR 25, BP 99/66, O_2 sat was 88% on RA, Lungs CTA bilat, CV tachy, ABD Soft, NT, ND, +BS, EXT no c/c/e
- ABG on 6L O_2 showed a pH 7.38 / PCO_2 29/ **PO_2 55** (metabolic acidosis with a superimposed respiratory alkalosis and hypoxemia)
- FiO2 was increased to 100% and the patient was transferred to ICU
- A stat portable CXR showed clear lung fields with bilateral central PA dilatation (dashed arrows) and abrupt PA tapering / oligemia (solid arrows) concerning for bilateral proximal pulmonary emboli (ie, saddle embolus)
- The patient then developed an SVT at 140 BPM, with a repeat ABG showing a **pH 7.22/ PCO_2 35**/ PO_2 66 (worsening metabolic acidemia with a new superimposed respiratory acidosis and shunt physiology)
- Followed immediately by a PEA cardiac arrest (narrow complex tachycardia), concerning for acute RV failure / fatal pulmonary embolism

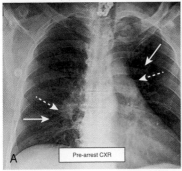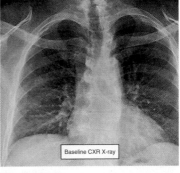

Cardiac Arrest One and Two

- ACLS was initiated, the patient was intubated, and ROSC was achieved 18 min later (presumably as the saddle emboli was fragmented and dislodged by CPR)
- Mechanical ventilation ensued (AC 20/500/p5/ FiO2 100%), **BUT** 4 minutes later O_2 saturation dropped, followed by HR (sinus bradycardia in the 60s, 50s, then 40s, 30s ...)
- Repeat ABG showed a **pH 6.90 / PCO_2 95**/ PO_2 38 (critical respiratory acidemia from extreme dead space physiology, with profound hypoxemia)
- $NaHCO_3$ IV was given, **minute ventilation (MV)** and PEEP were increased to 17.5 L /M and 10 cm H_2O (respectively)
- Despite this the patient suffered another PEA cardiac arrest (sinus bradycardia) from hypoxemia
- ACLS was reinitiated, and copious pink frothy secretions had to be emptied from the ET tube during manual bagging, until ROSC was achieved 3 min later
- Repeat ABG showed persistent respiratory acidemia, extreme dead space physiology and hypoxemia (pH 7.11 / PCO_2 103/ PO_2 50)
- PEEP was increased to 20 cm H_2O and a repeat chest x-ray and ABG were obtained

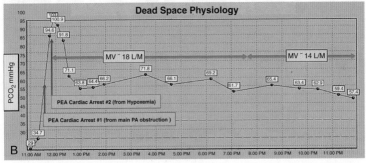

Fig. 15.1 Encapsulated case of a saddle pulmonary embolism causing an obstructive cardiac arrest with return of spontaneous circulation (ROSC) occurring after CPR dislodged and fragmented the clot, followed by a second cardiac arrest from hypoxemia, with ROSC occurring after improved oxygenation with increased positive end-expiratory pressure (PEEP). **(A)** Initial prearrest presentation demonstrates the classic features of PE, namely the patient's sense of impending doom, tachycardia, tachypnea, and arterial blood gas (ABG) showing a respiratory alkalosis with a significant A-a gradient. The respiratory alkalosis threatens to mask an underlying metabolic acidosis by normalizing the pH. This is easy to spot, acknowledging that a PCO_2 of 29 mm Hg (<35 mm Hg) is **low** and thus the pH should be **high** (>7.45). Instead, the acidemic pH reveals the underlying metabolic acidosis, which was secondary to lactate from developing cardiogenic shock (not something to be missed). The prearrest chest x-ray shows bilateral oligemia or Westermark's sign (solid arrows) and main pulmonary artery "sausage-like" dilation with rapid tapering or Palla's signs (dashed arrows). The patient's repeat ABG shows both shunt physiology and the development of a (relative) respiratory acidosis, as evidenced by a PCO_2 of 35 mm Hg (despite the fact that the value is in the normal range). Appropriate compensation for a metabolic acidosis yielding a pH of 7.22 is a PCO_2 of 22 mm Hg. Because the patient was tachypneic, attempting but unable to ventilate maximally impending hypercapnic respiratory failure should be anticipated. Shunt physiology is suggested by the PaO_2 of 66 mm Hg on 100% FiO2. **(B)** Development of lung failure occurring after ROSC, as evidenced by extreme dead space physiology with a $PCO_2 > 90$ mm Hg despite a minute ventilation >17.5 L/min and critical shunt physiology with a PaO_2 of 38 mm Hg despite mechanical ventilation with a FiO2 of 100% and a PEEP of 10 cm H_2O.

Continued

PEEP Sensitive Shunt Physiology After PE

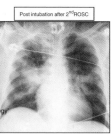
Post intubation after 2ndROSC

- Chest x-ray showed new patchy ground glass opacities and bilateral consolidations
- Repeat ABG showed a pH 7.00 / PCO_2 101/ PO_2 65 (persistent respiratory acidemia with extreme dead space physiology and shunt, with improved oxygenation after increased PEEP)
- Bedside echo was performed showing depressed RV systolic function (with preserved LV function), without evidence of intracardiac shunt (negative bubble study)
- Thrombolysis was considered, but held given recent c-spine surgery and a concern for a possible concomitant CVA, given a fixed deviated gaze at the time of his initial arrest
- The patient was empirically heparinized, **BUT** PO_2 fell again into the 50's requiring further increases in PEEP to 25 cm H_2O, which he responded to, demonstrating 'PEEP sensitive physiology'
- CT scan of the head and chest were obtained
- Head CT showed no abnormalities

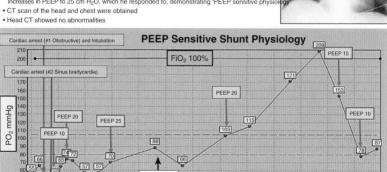

CTA Showing Bilateral Segmental and Subsegmental PE in ALL lobes (L>R)
NO Saddle Embolus

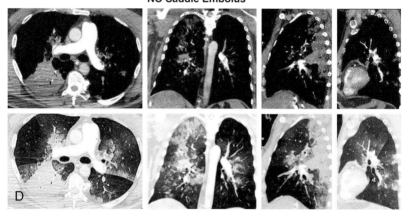

- Chest CTA showed bilateral segmental and subsegmental pulmonary emboli involving **ALL** lobes (L>R), with patchy areas of ground glass opacity (with septal thickening) and focal areas of consolidation/atelectasis (R>L), leading to transient **Lung Failure** (BOTH shunt and extreme dead space physiology)
- No saddle embolus identified, presumably because it was mechanically dislodged and fragmented by chest compressions
- An IVC filter was then placed (given the patients inability to tolerate recurrent emboli), and over the next 48 hours the patients lung function and hemodynamics returned to normal and the patient was extubated
- **He was discharged from the hospital 2 weeks later without permanent sequela from his cardiac arrests,** IVC filter was removed 4 weeks after discharge

Fig. 15.1, Cont'd (C) Initial management of the shunt physiology, (which was) attributed to pulmonary edema and atelectasis involved increasing PEEP. Though the high PEEP decreased venous return (evidenced by an increased HR and decreased BP), a priority was placed on maintaining the patient's $PaO_2 > 60$ mm Hg, given his prolonged cardiac arrest (for both CNS and RV protection). The shunt physiology resolved approximately 10 hours after its onset, as evidenced by a $PaO_2 > 200$ mm Hg. **(D)** CTA showing multiple subsegmental pulmonary emboli evident in all lobes (globally L > R) with atelectasis and ground glass opacities diffusely (R > L). The absence of a saddle embolus, or obstructing thrombus in either main PA, suggests that the saddle emboli seen on the prearrest chest x-ray was fragmented and mechanically dislodged during CPR. Although this saved the patient's life, it lead almost immediately to near fatal lung failure, which resolved in hours with supportive care, as intrinsic thrombolysis occurred and VQ matching improved.

Detail Showing the Parenchyma in Both Occluded and Non Occluded Segments

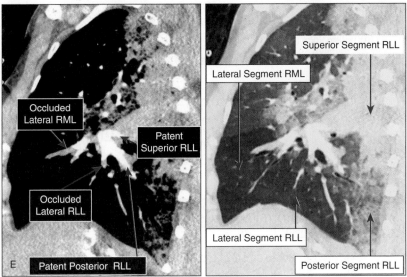

- Atelectasis and ground glass opacities occur in the unobstructed segments of the right lower lobe
- The parenchyma in the obstructed segments appears oligemic, creating mosaicism

Fig. 15.1, Cont'd (E) Detailed highlight of the mechanisms of extreme VQ mismatch and dead space. The **obstructed segments** receive the majority of the **ventilation but no perfusion** (ie, they become physiologic dead space), whereas the unobstructed segments receive all of the perfusion but no ventilation (because they are prone to flow-related edema and inflammatory atelectasis).

- VQ scan interpretation:
  - **High probability = two or more unmatched** segmental perfusion defects
  - **Intermediate probability = one unmatched** segmental perfusion defect
  - **Low probability = one matched** segmental perfusion defect
  - **Very low probability = no segmental** perfusion defects
- When clinical suspicion for PE is high, a low- or very low–probability VQ scan is required to suggest an alternate diagnosis
- PE (cardiopulmonary) signs and symptoms occurring **with** an edematous extremity is very suggestive of VTE
  - The initial step should be an ultrasound examination of the abnormal extremity that looks for DVT (as well as the contralateral side for good measure)
    - If a DVT is found, symptomatic PE is presumed (on clinical grounds)
      - Urgent CTA or VQ scan to confirm the diagnosis of PE in this setting is **not** indicated
        - VQ should eventually be done, at hospital discharge and/or shortly after therapy has begun, to establish an early "postinitiation of therapy" perfusion baseline (see initial management section)
    - If no DVT is found, a CTA (or VQ scan if CTA is contraindicated) should be performed
- When PE is diagnosed, risk stratification by looking for evidence of RV strain or injury is required to establish the appropriate therapy
  - PE kills by causing isolated RV failure:
    - Pulmonary obstruction increases RV afterload
    - As the RV fails to maintain CO, it dilates, increasing wall tension
    - As wall tension increases, subendocardial perfusion decreases, leading to catastrophic RV ischemia and failure, causing sudden cardiac death

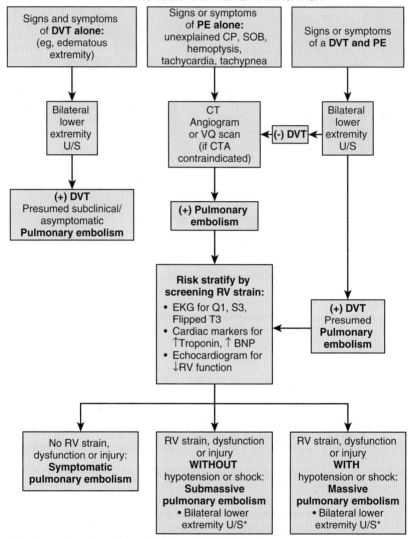

Fig. 15.2 Flow diagram outlining the diagnostic algorithms for venous thromboembolism (VTE) based on the presenting signs and symptoms (ie, deep vein thrombosis (DVT) alone, DVT and pulmonary embolism (PE), or PE alone). After diagnosis, patients should be risk stratified and classified as having an asymptomatic, symptomatic, submassive, or massive PE. Patients with a submassive or massive PE should have a bilateral lower extremity (LE) ultrasound performed (if not done as a part of the diagnosis) looking for significant residual thrombus (which may prompt IVC filter placement).

- RV strain, injury, or dysfunction is screened for by:
  - ECG looking for right axis deviation and/or RV strain pattern (Q1, S3, flipped T3)
  - Cardiac markers looking for RV ischemia (eg, troponins) and RV/RA dilation (eg, BNP)
  - Echocardiogram looking for evidence of increased right-sided pressure/decreased RV function

- Patients with PE and hypotension, or signs of systemic hypoperfusion (eg, lactate production, prerenal indices), are in cardiogenic shock from isolated right-sided heart failure and have a high mortality from either worsening RV failure or recurrent embolism
  - Dopamine is the inotrope of choice for isolated RV failure (based on expert clinical observations of efficacy)
- Ultimately, patients with VTE are divided into four categories:
  - **Asymptomatic/subclinical PE**
    - Every patient with a DVT
  - **Symptomatic PE**
    - Patients with PE and symptoms **not** caused by RV strain or injury (eg, tachypnea, pleuritic chest pain)
      - These symptoms are caused by increased dead space, parenchymal atelectasis, and/or pleural involvement
  - **Submassive PE**
    - Patients with PE and evidence of RV strain, dysfunction, or injury **without** cardiogenic shock
  - **Massive PE**
    - Patients with PE and evidence of RV strain, dysfunction, or injury **with** cardiogenic shock
- Patients with submassive or massive PE need a bilateral LE ultrasound (if not already done) to risk stratify by screening for a residual clot

INITIAL VTE MANAGEMENT (FIG. 15.3)

- The initial goals of VTE management are to prevent recurrent emboli and/or fatal RV-mediated cardiogenic shock
- **Anticoagulation** is the mainstay of therapy it because stabilizes and prevents extension of **the residual clot** in the deep venous system (the site of embolism), **not** the already embolized clot in the pulmonary vasculature
  - Relevant in situ thrombosis (ie, extension) of the already embolized acute clot (lodged in the pulmonary vasculature) is rare, and is **not** the main target of heparin therapy
    - Anticoagulation for VTE may be done with several different agents:
      - IV unfractionated heparin
        - Because of its short duration of action and ability to be reversed, IV heparin is the preferred mode of anticoagulation for:
          - Individuals at risk for clinical deterioration, ie, submassive or massive PE,
            - When PE patients develop cardiogenic shock, they often require additional procedures (eg, line placement, IVC filter placement, catheter-mediated embolectomy, surgical embolectomy), which all may be complicated by nonreversible anticoagulants
          - Individuals with an unclear/potential bleeding risk
        - Patients with a large clot burden often have very high heparin requirements, which decrease in 48–72 hours as the clot resolves
          - Clinically, this translates to initially subtherapeutic PTT values (despite weight-based dosing via protocol) followed by a period of therapeutic PTT values and then elevated PTT values (despite the same heparin dose)
        - IV heparin requires close monitoring (PTT every 6 hours) and is at risk for failing if patients are allowed to remain in a subtherapeutic PTT range
      - Low-molecular-weight heparin, fondaparinux, direct thrombin inhibitors, and direct factor Xa inhibitors have the general benefit of **not** requiring monitoring of their anticoagulant effect, **but** dosing may be less reliable in cases of obesity, gross volume overload, poor intestinal absorption, and/or renal insufficiency
      - The dosing of warfarin must commence **after** individuals have been therapeutic on heparin, and heparin must be continued for 5 days of overlap
      - Other oral anticoagulants do not require heparin overlap, but in general PE should be initially treated with at least 5 days of heparin (LMW or IV)

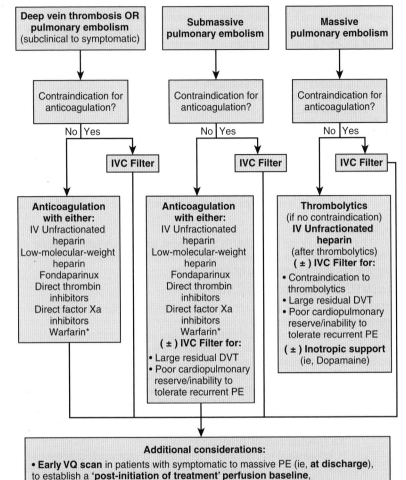

INITIAL VENOUS THROMBOEMBOLISM MANAGEMENT

Deep vein thrombosis OR pulmonary embolism
(subclinical to symptomatic)

Submassive pulmonary embolism

Massive pulmonary embolism

Contraindication for anticoagulation?

No | Yes

Contraindication for anticoagulation?

No | Yes

Contraindication for anticoagulation?

No | Yes

IVC Filter

IVC Filter

IVC Filter

Anticoagulation with either:
IV Unfractionated heparin
Low-molecular-weight heparin
Fondaparinux
Direct thrombin inhibitors
Direct factor Xa inhibitors
Warfarin*

Anticoagulation with either:
IV Unfractionated heparin
Low-molecular-weight heparin
Fondaparinux
Direct thrombin inhibitors
Direct factor Xa inhibitors
Warfarin*
(±) IVC Filter for:
• Large residual DVT
• Poor cardiopulmonary reserve/inability to tolerate recurrent PE

Thrombolytics
(if no contraindication)
IV Unfractionated heparin
(after thrombolytics)
(±) IVC Filter for:
• Contraindication to thrombolytics
• Large residual DVT
• Poor cardiopulmonary reserve/inability to tolerate recurrent PE
(±) Inotropic support
(ie, Dopamaine)

Additional considerations:
• **Early VQ scan** in patients with symptomatic to massive PE (ie, **at discharge**), to establish a **'post-initiation of treatment' perfusion baseline**, for comparison in case they re-present subacutely, with possible recurrent PE
• **IVC Filter removal** (if present) at 4–6 weeks **IF anticoagulation becomes possible** (eg, bleeding risk decreased)
• In general heparin (LMWH or IV unfractionated) should be given for 5 days prior to initinating non warfarin oral anticoagulants

* Warfarin should be given after therapeutic heparinization, with 5 days of heparin, warfarin overlap
‡ Unfractionated heparin (IV) is preferred for those at risk for deterioration

Fig. 15.3 Flow diagram outlining the initial management of venous thromboembolism (VTE), based on the classification and risk stratification. Individuals with a deep vein thrombosis (DVT) and/or pulmonary embolism (PE) (without right ventricular [RV] strain) require anticoagulation alone. Those who cannot be anticoagulated should receive an IVC filter. Individuals with submassive PE require anticoagulation, typically with IV heparin, given their risk for clinical deterioration (if the RV begins to fail). Individuals with submassive PE who have a large residual DVT or poor cardiopulmonary reserve should be considered for inferior vena cava (IVC) filter placement. Individuals with massive PE should receive thrombolytics (in the absence of contraindications). Those who are not candidates for thrombolysis should be offered catheter-based embolectomy, if available (center dependent), or be considered for open embolectomy by CT surgery via cardiopulmonary bypass. Patients with massive PE whose only option is IV heparin, should also have an IVC filter placed (given their inability to tolerate recurrent emboli). Dopamine (typically in the 5–12-mcg/kg/min range) is the inotrope of choice for isolated RV failure (based on expert opinion of its efficacy). Early VQ scanning should be considered in every patient with symptomatic to massive PE to establish an early post VTE baseline, or in any patient whose PE was diagnosed presumptively (ie, with the discovery of a DVT). This is extremely useful if the patient re-presents with signs and symptoms concerning for recurrent VTE, and/or to compare with the 6-month end of an anticoagulation VQ scan. If anticoagulation becomes feasible, IVC filter removal should be perused after 4–6 weeks.

- Patients unable to tolerate anticoagulation require IVC filter placement to prevent death from recurrent emboli
  - IVC filters prevent large recurrent emboli
  - Individuals whose contraindication to anticoagulation is temporary (eg, active bleeding) should be anticoagulated as soon as it is possible/safe, despite having an IVC filter
  - Most IVC filters should be removed when anticoagulation becomes possible, unless the patient has:
    - Recurrent emboli despite therapeutic anticoagulation
    - CTEPH
  - If the filter is **not** removable (by design or complication), anticoagulation should be pursued as soon as possible to:
    - Reduce the risk of postphlebitic syndrome (distal to the area of the DVT)
    - Maintain filter patency
      - IVC filters (in the absence of anticoagulation) may fill with clot, leading to:
        - IVC occlusion with collateral formation (ultimately restoring the risk of pulmonary embolism)
        - Bilateral LE postphlebitic syndrome (very morbid)
        - Clot formation and embolism from the occluded filter itself
- Despite limited data, many experts believe that IVC filters should be offered **with** anticoagulation to patients suffering from:
  - Massive PE who are not candidates for thrombolysis (or who remain in shock after thrombolysis) because of an inability to tolerate any recurrent emboli
  - Massive or submassive PE with a large residual DVT to prevent death from recurrent embolization of the already formed clot
  - Submassive PE with severe preexisting cardiopulmonary disease (ie, poor cardiopulmonary reserve) because of an inability to tolerate any recurrent emboli
- In patients tolerating anticoagulation, IVC filters should be removed after 4–6 weeks
- Thrombolytics should be used in patients with massive PE (and no contraindication)
  - Thrombolytics hasten clot lysis, resolving thrombus approximately 48 hours faster than the body's intrinsic fibrinolytic system
  - The rationale for their use in massive PE is to rapidly reduce RV afterload before RV ischemia can progress to RV infarct (and death)
  - Thrombolytics come with a real risk of major bleeding, especially intracranial hemorrhage
    - Patients require a thorough neurologic examination to ensure no concomitant acute paradoxical embolic CVA
      - Occurs when a PFO opens because of isolated RV-mediated cardiogenic shock, causing high right-sided pressure and low left-sided pressure, favoring right-to-left shunt and creating the risk of paradoxical embolization
      - Outside of a narrow time window (often missed in a massive PE presentation), thrombolytics increase the risk of hemorrhagic conversion associated with embolic stroke and are contraindicated
- Catheter-mediated embolectomy by interventional radiology (IR) and/or surgical embolectomy by CT surgery are center-specific interventions that may be considered (if available) for massive pulmonary embolism in patients with a contraindication to fibrinolytic therapy
- Surgical embolectomy may be the primary modality for a large, mobile RV thrombus (ie, large PE in transit)
  - These clots are found by echocardiogram often appearing to be trapped in the RV by their size (or tethered by a strand), raising the theoretical concern that thrombolysis will provoke embolization (before complete lysis occurs)
- **Pitfalls** in the **diagnosis** of **massive PE**
  - Shock from PE and RV failure is often diagnosed by an echocardiogram showing normal LV function, an elevated PAS pressure, and decreased RV function

- This constellation of findings is **not** pathognomonic for massive PE but instead is commonly seen in diastolic dysfunction, CTEPH, or severe parenchymal lung disease
- RV hypertrophy and/or extremely high PAS pressures imply chronicity and should call into question the acuity, and thus the etiology, of the RV failure
  - Importantly, biventricular failure from diastolic dysfunction and isolated right-sided heart failure from PE can look the same on an echocardiogram:
    - Small, underfilled, hyperdynamic LV, hypodynamic RV with a dilated RA
      - LA enlargement (if present) supports the alternate diagnosis of biventricular failure from diastolic dysfunction
  - Patients with CTEPH are often misdiagnosed as having an acute saddle emboli (receiving thrombolytics inappropriately for a chronic clot)
    - Consider CTEPH when the CTA reveals:
      - RV hypertrophy
      - Mosaicism (from heterogeneous perfusion)
      - Linear appearance to central thrombus
- Deterioration despite anticoagulation:
  - Patients being anticoagulated for a DVT and/or PE who become hemodynamically unstable must be urgently evaluated for acute **hemorrhage** (a complication of anticoagulation) vs **isolated right-sided heart failure** (recurrent emboli or progressive RV failure)
    - Best done by an echocardiogram
      - Small, underfilled ventricles bilaterally suggests acute hemorrhage
      - Dilated RV with a small underfilled LV suggests isolated right-sided heart failure
    - Acute hemorrhage requires cessation of anticoagulation, resuscitation, and IVC filter placement
    - Recurrent emboli and/or progressive RV failure requires inotropic support (eg, dopamine), IVC filter placement, and consideration of thrombolysis
- Role of early VQ scanning:
  - Early VQ scanning (ie, at discharge), to establish an "initiation of treatment" perfusion baseline, can be considered in every patient:
    - Extremely useful if the patient re-presents subacutely, with nonspecific symptoms, possibly related to recurrent emboli (eg, chest pain)
    - Especially in individuals with a significant proximal clot burden (eg, saddle emboli)
      - Specifically helping to separate Migration of a clot (proximal to distal) that may cause pleurisy **without** new perfusion defects (clinically insignificant) vs recurrent emboli/failed therapy **with** new perfusion defects (**very** clinically significant)
  - Early VQ scanning should be performed in patients with a DVT who were treated empirically for symptomatic PE (without a CTA or VQ scan) for future comparison:
      - In case of a subacute representation concerning for recurrent emboli
      - And to compare with the 6-month (end of anticoagulation) perfusion scan
        - Differentiating recurrent emboli (ie, failed anticoagulation), which is suggested by **new** perfusion defects on the 6-month VQ, from persistent perfusion defects (possible CTEPH)

ESTABLISHING THE DURATION OF ANTICOAGULATION AND FOLLOW-UP FOR A VTE (FIG. 15.4)

- **Small provoked VTE** with **transient risk factors** and **no comorbidities**:
  - Plan for **3 months of anticoagulation**
  - At 3 months, obtain a D-dimer and repeat any previously abnormal studies (eg, LE ultrasound, VQ)

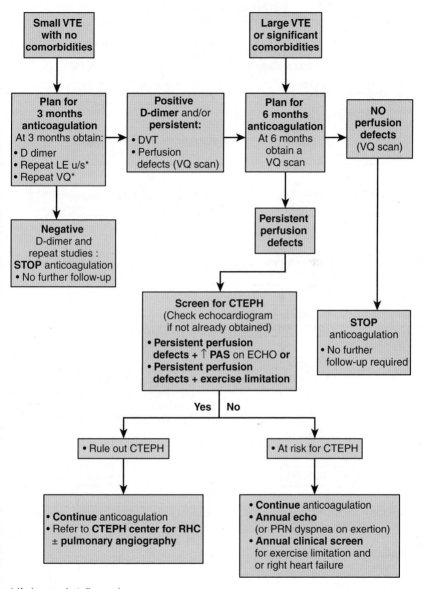

ESTABLISHING THE DURATION OF ANTICOAGULATION AND
FOLLOW UP FOR A PROVOKED VENOUS THROMBOEMBOLISM, ALL RISK FACTORS TRANSIENT

Small VTE with no comorbidities

Large VTE or significant comorbidities

Plan for 3 months anticoagulation
At 3 months obtain:
• D dimer
• Repeat LE u/s*
• Repeat VQ*

Positive D-dimer and/or persistent:
• DVT
• Perfusion defects (VQ scan)

Plan for 6 months anticoagulation
At 6 months obtain a VQ scan

NO perfusion defects (VQ scan)

Negative
D-dimer and repeat studies :
STOP anticoagulation
• No further follow-up

Persistent perfusion defects

Screen for CTEPH
(Check echocardiogram if not already obtained)
• Persistent perfusion defects + ↑ **PAS** on ECHO or
• Persistent perfusion defects + exercise limitation

STOP anticoagulation
• No further follow-up required

Yes | No

• Rule out CTEPH

• At risk for CTEPH

• **Continue** anticoagulation
• Refer to **CTEPH center for RHC** ± pulmonary angiography

• **Continue** anticoagulation
• **Annual echo** (or PRN dyspnea on exertion)
• **Annual clinical screen** for exercise limitation and or right heart failure

* If abnormal at diagnosis

A

Fig. 15.4 (A) Flow diagram outlining the duration of anticoagulation and appropriate follow-up after an individual suffers a provoked DVT with transient risk fractures (eg, a broken leg). Those with a small VTE event and no significant comorbidities may attempt 3 months of anticoagulation. However, if any residual abnormalities persist at 3 months (ie, positive D-dimer, nonocclusive LE thrombus, or a perfusion defect), anticoagulation should be continued for another 3 months. Individuals with a large VTE event or significant comorbidities should be anticoagulated for 6 months. All patients should have a VQ scan performed 6 months after their PE to ensure that their perfusion defects have resolved. Individuals with persistent perfusion defects should be screened for CTEPH by looking for PH and right-sided heart failure. Those with possible PH or right-sided heart failure should be referred to a CTEPH center of excellence for a formal evaluation. Those with a normal echocardiogram and exercise tolerance should be screened annually for the development of PH and/or right-sided heart failure.

Continued

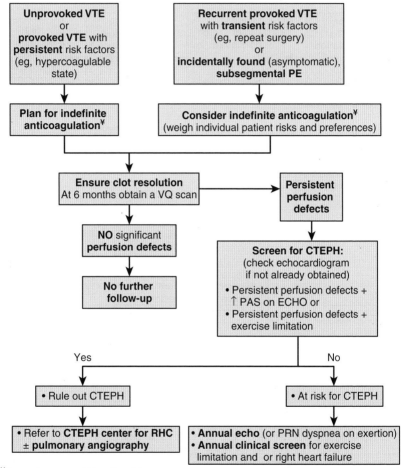

ESTABLISHING THE DURATION OF
ANTICOAGULATION AND FOLLOW-UP FOR:

Unprovoked VTE, provoked VTE (persistent risk factors),
provoked recurrent VTE (transient risk factors),
and **incidentally found**, asymptomatic, subsegmental PE

Unprovoked VTE
or
provoked VTE with
persistent risk factors
(eg, hypercoagulable
state)

Recurrent provoked VTE
with **transient** risk factors
(eg, repeat surgery)
or
incidentally found (asymptomatic),
subsegmental PE

**Plan for indefinite
anticoagulation**¥

Consider indefinite anticoagulation¥
(weigh individual patient risks and preferences)

Ensure clot resolution
At 6 months obtain a VQ scan

**Persistent
perfusion
defects**

NO significant
perfusion defects

Screen for CTEPH:
(check echocardiogram
if not already obtained)
• Persistent perfusion defects +
↑ PAS on ECHO or
• Persistent perfusion defects +
exercise limitation

**No further
follow-up**

Yes

No

• Rule out CTEPH

• At risk for CTEPH

• Refer to **CTEPH center for RHC**
± **pulmonary angiography**

• **Annual echo** (or PRN dyspnea on exertion)
• **Annual clinical screen** for exercise
limitation and or right heart failure

¥Assuming normal bleeding risk

B

Fig. 15.4, Cont'd (B) Flow diagram outlining the duration of anticoagulation and appropriate follow-up after an
individual suffers an unprovoked VTE, a provoked VTE with persistent risk factors, a provoked recurrent VTE (transient
risk factors), or an incidentally found PE. With varying degrees of evidence, all of these individuals should consider
indefinite anticoagulation. The plan for indefinite anticoagulation must always be reevaluated if patients develop
bleeding complications. When data are lacking, as in the incidentally found subsegmental PE, a discussion of risks
and benefits should be had with the patient, allowing their preferences to be weighed heavily. This makes any future
complications and/or undesired outcomes more palatable for the individual (and practitioner). All patients should have
a VQ scan performed 6 months after their PE, looking for persistent perfusion defects, as previously discussed in
panel A.

- Negative D-dimer (and repeat studies) means it is safe to stop anticoagulation
  - No further VTE follow-up required
- Positive D-dimer and/or persistent DVT or perfusion defects
  - Plan for 3 more months of anticoagulation (ie, 6 months total)
- **Small provoked VTE** with **significant comorbidities** or **large provoked VTE** with **transient risk factors**:
  - Plan for **6 months of anticoagulation**
- **Unprovoked VTE** or **provoked VTE with persistent risk factors** (eg, hypercoagulable state)
  - Plan for indefinite anticoagulation
- **Recurrent provoked VTE** with **transient risk factors** (ie, repeat surgery) or **incidentally found subsegmental PE**
  - Consider **indefinite anticoagulation** (vs 6 months), weighing individual patient risk for serious bleeding against the risk of death from recurrent VTE
  - Factor in patient priorities and preferences
- **After 6 months of anticoagulation, obtain a VQ scan** and repeat any previously abnormal VTE studies (ie, LE ultrasound and or echocardiogram)
  - Establish the presence or absence of persistent perfusion defects
    - **No perfusion defects**:
      - **Stop anticoagulation**; no further VTE follow-up is required
      - A persistent nonocclusive DVT is considered a chronic DVT
        - Management is based on the presence and severity of postphlebitic symptoms and ranges from compression stockings to more aggressive catheter-guided fibrinolytic or mechanical approaches
      - A persistently abnormal echocardiogram in the absence of perfusion defects is **not** related to VTE and should be worked up independently (eg, screen for occult left heart failure)
    - **Persistent perfusion defects**:
      - **Screen for CTEPH** with an echocardiogram
      - **Elevated PAS or RV failure** seen on **echocardiogram** or unexplained **exercise limitation**/right-sided heart failure signs and symptoms
        - **Continue anticoagulation**
        - **Refer to a CTEPH center for RHC and possible pulmonary angiography**
      - Normal **echocardiogram** and/or no exercise limitation/right-sided heart failure signs and symptoms
        - Patient is **at risk** for CTEPH
        - Though data is limited most experts continue anticoagulation in the face of significant persistent perfusion defects
        - Inform patient to report any change in exercise ability
      - Perform a yearly echocardiogram for 5 years (or indefinitely if the perfusion defects are extensive)

UPPER EXTREMITY DVTS

- Upper extremity DVTs occur in two different circumstances, each with very different inciting factors, management approaches, and overall prognoses:
  - **Inpatients,** as a **complication of hospitalization with central line use**
  - **Outpatients,** as a **spontaneous event**
- Upper extremity DVT as a complication of hospitalization:
  - Majority associated with central line/PICC use AND malignancy
    - Often nonocclusive
    - Have low rates of symptomatic pulmonary embolism and postphlebtic syndrome
    - Are managed with line removal and anticoagulation

- Upper extremity DVTs occurring spontaneously in outpatients:
  - Majority are related to upper extremity effort (Paget-Schroetter syndrome), thoracic outlet syndrome, or upper extremity trauma
    - Often the clot is extensive and occlusive
    - High rates of symptomatic pulmonary embolism and postphlebitic syndrome
      - Brachial plexus injury and complex regional pain syndrome are both extremely morbid potential consequences
    - Should be managed in consultation with vascular surgery or vascular IR, so that catheter mediated thrombectomy or local instillation of tPA may be considered

COMMON QUESTIONS GENERATED BY THIS TEACHING

1. Where is the DVT in an individual with a pulmonary embolism **and** negative bilateral lower extremity Dopplers?
   The majority of DVTs not occurring in the lower extremities arise in the pelvis and are difficult to screen for (usually requiring venography) and thus are typically presumed.
2. If there were an ultrasound-proven DVT and it completely embolized (repeat ultrasound negative at time of PE), would I still need to use heparin?
   Yes. Even though most of the clot has embolized, one must presume an injured vascular surface remains, where residual thrombus is ready to extend, break off, and cause a recurrent embolus.
3. What is the preferred approach to a PE diagnosed "in transit" (ie, thrombus found trapped in the RV during an echocardiogram)?
   Expert opinion favors CT surgery intervention with open cardiac embolectomy (performed on cardiopulmonary bypass). Assuming no contraindication, thrombolytics may be used if a CT surgical intervention is not possible or safe, given comorbidities or lack of resources.

CHAPTER 16

PNEUMOTHORAX AND BRONCHOPLEURAL FISTULAS: AIR IN THE PLEURAL SPACE

COMMON MISCONCEPTIONS AND MISTAKES

- The proper way to screen for a pneumothorax (PTX) is by looking for areas on the chest x-ray (CXR) that do not have lung markings

- A pneumothorax (PTX) occurring after an uncomplicated/successful thoracentesis likely represents air entrained around the needle/catheter

- A chest tube should always be placed on suction to physically suck the visceral pleura up against the chest wall (ie, to maintain pleural apposition) when a BPF exists

  - Thinking that a PTX is synonymous with a bronchopleural fistula (BPF)

APPROACH TO THE PNEUMOTHORAX

- A PTX means air in the pleural space

- Commonly detected in three situations, when a chest radiograph is obtained to evaluate:
  1. Chest pain (pleura innervated with pain fibers) and/or SOB
  2. Elevated airway pressure in a mechanically ventilated patient
  3. For possible postprocedure complication (after thoracentesis, central line or chest tube placement)

- A PTX should be screened for (and is usually detected by) demonstration of a visceral pleural edge (separated from the parietal pleura and chest wall) appearing as an *unexpected line:*
  - Often at the apex, because air will rise in a normal upright thorax (Fig. 16.1)
  - Supine patients (like those requiring mechanical ventilation) will have air rise and accumulate at the base of the lung (deep sulcus sign) because the apex is more dependent when supine (Fig. 16.2)
  - Although an absence of lung markings is also apparent when a PTX is large, this finding is less reliable in detecting a small PTX at the apex
    - Especially with apical bullous disease, where lung markings are sparse
  - Additionally, individuals with pleural parenchymal scarring may have a loculated PTX:
    - The unexpected pleural line may **not** be apical if the apex is scarred
    - A loculated PTX may have lung markings visible past the visceral pleural edge as aspects of the lung are tethered to the chest wall (Fig. 16.3)

- Initial evaluation of the PTX should assess the size as **small** or **large**:
  - **Small**: $<\sim3\,cm$ between the chest wall and the visceral pleural line (at any point)
  - **Large**: $>\sim3\,cm$ between the chest wall and the visceral pleural line (at any point)
  - Very large PTXs (like those causing tension physiology) should be obvious on physical examination (absent breath sounds over a hemithorax) and imaging (no lung markings)

Apical Pneumothorax

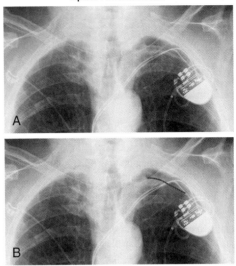

Fig. 16.1 (A) Left apical pneumothorax evidenced by an unexpected apical line (visceral pleural edge), (B) outlined in red. **Note:** A pacemaker with leads complicates the visual field.

Deep Sulcus Sign

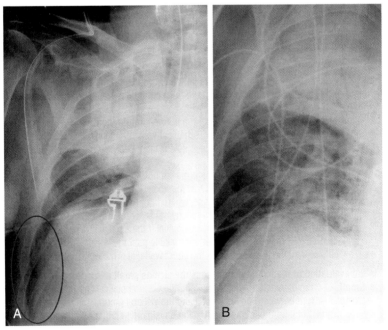

Fig. 16.2 (A) Right basilar deep sulcus sign. Note that the area of the sulcus appears excessively black (ie, as black as air outside of the chest) (B) Close-up.

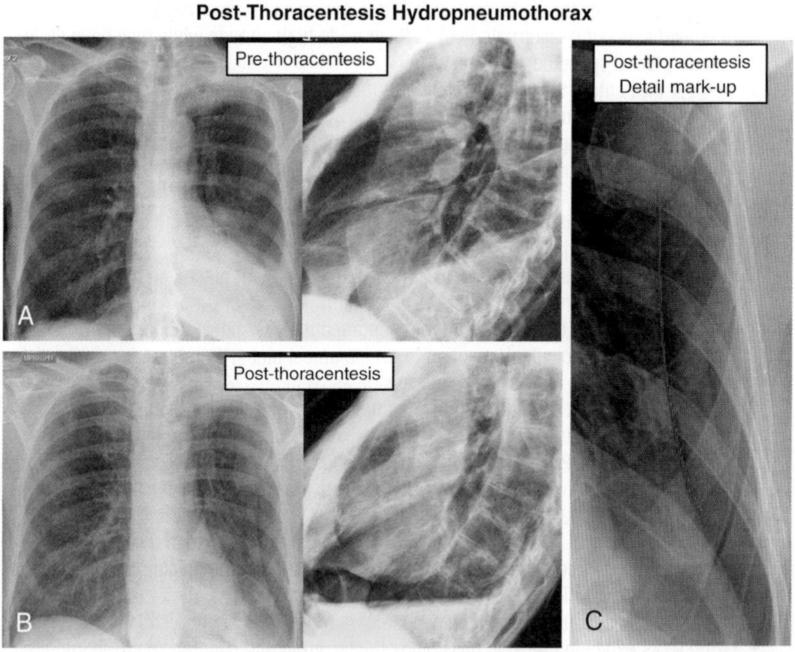

Post-Thoracentesis Hydropneumothorax

Fig. 16.3 (A) Posteroanterior (PA) and lateral chest x-ray showing a left-sided pleural effusion. (B) Repeat PA and lateral chest x-ray after thoracentesis, showing a left hydropneumothorax as evidenced by a straight line (air-fluid interface) on the lateral film. (C) Close inspection of the frontal x-ray demonstrates a loculated pneumothorax (PTX) evidenced by a lateral pleural edge, with lung markings visible beyond it. The PTX was loculated because the patient had had radiation therapy for left upper lobe lung cancer (note the opacified left apex with left hilar retraction, indicating scarring and volume loss).

- **Large PTXs should be screened for signs of tension (eg, mediastinal shift away from the PTX; see Chapter 4)**
  - Tension physiology occurs when a persistent bronchopleural fistula (BPF) develops a check valve-like behavior:
    - Inspiration generates negative intrathoracic pressure, which expands the lungs, opens the bronchi, and promotes airflow from the tracheobronchial tree through the BPF and into the pleural space
    - Exhalation generates positive intrathoracic pressure, which collapses the bronchi, decreasing airflow through the BPF, thus trapping air in the pleural space
    - Each respiratory cycle progressively increases the volume of air in the pleural space, increasing intrathoracic pressure and eventually decreasing venous return to the right atrium
      - The right ventricle (RV), in the face of decreased preload (and diminished filling), attempts to maintain cardiac output (CO) by becoming tachycardic
      - Eventually RV stroke volume and CO fall, leading to decreased left ventricle (LV) CO and systemic hypotension (cardiogenic shock)
      - If unchecked, this process will lead to PEA cardiac arrest as venous return to the right atrium effectively falls to zero and the heart fails to fill
    - Tension physiology mandates urgent decompression, or venting of the thorax

- Observation vs. small-bore **chest tube placement**
  - Small PTXs in patients **not** requiring mechanical ventilation should be observed
    - A repeat CXR in 4 to 6 hours demonstrating stability or decrease in size of the PTX suggests resolution of the BPF

- Any residual air should be reabsorbed in a matter of hours or days
  - Patients should be instructed not to fly or go to high altitude while they have air in their pleural space because:
    - Air that enters the pleural space at atmospheric pressure will expand when ambient pressure drops
- Small PTXs occurring in patients placed on mechanical ventilation can rapidly expand and create tension physiology such that the vast majority will require chest tube placement
  - Repeat imaging (if indicated by extremely small initial size) should be done at short time intervals initially (30–60 minutes)
- Large PTXs, expanding PTXs, or PTXs occurring in a patient placed on mechanical ventilation typically require chest tube placement
  - Patients **without COPD** (ie, primary spontaneous PTX) should be nonemergently evaluated for surgical intervention to excise apical blebs, thereby reducing the risk of recurrence (often on the contralateral side as well)
    - These patients should be counseled never to scuba dive (without surgical intervention bilaterally)
  - Patients **with COPD** (ie, secondary spontaneous PTX) also have high recurrence rates:
    - The decision to intervene surgically involves many factors:
      - Benign vs catastrophic nature of the initial presentation
      - Morbidity of VATS in patients with severe parenchymal lung disease
      - Difficulty finding normal lung to staple through (thereby risking the creation of additional BPFs)
    - Recurrence is the most definitive indication for surgical intervention
- Large PTXs exhibiting tension physiology (tachycardia and hypotension from impaired venous return) should be urgently decompressed:
  - 18-gauge needle (of appropriate length to reach the pleural space) blindly inserted into the anterior second intercostal space at the midclavicular line
    - Leading to an audible/tactile evacuation of air from the thorax
  - This stabilizes the patient allowing for more definitive chest tube placement
    - Required to prevent recurrent PTX and tension physiology as the BPF continues its check valve behavior

- **A PTX occurring after uncomplicated thoracentesis or chest tube insertion** for drainage of a pleural effusion is typically an **ex-vacuo** phenomenon, representing a vacuous space (ie, created by a vacuum) and not actually "air" occurring when:
  - Fluid removal fails to lead to lung reexpansion because of a stiff, noncompliant, diseased visceral pleura, which encases the lung and prevents reexpansion
    - Pleura may be visibly thickened on CT scan
  - Lung entrapment vs trapped lung can only be determined over time, based on whether or not the lung ultimately reexpands
  - The lung is said to be "entrapped" if over time it ultimately reexpands, implying that the pleural disease represented an acute inflammatory process (Fig. 16.4)
  - The lung is said to be "trapped" if it never reexpands, usually as a result of postinflammatory scarring or malignancy
  - When the lung is trapped the effusion will reaccumulate, filling the ex-vacuo space over time (days to weeks) (Fig. 16.5)
    - The ex-vacuo pleural collection, with its more negative pressure, gradually draws a serous (transudative) fluid into the space until it fills (equalizing the pleural and tissue pressures)
    - Repeated thoracentesis in this situation only makes sense if the patient's effusion recurs **and then** extends beyond the trapped lung edge, producing symptoms by compressing normal lung, as occurs with ongoing exudative pathology (eg, pleural infection or malignancy)

Lung Entrapment

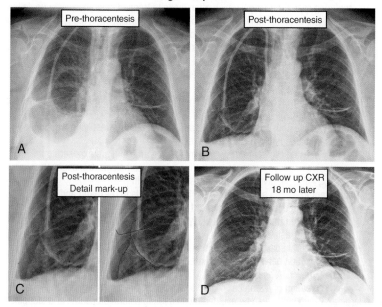

Fig. 16.4 (A) Frontal view of the chest shows a loculated right-sided pleural effusion. (B) Repeat frontal view of the chest after an uncomplicated thoracentesis shows a loculated right basilar hydropneumothorax. (C) Close-up panel shows several abnormal pleural lines (outlined in red). (D) Repeat chest x-ray (CXR) 18 months later shows lung reexpansion with only slight pleural thickening remaining.

Trapped Lung

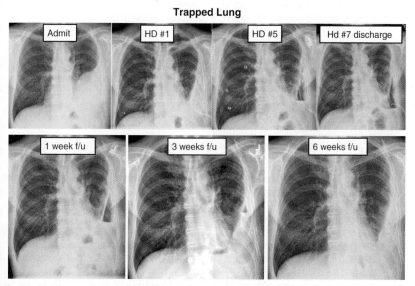

Fig. 16.5 Frontal views of the chest demonstrate a left-sided, loculated pleural effusion on admission. Small-bore chest tube drainage resulted in a hydropneumothorax. Serial imaging demonstrates that the lung is trapped by visceral pleural scarring such that it never reexpands. Instead, the ex-vacuo space fills over time with a transudative effusion.

- Malignant pleural effusions are commonly recurrent, large, and symptomatic requiring repeat drainage, which often leads to trapped lung physiology (ie, failure of the lung to completely reexpand with drainage, which often leads to trapped lung physiology (ie, failure of the lung to completely reexpand with drainage))
  - Because the trapped lung prevents pleural apposition, pleurodesis is impossible
  - In this situation, a tunneled pleural catheter may allow for intermittent pleural drainage, just to the point of lung entrapment, relieving symptoms without causing an ex-vacuo space
- One should attempt to avoid the creation of a large ex-vacuo (negative pressure) space during thoracentesis for two reasons:
  1. It may cause chest pain as the pleura is tugged on (only resolving when fluid reaccumulates and pressure increases)
  2. It may cause a BPF as relatively normal pleura and lung are exposed to the excessive negative pressure, promoting a large, pathologic, transpulmonary gradient ($P_{airways} - P_{pleura}$), favoring overexpansion and tearing
- A persistent ex-vacuo space, where the lung both fails to reexpand and fails to reaccumulate fluid, implies a **persistent BPF**
  - In this situation the patent is not likely to develop further lung collapse or tension (the trapped lung resists collapse)
  - But the pleural space is vulnerable to recurrent infection because of ongoing communication between contaminated airway secretions and the sterile pleural space (Fig. 16.6A and B)
- While the creation of a small ex-vacuo space post thoracentesis may be inevitable, a large ex-vacuo space can be avoided by measuring pleural pressures and stopping fluid removal when patients develop negative pressures in excess of -15 to -20 cm H_2O

PATHOPHYSIOLOGY OF BRONCHOPLEURAL FISTULAS

- **Air can only enter the pleural space in two ways:**
  - Through the tracheobronchial tree via a BPF (**very common**) or
  - Through the chest wall via a hole caused by penetrating trauma or a transthoracic procedure where the thorax is accidentally left open to air (**rare**)

- BPFs occur in four situations:
- Blunt chest wall trauma (eg, broken rib lacerates visceral pleura and bronchi)
- **Iatrogenically**, after a thoracic procedure (eg, central line placement, thoracentesis, transbronchial biopsy, transthoracic lung biopsy)
- As a **"secondary"** complication in patients with underlying lung disease (mainly chronic obstructive pulmonary disease [COPD]) or
- As a **"primary,"** spontaneous event occurring in an individual without recognized lung disease (typically tall young men with long thoraces/apical blebs)

- **Iatrogenic BPFs** occurring as a procedural complication in normal lung tissue from a needle are commonly **small** and **transient,** requiring observation only (to ensure no active BPF):
  - Typically cause a small PTX (<3 cm between the chest wall and visceral pleural line)
  - Asymptomatic; detected on routine postprocedure CXR
  - Occur during needle insertion when visceral pleura, alveolar tissue, and terminal bronchi are crossed (intentionally in the case of an IR-guided lung Bx or unintentionally during central line placement), leading to a transient release of air from the tracheobronchial tree into the pleural space
  - Injured alveolar air sacs collapse and normal surrounding lung expands to fill the space and seal the defect
    - The immediate postprocedure CXR demonstrates a small PTX

Persistent BP fistula with Trapped Lung Complicated by Recurrent Pleural Infection

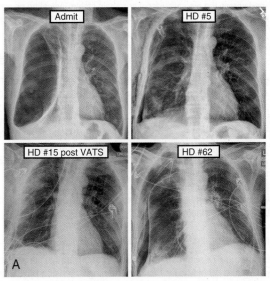

Persistent large air leak requiring continuous suction, despite VATS (blebectomy & pleurodesis)
ultimately requiring endobronchial valve placement (eventually allowing chest tube removal)

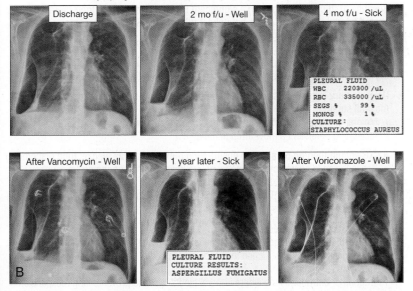

Fig. 16.6 (A) Frontal view of the chest shows a large, right-sided pneumothorax on admission, evacuated with a surgical chest tube. A persistent, large air leak requiring continuous suction prompts a video-assisted thoracic surgery (blebectomy and pleurodesis), which fails, ultimately necessitating endobronchial valve placement (eventually allowing chest tube removal). (B) Frontal view of the chest shows a right-sided hydropneumothorax increasing after discharge suggesting trapped lung with an ex-vacuo space passively filling with a transudative process, until the patient re-presented 4 months later, febrile, with a thoracentesis showing methicillin-resistant *Staphylococcus aureus* infection, (suggesting persistent bronchopleural fistula [BPF] occurring with trapped lung) in addition to trapped lung. The effusion decreases and the patient defervesces after vancomycin treatment, only to re-present 1 year later, febrile, with a repeat thoracentesis aspirate growing aspergillus. Again the effusion decreases, and the patient defervesces after treatment. The lung never reexpands, because it is trapped, yet it does not fill with fluid, because of a persistent BPF. Increasing fluid in this individual actual reflected recurrent infection.

- After 4 hours, a follow-up CXR will either show improvement (as the air is passively reabsorbed across the pleural surface) or remain stable, indicating no active/ongoing BPF
- Because the pleural air collection is ~80% nitrogen, placing the patient on 100% oxygen (for the 4-6 hours while waiting for the repeat CXR) can "wash" nitrogen out of the blood
  - Replacing all the dissolved nitrogen in the blood with oxygen creates a strong gradient for nitrogen gas to exit the pleural space and enter the bloodstream

- **Spontaneous BPFs** are associated with a ruptured bleb or bullae occurring as a complication of underlying lung disease (mainly COPD) or as a primary disease in the predisposed (typically young males with long thoraces and apical blebs)
  - Spontaneous BPFs represent a primary failure of lung parenchymal integrity
  - Secondary, spontaneous BPFs (as seen in COPD) are often **large** and persistent because:
    - The defects are large (abnormally compliant lung tears) and
    - There is a paucity of normal surrounding lung tissue to expand and close defects
    - Secondary spontaneous BPFs:
      - May take days or weeks to heal
      - Have high recurrence rates, occasionally requiring surgical intervention (blebectomy and pleurodesis) (Fig. 16.7A and B)

MANAGEMENT OF PERSISTENT BRONCHOPLEURAL FISTULAS:

- A large or expanding PTX suggests the presence of an "active" or persistent BPF at risk for behaving in a "check valve" fashion, leading to tension physiology (previously described)

- Because of this individuals with a significant BP fistula must have their thorax urgently vented by placement of a small-bore chest tube via the Seldinger technique

- Initial chest tube insertion should be followed by a rush of air out of the thorax

- To facilitate complete air evacuation, the chest tube should be connected to a dry-suction water seal system and placed on suction initially

- Unless a very large BPF is suspected, the patient should then be placed on water seal (no wall suction)
  - Maintaining large negative pleural pressures with suction may hinder BPF healing by facilitating persistent airflow through the defect

- A CXR should then be obtained to ensure lung reexpansion (as well as tube placement)
  - Reexpansion is proven by demonstrating pleural apposition on the postevacuation CXR (resolution of the visceral pleural line)
  - Reexpansion promotes BPF closure (allowing uninjured lung to expand, helping to close defects)

- **Failure to reexpand implies either a:**
  - Large BPF (obvious, large, continuous air leak treated with continued suction)
  - Concomitant airway obstruction (tumor or foreign body), which prevents the atelectatic lobe from reinflating
  - Trapped or entrapped lung where visceral pleural disease prevents lung reexpansion

- A persistent BPF (failing to heal in days or weeks) may require surgical resection, where a staple line is created in an area of relatively normal lung between the BP fistula and the hilum, subanatomically resecting an area with blebs and bullae (where the BPF is believed to be located)
  - This can be difficult or impossible in patients with significant parenchymal disease (no normal lung to staple through)
  - Endobronchial valves may have an off-label role in this situation, allowing for decreased airflow, promoting healing (although BPF localization can be extremely difficult)

Recurrent Secondary Spontaneous Pneumothorax

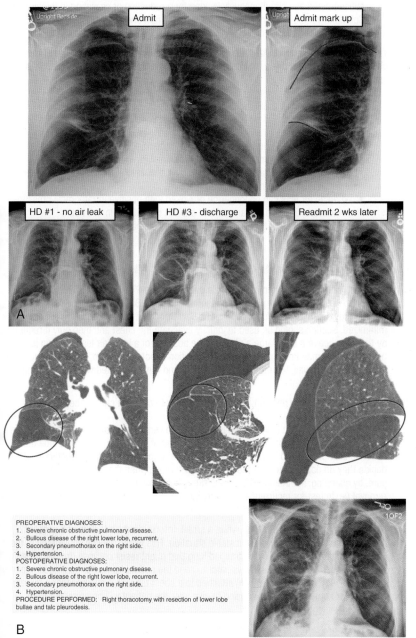

PREOPERATIVE DIAGNOSES:
1. Severe chronic obstructive pulmonary disease.
2. Bullous disease of the right lower lobe, recurrent.
3. Secondary pneumothorax on the right side.
4. Hypertension.
POSTOPERATIVE DIAGNOSES:
1. Severe chronic obstructive pulmonary disease.
2. Bullous disease of the right lower lobe, recurrent.
3. Secondary pneumothorax on the right side.
4. Hypertension.
PROCEDURE PERFORMED: Right thoracotomy with resection of lower lobe bullae and talc pleurodesis.

Fig. 16.7 (A) Frontal view of the chest on admission shows a large, right-sided pneumothorax (PTX), evacuated with a small-bore chest tube, achieving lung reexpansion and bronchopleural fistula closure (no air leak). The patient was then readmitted 2 weeks later with a recurrent right-sided PTX. (B) A chest computed tomography scan shows right lower lobe bullae and subpleural blebs amenable to surgical intervention. A frontal-view chest x-ray shows right lower lobe linear scarring and staples after a successful video-assisted thoracic surgery blebectomy and pleurodesis.

- Endobronchial localization is attempted by individually balloon-occluding airway subsegments and simultaneously looking for a reduction or cessation in the air leak
- Collateral ventilation, where air passes directly from one adjacent lung segment to another via pores, can make this process less sensitive (and less satisfying)

- **The presence and relative size of a BPF is determined by the air leaking out of the chest from the pleural drain (not based on imaging because the defect is usually too small to see)**
  - BPFs do not behave in a binary fashion (ie, open or closed)
  - The air leak caused by a BPF tends to:
    - Start out continuous (as air is evacuated from the chest) and stay continuous if the BPF is large
    - As healing begins The air leak becomes intermittent, associated with exhalation alone, and then it becomes infrequent, only seen with forceful cough
      - Before concluding that a BPF is healed, one should look for the presence of an air leak during a forced maximal cough
      - When an air leak can no longer be provoked with positive intrathoracic pressure maneuvers, the tube is clamped and an CXR is obtained in 4-6 hours
        - No recurrence of the PTX means the BP fistula has healed and the tube should be removed

COMMON QUESTIONS GENERATED BY THIS TEACHING

1. **Is suction good or bad when managing a patient with a PTX from a BPF? Do I need suction to ensure/maintain pleural apposition while the BPF heals?**
   Suction may serve to perpetuate continuous flow through a BPF and thus should be minimized. Suction should be used to initially evacuate the chest and then only if required by the presence of a **very** large air leak. In the absence of a large air leak, suction is **not** required to maintain pleural apposition. Suction is **not** required to "suck the lung up against the chest wall." Normal lungs will inflate and remain inflated without requiring additional force.

2. **During my CT surgery rotation, I was taught never to clamp a chest tube (question implied by tone).**
   Philosophically speaking a chest tube is designed to vent the thorax. If you clamp a chest tube, it can no longer vent the thorax. So, in the mind of a surgeon, any chest tube that could be clamped should just be removed. Practically speaking medicine doctors tend to decide they do not need to vent the thorax any more, but then they check, just to make sure, by clamping. In other words, a chest tube should **only** be clamped in preparation for removal (ie, to test for recurrence or worsening of the PTX when the thorax is closed yet still easy to open again—by simply unclamping the tube).

3. **Should I ever clamp a chest tube while a small, intermittent air leak is still present?**
   No. This represents an inherently unstable situation. This would only be considered in the case of both a persistent BPF and trapped lung that might resist collapse (from scarring involving the chest wall). It is always safer to send the patient home (for continued healing) with a one-way valve (eg, Heimlich) attached to a chest tube. This ensures that if forceful coughing at home causes an adhesion to give way, the patient will be protected from tension physiology.

4. **How do I know when to take the chest tube out?**
   Under most circumstances, when a patient tolerates clamping for 4 to 6 hours.

CHAPTER 17

DIFFUSE PARENCHYMAL LUNG DISEASE AND ITS MIMICS

COMMON MISCONCEPTIONS AND MISTAKES

- Bronchoscopy with transbronchial biopsies are usually indicated and helpful in the evaluation of diffuse parenchymal lung disease
- Video-assisted thoracoscopic surgery (VATS) lung biopsy is always required to confirm the diagnosis of usual interstitial pneumonia (UIP)/idiopathic pulmonary fibrosis (IPF)
- Bronchial alveolar lavage is **always** the initial step in the evaluation of diffuse parenchymal lung disease (DPLD)
- Prematurely celebrating a steroid response in a patient with hypoxemic respiratory failure secondary to DPLD
- Advising a patient with respiratory failure and DPLD to be do not intubat (DNI) because they "will never be able to be extubated"

DIFFUSE PARENCHYMAL LUNG DISEASE

- Describes a diverse group of conditions that share the common pathologic feature of diffuse interstitial and/or alveolar inflammation, cellular infiltration, and/or fibrosis
  - Fibrosis may exist alone, as in UIP, or with an inflammatory cellular infiltrate, as in nonspecific interstitial pneumonia (NSIP)
- The radiographic patterns exist on a spectrum from specific—as in UIP, where a "definite UIP" scan can obviate the need for biopsy—to diffuse ground glass (broad differential)
- Several DPLD entities have classic, characteristic CT scan patterns (eg, chronic eosinophilic pneumonia [CEP], cryptogenic organizing pneumonia [COP], respiratory bronchiolitis-associated interstitial lung disease/desquamative interstitial pneumonia [RB-ILD/DIP]), recognition of which is key to appropriate evaluation and management
- The clinical presentations are diverse and can be broadly divided into three categories:
  - **Asymptomatic**
    - Incidental finding in chest x-ray films and/or CT imaging
  - **Subacute**
    - Progressive dyspnea on exertion (weeks to months)
    - Often with cough, night sweats, and fatigue
    - Pulmonary function tests (PFTs) show restriction with a reduced diffusing capacity of the lung for carbon monoxide (DLCO) (may show isolated low DLCO initially)
  - **Acute hypoxemic respiratory failure** (days to weeks)
    - Often progresses over days
    - May require 100% O_2 (high flow), bilevel positive airway pressure (BiPAP), or mechanical ventilation with high positive end-expiratory pressure (PEEP)
    - In the case of an acute exacerbation of UIP/IPF, it is often fatal
- **Cardiogenic pulmonary edema** (ie, heart failure) and **atypical pneumonia** (eg, pneumocystis jiroveci pneumonia [PJP], nontuberculous mycobacteria [NTM], viral) are important, common mimics
- Presumptive diagnosis of DPLD requires integrating the clinical presentation with the CT scan radiographic pattern
  - Often made **after** empirically treating and/or ruling out heart failure and atypical pneumonia

- Definitive diagnosis often requires a lung biopsy (not always practical or feasible) and a compatible clinical scenario
  - Adequate biopsy requires VATS, with multiple areas sampled (avoiding clearly fibrotic "burned out" areas)
  - Patients with fibrosis are at high risk for developing a persistent BP fistula after VATS, leading to:
    - Prolonged hospitalization (initially tethered to suction)
    - Discharge from the hospital with a chest tube and one-way valve (eg, Heimlich)
  - Occasionally patients experience accelerated fibrosis after VATS, leading to refractory/persistent hypoxemic respiratory failure, necessitating terminal extubation
- The **role of bronchoscopy** in diffuse parenchymal lung disease is to:
  - **Rule out atypical infection** (mainly):
    - PJP
    - NTM
    - Viral pneumonia (via polymerase chain reaction [PCR] testing)
  - **Make the diagnosis of:**
    - Diffuse alveolar hemorrhage (DAH)
      - Progressively bloodier alveolar lavage
    - Acute and chronic eosinophilic pneumonia
      - Bronchoalveolar lavage (BAL) eosinophilia >25% (often >60% in CEP)
    - Sarcoidosis (via endobronchial ultrasound–guided transbronchial needle aspiration)
      - Noncaseating granuloma, with no organism or material identified
    - Lymphangitic spread of tumor (via transbronchial biopsy)
      - Malignant cells identified by surgical pathology
    - Pulmonary alveolar proteinosis
      - Periodic acid shift (PAS) positive; milky, granular fluid recovered at BAL
  - **Support the diagnosis of:**
    - Cryptogenic organizing pneumonia
      - >25% lymphocyte cell count by BAL
    - Acute interstitial pneumonia
      - >25% (often >60%) neutrophil count by BAL
    - Pulmonary Langerhans cells
      - CD1a-positive Langerhans (>5%) cells
- Diagnostic and therapeutic approaches to diffuse parenchymal lung disease hinge on integrating the clinical presentation and CT scan pattern (Table 17.1)

ASYMPTOMATIC DIFFUSE PARENCHYMAL LUNG DISEASE PATTERN INCIDENTALLY FOUND BY CHEST CT IMAGING

- PFTs are normal, mildly restricted, or show an isolated low DLCO
- **Chest CT** scan **suggests:**
  - **Definite to possible UIP, NSIP, or hypersensitivity pneumonitis (HP)**
    - Classic imaging features shared by all three entities (Fig. 17.1):
      - Diffuse subpleural reticular infiltrate
      - Ground-glass opacities
      - Traction bronchiectasis
    - Diagnostic workup involves a clinical and/or immunologic **screen** for:
      - Hypersensitivity (eg, farmer's lung) and pneumoconiosis (eg, asbestosis)
        - Query exposures to birds, asbestos, silica, and environments that produce (or have produced in the past) respiratory symptoms for the patient
        - Check a hypersensitivity panel
      - Connective tissue disease
        - Examination for skin, muscle, and joint disease
        - Serology for RF, ANA, and ESR

Table 17.1 Restrictive Pattern on Pulmonary Function Testing (PFT)

CT SCAN PATTERN / PREDOMINANT FINDING	*Clinical Presentation*			
	ASYMPTOMATIC	SUBACUTE PRESENTATION	ACUTE PRESENTATION	
	Incidental Finding	Progressive DOE ± Dry Cough	Hypoxemic Respiratory Failure	
Usual Interstitial Pneumonia (UIP) Pattern: • Diffuse Subpleural Reticular Infiltrate • Lower lobe predominance • ≥ 2 rows of 'Honey Combing' • Traction Bronchiectasis **Minimal or NO:** Ground Glass, Nodules, Cysts, Adenopathy	Idiopathic Pulmonary Fibrosis (i.e. UIP) • Drug Induced • Connective tissue disease related Pneumoconiosis Post-Inflammatory	Idiopathic Pulmonary Fibrosis (i.e. UIP) • Drug Induced • Connective tissue disease related Pneumoconiosis	Idiopathic Pulmonary Fibrosis (i.e. UIP) • Drug Induced • Connective tissue disease related	
Non-specific Interstitial Pneumonia Pattern: • Multifocal Ground Glass Opacities • Scattered Subpleural Reticular Infiltrate • Traction Bronchiectasis **Minimal or NO:** Honeycomb Cysts	Non-specific Interstitial Pneumonia • Drug Induced • Connective Tissue Disease associated Pneumoconiosis	Non-specific Interstitial Pneumonia • Drug Induced • Connective Tissue Disease associated Pneumoconiosis Chronic Hypersensitivity Pneumonitis (upper lobe)	Non-specific Interstitial Pneumonia • Drug Induced • Connective Tissue Disease associated Acute Hypersensitivity Pneumonitis (upper lobe)	
Ground Glass Opacities alone	Respiratory Bronchiolitis-associated ILD Simple Pulmonary Eosinophilia	Desquamative Interstitial Pneumonia Pneumocystis Jiroveci Pneumonia Respiratory Bronchiolitis-associated ILD Simple Pulmonary Eosinophilia	Acute Respiratory Distress Syndrome Cardiogenic Pulmonary Edema (effusions) Diffuse Alveolar Hemorrhage Pneumocystis Jiroveci Pneumonia	
Ground Glass Opacities with Dense Consolidations ± Traction Bronchiectasis	Cryptogenic Organizing Pneumonia (Reverse Halo) Nontuberculous Mycobacteria (Tree & Bud) Chronic Aspiration	Cryptogenic Organizing Pneumonia (Reverse Halo) Chronic Eosinophilic Pneumonia (peripheral) Nontuberculous Mycobacteria (Tree & Bud)	Acute Eosinophilic Pneumonia Acute Interstitial Pneumonia Acute Respiratory Distress Syndrome Cardiogenic Pulmonary Edema (effusions) Cryptogenic Organizing Pneumonia (Reverse Halo) Severe Bacterial Pneumonia	

(Continued)

Table 17.1 Restrictive Pattern on Pulmonary Function Testing (PFT)—cont'd

CT SCAN PATTERN / PREDOMINANT FINDING	Clinical Presentation			
	ASYMPTOMATIC	SUBACUTE PRESENTATION	ACUTE PRESENTATION	
	Incidental Finding	Progressive DOE ± Dry Cough	Hypoxemic Respiratory Failure	
Nodules (Bronchovascular & Perilymphatic) with: • Hilar and mediastinal adenopathy • Conglomerate masses / Dense consolidations • ± Ground Glass	Sarcoidosis Stage II – III Lymphangitic / Metastatic Spread of Tumor	Sarcoidosis Stage II – III Lymphangitic/ Metastatic Spread of Tumor	Sarcoidosis Stage II – III Lymphangitic/ Metastatic Spread of Tumor	
Nodules (Centrilobular)	Nontuberculous Mycobacteria (Tree & Bud) Early Pulmonary Langerhans (Cavitary)	Nontuberculous Mycobacteria (Tree & Bud) Early Pulmonary Langerhans (Cavitary)	***	
Crazy Paving	Alveolar Proteinosis	Alveolar Proteinosis Cardiogenic Pulmonary Edema Lymphangitic Spread of Tumor	Cardiogenic Pulmonary Edema (effusions) Viral Pneumonia	
Cysts	Lymphocytic Interstitial Pneumonia	Lymphocytic Interstitial Pneumonia Lymphangioleiomyomatosis Late Pulmonary Langerhans (large, thicker walled)	Lymphocytic Interstitial Pneumonia Lymphangioleiomyomatosis	

Obstructive or Mixed Obstructive Restrictive Pattern on PFT

CT SCAN PATTERN / PREDOMINANT FINDING	Clinical Presentation			
	ASYMPTOMATIC	SUBACUTE PRESENTATION	ACUTE PRESENTATION	
	Incidental Finding	Progressive DOE ± Dry Cough	Respiratory Failure	
Ground Glass opacities alone	Respiratory Bronchiolitis-associated ILD	Respiratory Bronchiolitis-associated ILD	Cardiogenic Pulmonary Edema (effusions)	
Nodules (Bronchovascular & Perilymphatic) with: • Hilar and mediastinal adenopathy • Conglomerate masses / Dense consolidations • ± Ground Glass	Sarcoidosis (Stage II – III)	Sarcoidosis (Stage II – III)	Sarcoidosis (Stage II – III)	
Mosaicism from Air Trapping (Tree & Bud)	Bronchiolitis Obliterans	Bronchiolitis Obliterans	Bronchiolitis Obliterans	
Diffuse Cysts	Lymphangioleiomyomatosis	Lymphangioleiomyomatosis	Lymphangioleiomyomatosis	
Cavitary Nodules and Large Cysts	Pulmonary Langerhans	Pulmonary Langerhans	*******************************	

Types of Diffuse Parenchymal Lung Disease Opacities

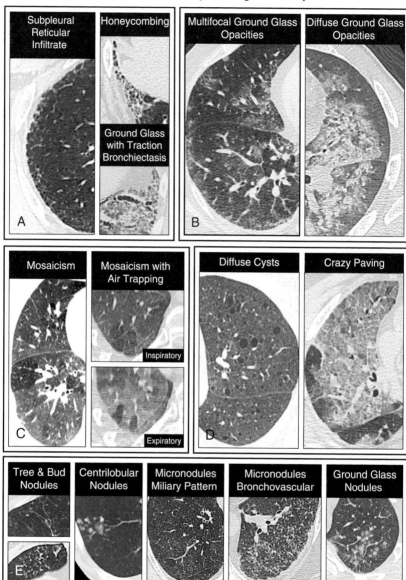

Fig. 17.1 Cropped chest computed tomography (CT) images of patients with diffuse parenchymal lung disease (and/or mimics), showing the most commonly seen types of opacities. **(A)** The opacities commonly seen in usual interstitial pneumonia, specifically a diffuse subpleural reticular infiltrate, basilar honeycombing, and traction bronchiectasis. **(B)** Both multifocal and diffuse ground-glass opacities are commonly seen in nonspecific interstitial pneumonia and mimics, like atypical infection, cardiogenic edema, and alveolar hemorrhage. **(C)** Mosaicism describes the juxtaposition of areas of increased attenuation with areas of decreased attenuation. The challenge is to establish whether the lower attenuation lung represents normal parenchyma, and the higher attenuation lung ground glass opacities, or whether the higher attenuation lung represents normal parenchyma and the lower attenuation lung represents disease; either trapped air (as seen in asthma with active bronchospasm or bronchiolitis obliterans) or decreased perfusion (as seen in chronic thromboembolic disease). Air trapping is demonstrated during expiratory CT imaging, which shows that the areas of decreased attenuation in the inspiratory film remain dark, whereas the areas of normal lung attenuation become whiter. If, on the other hand, the areas of decreased attenuation whiten with exhalation, then the low attenuation areas are normal, and the areas of increased attenuation on the inspiratory film actually represent ground glass. **(D)** Diffuse cysts (as seen in lymphangiomyomatosis and lymphocytic interstitial pneumonia) and crazy paving (as seen in cardiogenic edema, atypical infection, lymphangitic spread of tumor, and alveolar proteinosis). **(E)** Multiple nodules in varying distributions (as seen in granulomatous disease and atypical lung infection).

- Medications associated with DPLD (eg, Amiodarone, biologics, methotrexate, chemotherapeutics)
- A history of inhalation injuries (eg, chlorine fumes) or acute respiratory distress syndrome (ARDS)
- Cigarette smoking
- Management:
  - Serial PFTs and clinical screen for symptoms (± imaging)
    - Every 3–12 months based on concern (pattern and extent of disease) until 3–5 years of stability is demonstrated
  - Advise avoidance of environments that produce respiratory symptoms
  - Advise bird fanciers to get rid of their birds (surprisingly difficult and/or impossible)
    - The allergy can be to thermophilic bacteria that live in the bird guano such that individuals may be exposed via bird droppings on a balcony or window ledge
  - Individuals with a positive physical or immunologic screen for connective tissue disease should be evaluated by rheumatology
  - Stop any and all possible inciting medications
    - These are **not** appropriate drugs for an individual with a DPLD pattern on by imaging
  - Smokers should be aggressively counseled about cessation
- **Nontuberculous mycobacteria (NTM)** (Fig. 17.2)
  - Special features:
    - NTM are ubiquitous in soil and water, with infection occurring after inhalation, commonly during showering
    - Predilection for individuals with a long, thin thorax (same phenotype as primary spontaneous pneumothorax [PTX])
  - Classic imaging features:

Nontuberculous Mycobacterial Infection Pattern

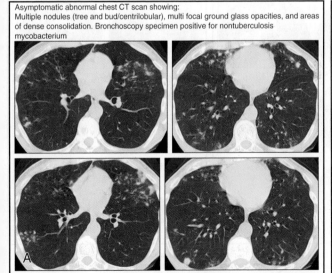

Asymptomatic abnormal chest CT scan showing:
Multiple nodules (tree and bud/centrilobular), multi focal ground glass opacities, and areas of dense consolidation. Bronchoscopy specimen positive for nontuberculosis mycobacterium

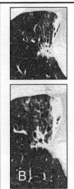

Different Patient with NTM showing classic RML traction bronchiectasis, consolidation and tree and bud nodules

Fig. 17.2 (A) Computed tomography (CT) imaging of a patient with nontuberculous mycobacteria (NTM) infection. Multiple centrilobular nodules can be seen existing on a size spectrum, from micronodules in a tree and bud distribution (≤5 mm), to ground-glass nodules (5 mm to 1 cm), to solid nodules >1 cm. There are also small peripheral dense consolidations in the left upper lobe with traction bronchiectasis. **(B)** A different patient with NTM and classic involvement/destruction of the right middle lobe with dense consolidation, volume loss, traction bronchiectasis, and tree and bud nodules.

- Tree and bud nodules
- Airway-associated consolidations and ground-glass opacities
  - Areas of dense consolidation accompanied by traction bronchiectasis and volume loss
  - Classically involving the right middle lobe
  - Subcentimeter nodules and/or calcified granuloma are also common
- Diagnostic workup involves screening for symptoms—mainly productive cough, weight loss, and night sweats
  - If the patient has a productive cough, send at least three specimens for acid-fast bacilli (AFB) stain and culture
- Management involves serial PFTs, a clinical screen for symptoms, and imaging
  - Every 3–12 months based on concern (extent of disease on imaging) until 3–5 years of stability is demonstrated
    - Stability in NTM may be interpreted as waxing and waning nodules as long as there is no net increase in parenchymal destruction and bronchiectasis over time
- **Chronic aspiration** (Fig. 17.3)
  - Special features:
    - Associated with sedative/hypnotic use at bedtime
  - Classic imaging features:
    - Dynamic basilar/dependent dense consolidations and ground-glass opacities
    - Nonspecific areas of fibrosis

Chronic Aspiration

48-year-old smoker with an incidental finding on a chest x-ray obtained for right upper quadrant pain, better characterized with a CT scan showing:
- Dense right upper lobe consolidation
- Right middle lobe ground glass opacities with focal areas of subpleural reticular markings and linear scarring

Follow-up CT scan 6 weeks later showing:
- Improved right upper lobe consolidation and right middle lobe ground glass opacities
- New, dense, right lower lobe consolidation with ground glass opacities and holes, which are actually preexisting emphysema masquerading as necrosis and fibrosis
- Patient using chlorohydrate for sleep

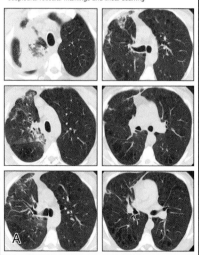 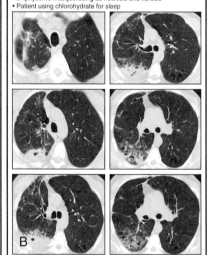

Fig. 17.3 **(A)** The initial computed tomography (CT) scan of a 48-year-old smoker who was incidentally found to have an abnormal chest x-ray and follow-up CT scan demonstrating a dense right upper lobe consolidation with right middle lobe ground glass and focal subpleural reticular scarring (sparing the base). The patient was treated with clindamycin for 1 month, and a repeat CT scan was obtained. **(B)** Follow-up CT scan (6 weeks later) demonstrating improvement in the right upper and middle lobes, with a new dense right lower lobe consolidation and possible abscess vs preexisting emphysematous hole. Further questioning of the patient revealed his nightly use of chlorohydrate for insomnia. The patient's recurrent aspiration resolved after chlorohydrate was discontinued.

- Diagnostic workup involves screening for gastroesophageal reflux disease (GERD) symptoms, choking on food, and/or nocturnal arousals associated with forceful coughing/choking episodes
- Management involves:
  - Proton pump inhibitor and treating reflux maximally if present (eg, elevation of the head of the bed, diet modification)
  - Screen for, and advise against, the use of sedative and/or alcohol use at bedtime (explain the importance of falling asleep vs passing out)
  - Antibiotics covering oral anaerobes should be used in most situations
    - The presence of an air fluid level within a consolidation is worrisome for necrosis (ie, lung abscess), which requires 1–3 months of oral anaerobic coverage until the air fluid level resolves
    - Occasionally, preexisting bullae partially fill with infected/inflammatory material, mimicking a lung abscess (CH 11)
  - Short-interval serial imaging and clinical follow-up:
    - Chest x-ray every 1–3 months, anticipating complete resolution of ground-glass and dense consolidations
    - Occasionally, new opacities appear as old ones resolve, necessitating continued imaging and interventions aimed at reducing aspiration
      - Any residual/persistent x-ray opacities should be evaluated by CT scan to ensure all findings are compatible with scarring (and not worrisome for malignancy)
- **Stage II and/or III sarcoidosis** (Fig. 17.4)
  - Special features:
    - Affects African Americans more than Caucasians and women more than men

Stage II-III Sarcoidosis

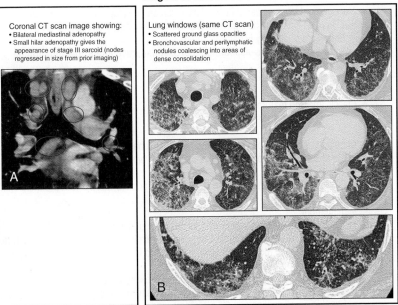

Coronal CT scan image showing:
- Bilateral mediastinal adenopathy
- Small hilar adenopathy gives the appearance of stage III sarcoid (nodes regressed in size from prior imaging)

Lung windows (same CT scan)
- Scattered ground glass opacities
- Bronchovascular and perilymphatic nodules coalescing into areas of dense consolidation

Fig. 17.4 **(A)** Bilateral paratracheal, hilar, and subcarinal adenopathy. The small size of the hilar adenopathy suggests stage III sarcoid (smaller from the previous scan [not shown]). **(B)** Classic parenchymal changes associated with stage II - III sarcoidosis—namely diffuse micronodules in a bronchovascular and perilymphatic distribution, coalescing into areas of dense consolidation, with multifocal ground-glass opacities.

- Common symptoms include cough and shortness of breath ± pleuritic chest pain
- The majority of the time, pulmonary sarcoidosis runs its course (and remits) irrespective of therapy
  - ~50% in 3 years, ~75% within 10 years
- Recurrence after 1 year of remission is rare (<5%)
- Nodular sarcoidosis progresses to a fibrotic pattern in 20–25% of cases (regardless of therapy)
  - Fibrotic progression is most common in poor African Americans who suffer disease onset later in life
- Classic imaging features:
  - Bilateral hilar and mediastinal lymphadenopathy
  - Bronchovascular and perilymphatic micronodules, often coalescing into
    - Macro nodules and dense consolidations
  - Ground-glass opacities
  - Scattered areas of subpleural reticular change
- Diagnostic workup involves:
  - PFTs
    - May show restriction **or** mixed obstructive-restrictive disease, with a decreased DLCO
  - Chronic granulomatous disease immunologic screen:
    - Interferon gamma release assay testing for TB exposure
    - Antigen/antibody testing for endemic fungal infection
  - Endobronchial ultrasound-guided transbronchial needle aspiration of any hilar and/or mediastinal lymphadenopathy
    - Transbronchial lung biopsies should be performed in the absence of adenopathy (also high yield)
- Management involves serial PFTs, clinical screen for symptoms, and ± imaging
  - Every 3–12 months based on concern (extent of disease on imaging) until 3–5 years of stability is demonstrated
- **Respiratory bronchiolitis-associated ILD/desquamative interstitial pneumonia** (Fig. 17.5)
  - Special features:
    - Active smokers
  - Classic imaging features:
    - Diffuse ground-glass opacities
      - Often faint/subtle
  - Diagnostic workup involves screening for active tobacco use
  - In the absence of tobacco use, individuals should be treated like **suspected HP/NSIP**
    - Early HP and NSIP may be hard to distinguish form RB-ILD/DIP (but are more likely to cause symptoms)
  - Management:
    - Smokers should be aggressively counseled about cessation
      - They should be informed that they have a relatively unusual allergy to cigarette smoke (unlike most people who only need to fear COPD and lung cancer) and that they are actively scarring their lungs
        - Patients should leave the office with a prescription for smoking cessation therapy (emphasizing the medical necessity of quitting)
    - Serial PFTs, clinical screen for symptoms, and ± imaging
      - Every 3–12 months based on concern (pattern and extent of disease on imaging) until 3–5 years of stability is demonstrated
    - Nonsmokers are managed like suspected HP/NSIP

Respiratory Bronchiolitis-Interstitial Lung Disease and Desquamative Interstitial Pneumonia

Smoker with cough and an abnormal chest x-ray followed by a CT scan showing:
- Faint diffuse ground glass opacities (basilar predominant)
- Clinically and radiographically suggestive of respiratory bronchiolitis-interstitial lung disease/desquamative interstitial pneumonia

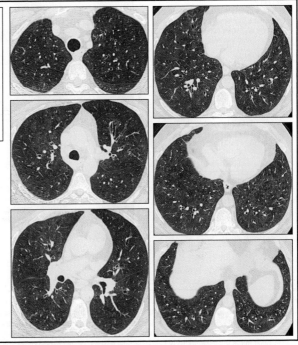

Fig. 17.5 Computed tomography (CT) imaging of the chest reveals a subtle, diffuse, ground-glass opacification, with probable areas of air trapping (no expiratory imaging available for conformation), in a smoker with a chronic cough and no change in exercise ability. Pulmonary function tests showed mixed obstructive-restrictive disease with a mildly decreased diffusing lung capacity for carbon monoxide. The clinical radiographic scenario is very suggestive of respiratory bronchiolitis-interstitial lung disease.

SUBACUTE DYSPNEA ON EXERTION WITH A DIFFUSE PARENTCHYMAL LUNG DISEASE PATTERN FOUND ON BY CHEST CT IMAGING

- PFTs show a restrictive pattern, with a reduced DLCO or an isolated low DLCO
- Patients may complain of a dry cough and/or systemic symptoms (eg, fevers, night sweats)
- Patients with DPLD, dyspnea, and restrictive PFTs deserve a screen for desaturation with exercise if they demonstrate any of the following:
  - Resting O_2 saturation <95% on RA
  - Moderately to severely reduced DLCO
  - Severe exercise limitation
- **Chest CT scan suggests:**
  - **Definite UIP** (Fig. 17.6)
    - Special features:
      - Idiopathic disease of polyclonal fibroblast proliferation in the pulmonary interstitium
      - Leads to progressive respiratory failure from hypoxemia and restrictive physiology
        - Median survival of 3 years
      - Tends to progress in a stepwise fashion with times of stable disability punctuated by episodes of precipitous decline
        - Often in the setting of, or triggered by, a respiratory infection
      - A rare familial form also exists

Usual Interstitial Pneumonia Pattern

Must Have:
• Diffuse subpleural reticular infiltrate
• Lower lobe predominance
• ≥ 2 rows of "honey combing"
• Traction bronchiectasis

Minimal or No:
• Ground glass, nodules, cysts, adenopathy

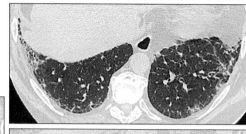

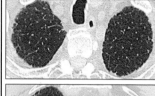

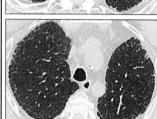

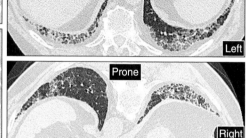

Fig. 17.6 Computed tomography (CT) imaging showing the pathognomonic "DEFINITE UIP" scan. A definite usual interstitial pneumonia scan must have a diffuse subpleural reticular infiltrate with a lower-lobe predominance and architectural distortion as evidenced by at least two rows of honeycomb cysts with traction bronchiectasis. The scan should also have little or no ground glass, nodules, cysts, or adenopathy. Those findings are associated with, and can be seen in, other (more treatable) forms of interstitial lung disease. Prone imaging shows that some of the left basilar ground-glass opacification clears (and thus was dependent atelectasis), whereas the honeycombing persists.

- Classic imaging features:
  - Diffuse subpleural reticular infiltrate
  - Lower-lobe predominance
  - Greater than or equal to two rows of "honeycombing" (ie, architectural distortion)
  - Traction bronchiectasis
  - Minimal or no:
    - Ground glass
    - Nodules
    - Adenopathy
    - Cysts (other than honeycombing)
- Diagnostic workup involves a clinical and/or immunologic screen for other, nonidiopathic causes:
  - Hypersensitivity and pneumoconiosis
  - Connective tissue disease
  - Medications associated with DPLD
  - Cigarette smoking
- **Management of definite UIP (CT scan pattern)/IPF (no cause found during workup)**
  - Explain to the patient the disease and the prognosis in understandable terms, hitting the key points:
    - IPF is a poorly understood disease involving scarring of the lungs
    - It often progresses in a stepwise fashion (times of stability punctuated by acute exacerbations, without return to previous baseline)

- It threatens possible death from respiratory failure over a 3–5-year period
- New medications are available that may slow the disease process
- Lung transplant may be required
- Consider:
  - Referral to an end-stage lung disease clinic as a part of the lung transplant evaluation process
  - Starting a proton pump inhibitor (supported by retrospective data)
  - Starting pirfenidone or nintedanib (choose based on cardiac disease or side effect profile)
    - Nintedanib has a "black box" warning for ischemic heart disease and is more likely to cause lower-GI side effects
    - Pirfenidone does not carry a cardiovascular warning and causes upper-GI side effects
    - Intolerance of both of these medications is relatively common
  - Ensuring/maintaining euvolemia (ie, no edema) with loop diuretics as necessary
    - Both left- and isolated right-sided heart failure complicate UIP/IPF, decreasing exercise tolerance
  - Serial PFTs every 3 months with a clinical screen for symptom progression, superimposed heart failure, and medication intolerance
- **Management of definite UIP (CT scan pattern) with possible cause found during workup**
  - Treat as **possible UIP/NSIP/HP**
- **Possible UIP, NSIP, HP or LIP**
  - Special features:
    - All four entities have very different prognoses, with UIP being the worst and HP being the best
    - Apical predominant disease distribution helps differentiate UIP from NSIP/HP
    - Diffuse cysts suggests LIP
    - UIP and NSIP are often associated with connective tissue disease (especially Rheumatoid arthritis) and/or an adverse reaction to a medication (eg, amiodarone)
    - HP is often associated with exposures (eg, farmer's lung, bird fancier's lung)
  - Classic imaging features:
    - Diffuse subpleural reticular infiltrate
    - Ground-glass opacities
    - Traction bronchiectasis
    - Apical predominance or even distribution throughout the lung
    - Varying degrees of nodules and cysts
  - Diagnostic workup involves a clinical and/or immunologic screen for:
    - Hypersensitivity/pneumoconiosis
      - Query exposures to birds, asbestos, silica, and environments that produce respiratory symptoms for the patient
      - Check a hypersensitivity panel
      - Connective tissue disease screen
        - Examination for skin, muscle, and joint disease
        - Serology for RF, ANA, and ESR
      - Medications associated with DPLD (eg, Amiodarone, biologics, methotrexate, chemotherapeutics)
      - Cigarette smoking
  - Management:
    - Advise avoidance of environments that produce respiratory symptoms
    - Advise bird fanciers to get rid of their birds (and any piles of bird guano)
    - Individuals with possible connective tissue disease should be evaluated by rheumatology
    - Stop any and all possible inciting medications

- **Not** appropriate drugs for individuals with symptomatic DPLD
- Smokers should be aggressively counseled about cessation
- Consider a lung biopsy (via VATS) to establish the diagnosis (UIP vs not UIP)
  - All non-UIP entities **might** respond to steroids
- Consider a trial of prednisone if VATS is too dangerous or the patient is unwilling
  - Obtain baseline imaging and PFTs
  - Give 40–60 mg of prednisone daily for 4 weeks
  - Reevaluate for response with imaging, PFTs, and clinical reassessment
  - If the patient has an objective response:
    - Consider continuing at a 20–40 mg dose (based on side effects) for an additional 2 months
      - Start PCP prophylaxis and consider vitamin D/calcium supplementation
    - Reevaluate for continued objective improvement and consider taper steroids if and when improvement plateaus
    - If the taper fails, consider adding azathioprine (as a steroid sparring agent) and then reattempt a taper
    - Obtain serial PFTs every 3–6 months for 3–5 years with a clinical screen for symptom progression
  - If the patient fails to respond, taper steroids and treat like **definite UIP/IPF**
- **Pulmonary Langerhans** (Fig. 17.7)
  - Special features:
    - Disease affecting young smokers (20–40 years old), in which pathologic S100, CD1a-positive Langerhans dendritic cells provoke pulmonary inflammation (involving all inflammatory cell lines)
    - Common symptoms include cough and shortness of breath
    - Characterized by multiple ground-glass opacities and **cavitary nodules** (early Langerhans) that enlarge and coalesce into giant, bizarrely shaped cysts (late Langerhans)
  - Classic imaging features:
    - Ground glass
    - Cavitating centrilobular nodules
    - Large, bizarrely shaped, confluent cysts with a slightly thickened wall
    - Upper lobe predominant
    - Spares the bases
  - Diagnostic workup involves screening for active tobacco use (nearly universal in pulmonary Langerhans), and in its absence, hypersensitivity triggers/exposures (ie, pet birds, exposure to environments that produce respiratory symptoms)
    - HP and early pulmonary Langerhans may be indistinguishable radiographically
      - Consider checking a hypersensitivity panel
  - Management:
    - Smokers should be aggressively counseled about cessation
      - They should be informed that they have an allergy to cigarette smoke (unlike most people who only need to fear COPD and lung cancer) and that they are actively making giant holes in their lungs (show them their scan)
      - Patients should leave the office with a prescription for smoking cessation therapy (emphasizing the medical necessity of quitting)
    - Patients who remain symptomatic despite smoking cessation (and nonsmokers) may deserve a trial of prednisone, as previously outlined under management of symptomatic **possible UIP/NSIP/HP**
    - Nonsmokers should be treated like possible HP
- **Nontuberculous mycobacteria** (see previously discussed details under asymptomatic NTM presentation)

Pulmonary Langerhans

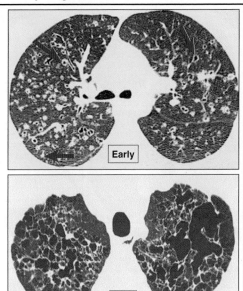

Upper lobe chest CT scan images showing:
- Early pulmonary Langerhans (top panel) with multiple caveating nodules
- Arrows highlighting various stages of cavitation
- Late pulmonary Langerhans (bottom panel) showing how cavitary nodules have grown and coalesced into bizarre shaped cysts
- Only the upper lobe is shown since this disease uniformly spares the bases

Fig. 17.7 Upper-lobe computed tomography (CT) imaging of two different individuals with pulmonary Langerhans. The top panel shows early pulmonary Langerhans characterized by multiple cavitary nodules. Red arrows highlight the various stages of necrosis. The cavities can be difficult to distinguish from airways with thickened walls (on a single CT scan slice). The bottom panel shows late pulmonary Langerhans, characterized by multiple large, bizarrely shaped cysts with a slightly thickened wall. Lower-lobe CT images are not included because this disease uniformly spares the bases.

- Special features:
  - Common symptoms include cough (often productive), night sweats, and weight loss
  - Shortness of breath and exercise limitation are not common unless patients have underlying COPD or restrictive physiology/end-stage fibrosis related to long standing NTM infection
- Diagnostic workup for suspected symptomatic NTM infection involves:
  - Obtaining at least three specimens for AFB stain and culture (if the patient has a productive cough)
  - If the patient does not have a productive cough and/or sputum samples are inadequate or persistently negative, consider bronchoscopy with BAL to increase the likelihood of recovering NTM
- Management involves considering treating patients who grow a pathogenic organism (ie, MAC) and who are suffering from a compatible clinical radiographic syndrome
  - Treatment typically involves three to four antimycobacterial medications for 12–24 months
- **Cryptogenic organizing pneumonia** (Fig. 17.8)
  - Special features:
    - Often occurs after an episode of typical bacterial pneumonia
    - Cough, dyspnea, and fever are common
    - Associated with rheumatologic disease (eg, rheumatoid arthritis) and lymphoma (eg, chronic lymphocytic lymphoma [CLL])

Cryptogenic Organizing Pneumonia Pattern

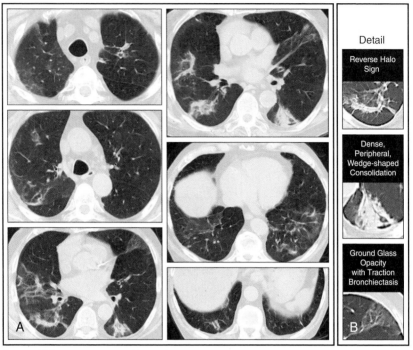

Fig. 17.8 **(A)** Computed tomography (CT) scan of a patient with cryptogenic organizing pneumonia, demonstrating all of the classic radiographic findings. Multifocal, peripheral, wedge-shaped opacities (both dense consolidations and ground glass) with traction bronchiectasis are visible in all lobes. Several of the opacities demonstrate the "reverse halo sign," in which semicircular band-like dense consolidations surround areas of ground glass. **(B)** Detailed close up of each finding previously described.

- Classic imaging features:
  - Circular or semicircular, band-like consolidations with ground-glass opacities in the center (reverse halo sign)
  - Peripheral wedge-shaped, dense consolidations
  - Ground-glass opacities
  - Traction bronchiectasis
- Diagnostic workup involves screening for a compatible history:
  - Weeks to months of pneumonia symptoms with persistent or worsening infiltrates despite antibiotic therapy
  - Consider bronchoscopy with BAL, looking for >25% lymphocytes (supportive)
- Management involves prednisone:
  - ~80% response rate (60% complete response)
  - Obtain baseline imaging and PFTs
  - Start PJP prophylaxis and consider vitamin D/calcium supplementation
  - Give prednisone 40–60 mg per day for 1–2 months and reevaluate with imaging, PFTs, and clinical reassessment
  - If the patient is stable or improved, attempt to decrease the dose to the 20–40-mg range for another 1–2 months
  - After 3–6 months, prednisone should be tapered off completely
  - Relapse is common

Chronic Eosinophilic Pneumonia Pattern

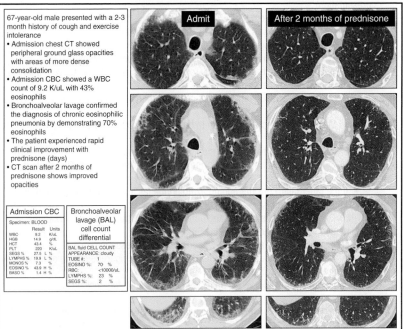

67-year-old male presented with a 2-3 month history of cough and exercise intolerance
- Admission chest CT showed peripheral ground glass opacities with areas of more dense consolidation
- Admission CBC showed a WBC count of 9.2 K/uL with 43% eosinophils
- Bronchoalveolar lavage confirmed the diagnosis of chronic eosinophilic pneumonia by demonstrating 70% eosinophils
- The patient experienced rapid clinical improvement with prednisone (days)
- CT scan after 2 months of prednisone shows improved opacities

Admission CBC		
Specimen: BLOOD		
	Result	Units
WBC	9.2	K/uL
HGB	14.9	g/dL
HCT	43.4	%
PLT	220	K/uL
SEGS %	27.5 L	%
LYMPHS %	19.9 L	%
MONOS %	7.3	%
EOSINO %	43.9 H	%
BASO %	1.4 H	%

Bronchoalveolar lavage (BAL) cell count differential

BAL fluid CELL COUNT		
APPEARANCE: cloudy		
TUBE #:	1	
EOSINO %:	70	%
RBC:	<10000/uL	
LYMPHS %:	23	%
SEGS %:	2	%

Fig. 17.9 Encapsulated case of a patient with chronic eosinophilic pneumonia. Although extreme bronchoalveolar lavage eosinophilia (in the correct clinical/radiographic scenario) is diagnostic, the peripheral eosinophil count is often normal or only slightly elevated.

- **Chronic eosinophilic pneumonia** (Fig. 17.9)
  - Special features:
    - Patients complain of months of cough, fevers, night sweats, and variable exercise limitation
  - Steroid response is prompt (24–48 hours)
  - Classic imaging features:
    - Peripheral ground-glass opacities (a.k.a. "reverse cardiogenic pulmonary edema pattern")
    - Peripheral areas of dense consolidations
  - Diagnostic workup
    - CBC may show peripheral eosinophilia
    - BAL
      - BAL with >25% eosinophils is suggestive and >40% is diagnostic (in the appropriate clinical/radiographic setting)
  - Management involves prednisone
    - A rapid response to prednisone (48 hours to 2 weeks) is anticipated, and failure suggests and alternate diagnosis
    - Give 40–60 mg of prednisone daily, and reevaluate with imaging, PFTs, and a clinical reassessment in 2–4 weeks
      - Start PJP prophylaxis and consider vitamin D/calcium supplementation
      - Continue high-dose prednisone until symptoms resolve and imaging improves (usually 4–6 weeks)
      - Then attempt a slow taper over an additional 1–2 months
      - Relapse is very common

- **Stage II and/or III sarcoidosis** (see previously discussed details under asymptomatic presentation)
  - Management of symptomatic sarcoidosis involves prednisone:
    - Response to therapy is typically slow/difficult to appreciate
    - Obtain baseline imaging and PFTs
    - Start PJP prophylaxis, and consider vitamin D/calcium supplementation
    - Give 40–60 mg of prednisone daily for 2–3 months, and reevaluate with imaging, PFTs, and clinical reassessment:
      - Continue prednisone for an additional 2–3 months (to prevent relapse, which is common)
      - May consider decreasing dose to the 20–40-mg range (in an effort to minimize side effects)
        - Patients who have responded (after 3–6 months of therapy) should have their prednisone tapered to the lowest effective dose (or off entirely if possible)
    - If the taper fails, consider adding azathioprine (as a steroid sparring agent) and then reattempt a taper
- **RB-ILD/DIP** (see previously discussed details under asymptomatic presentation)
  - Management of symptomatic RBILD/DIP:
    - Smokers should be aggressively counseled about cessation
      - They should be informed that they are allergic to cigarette smoke and that they are actively scarring their lungs
        - Patients must leave the office with a prescription for smoking cessation therapy
    - Patients who do not improve with smoking cessation alone, warrant a trial of prednisone
    - Nonsmokers should be evaluated and managed as previously described, under **possible NSIP/HP**
- **Lymphocytic interstitial pneumonia** (Fig. 17.10)
  - Special features:
    - Occurs as an HIV- or non–HIV-associated disease
    - Caused by a polyclonal proliferation of lymphocytes possibly triggered by viral infection
    - Also associated with Sjögren's syndrome
  - Classic imaging features:
    - Multiple cysts
    - Ground glass
    - Basilar predominance
  - Diagnostic workup involves VATS lung biopsy
    - Management involves prednisone and/or other immunosuppressants
- **Lymphangioleiomyomatosis** (Fig. 17.11)
  - Special features:
    - Affects women of childbearing age
    - Often presents with a pneumothorax and/or a chylothorax
  - Classic imaging features:
    - Multiple cysts
    - Pneumothoraces (occasionally loculated)
  - Diagnostic workup involves:
    - PFTs (often showing an isolated low DLCO [ie, preserved volumes]) or mixed obstructive-restrictive disease
    - VATS lung biopsy
  - Management involves prednisone and/or other immunosuppressants

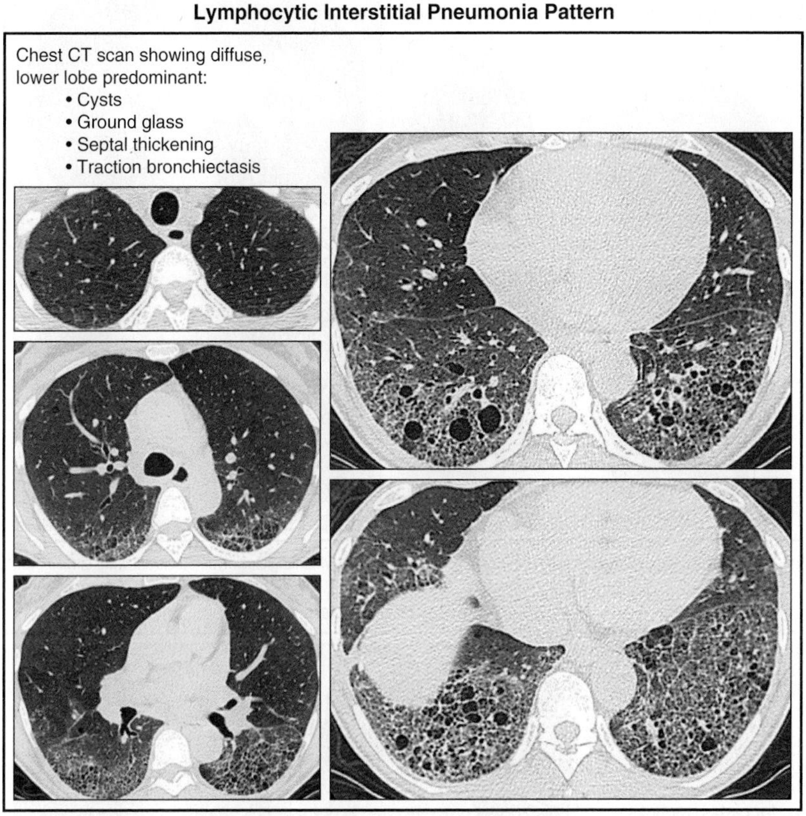

Lymphocytic Interstitial Pneumonia Pattern

Chest CT scan showing diffuse, lower lobe predominant:
- Cysts
- Ground glass
- Septal thickening
- Traction bronchiectasis

Fig. 17.10 Chest computed tomography (CT) imaging of a patient with lymphocytic interstitial pneumonia, showing basilar predilection and dominant cystic appearance, with septal thickening, ground-glass opacities, and traction bronchiectasis. Note that the cysts are much larger than the honeycomb cysts of usual interstitial pneumonia.

- **Alveolar proteinosis** (Fig. 17.12)
  - Special features:
    - Congenital and acquired impaired lung surfactant processing and clearance
      - Possibly autoimmune
    - Leads to the deposition of PAS-positive material in alveolar spaces
  - Classic imaging features:
    - Diffuse crazy paving
  - Diagnostic workup involves:
    - BAL analysis:
      - Macroscopic examination shows a cloudy/turbid fluid with granular sand-like material deposited at the bottom of the collection chamber
      - Microscopic examination reveals alveolar macrophages filled with PAS-positive material
    - Elevated anti-GM CSF antibody titer common
  - Management involves periodic whole-lung lavage
    - One whole-lung lavage (each lung done separately during the same hospital stay) can provide a durable remission

Lymphangioleiomyomatosis Pattern

Chest CT scan of a patient with lymphangioleiomyomatosis showing diffuse cysts

Fig. 17.11 Chest computed tomography (CT) imaging of a patient with lymphangioleiomyomatosis showing diffuse cysts.

Alveolar Proteinosis

Clinical scenario:
- Subacute dyspnoea on exertion
- Hypoxemia
- Restricted pulmonary function tests / low diffusing lung capacity for carbon monoxide
- Diffuse crazy paving

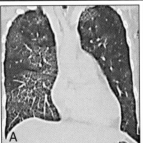
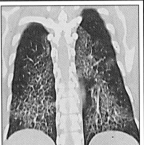

Whole lung lavage showing:
- Cloudy/turbid fluid with granular sand like material deposited at the bottom of the collection chamber
- Microscopic exam reveals alveolar macrophages filled with periodic acid-Schiff-positive material

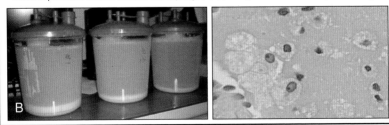

Fig. 17.12 (A) Typical clinical radiographic presenting scenario of alveolar proteinosis, namely progressive dyspnoea on exertion with restrictive/low diffusing lung capacity for carbon monoxide on pulmonary function testing, hypoxemia, and computed tomography (CT) imaging demonstrating diffuse "crazy paving" (ie, ground-glass and septal thickening). **(B)** Macroscopic and microscopic results of a therapeutic, whole-lung lavage in an individual with alveolar proteinosis. Macroscopically, a sand-like material can be seen settling at the bottom of the suction chambers (that are filled with a cloudy fluid). Microscopically, alveolar macrophages filled with periodic acid-Schiff-positive material can be seen.

- **PJP**
  - Special features:
    - Only occurs in immunosuppressed individuals:
      - HIV (CD 4^+ <200)
      - Prednisone use ($\geq$20 mg daily for >1 month)
      - Hematologic malignancy (eg, CLL)
    - O_2 desaturation with exercise is common
  - Classic imaging features:
    - Diffuse ground-glass opacification (nonspecific)
      - Chronic PJP often has upper-lobe cysts
  - Diagnostic workup involves:
    - BAL with silver stain ($\pm$ direct fluorescent antibody testing for PJP and beta–d-glucan) is the gold standard for the diagnosis
      - High yield, especially in HIV-associated disease
      - BAL Beta–d-glucan has excellent negative predictive value
  - Management involves sulfamethoxazole with trimethoprim (and prednisone for the hypoxemic)
- **Cardiogenic pulmonary edema**
  - Classic imaging features:
    - Bilateral pleural effusion
    - Ground-glass opacities (often perihilar) may coalesce into areas of more dense consolidation
    - Septal thickening
  - Diagnostic workup involves:
    - Screen for weight gain
    - Survey for generalized edema
    - Echocardiogram showing heart failure with preserved ejection fraction (HFpEF) or heart failure with reduced ejection fraction (HFrEF):
      - Unexplained HFpEF should be screened for obstructive sleep apnea (OSA)
      - Unexplained HFrEF should be screened for ischemic cardiomyopathy
  - Management:
    - Loop diuretic administration until euvolemia
    - 2 g daily sodium restriction
- **Lymphangitic spread of tumor**
  - Special features:
    - Often related to breast or lung adenocarcinoma
  - Classic imaging features:
    - Crazy paving
    - Focal pleural thickening
  - Diagnostic workup involves screening for an individual history of adenocarcinoma
    - Transbronchial biopsies are high yield
  - Management involves specific therapy based on tumor type
- **Obstructive or mixed obstructive-restrictive pattern during pulmonary function testing**
  - **Bronchiolitis obliterans** (Fig. 17.13)
    - Special features:
      - Occurs after bone-marrow transplant (BMT) as a part of graft-versus-host disease (GVHD)
      - Seen in diffuse panbronchiolitis (80% of cases occur in Asians)
      - Associated with "burn pit" exposure among veterans deployed to the Middle East
    - Classic imaging features:
      - Diffuse mosaicism/air trapping
      - Tree and bud nodules (nonmigratory)

Bronchiolitis Pattern

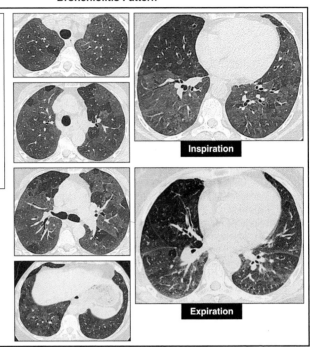

- Diffuse mosaicism
- Air trapping confirmed on expiratory imaging
- Low attenuation areas on the expiratory imaging correspond to trapped air
- Right middle lobe demonstrates air trapping and oligemia (possibly from hypoxemic vasoconstriction)

Inspiration

Expiration

Fig. 17.13 Chest computed tomography (CT) imaging shows diffuse mosaicism (ie, alternating areas of both low and high attenuation). Air trapping, in which low attenuation areas are caused by trapped air, is suggested on the inspiratory images by the clearly demarcated borders between low and high attenuation zones (less common with ground glass). Air trapping is then confirmed by expiratory images, as low attenuation areas persist despite exhalation. This can be seen in asthma if the CT is obtained during an asthma attack or in bronchiolitis obliterans (BO), where the severe obstruction is fixed. Areas of trapped air associated with BO may also display oligemia or smaller-than-normal vessel caliber, secondary to pulmonary artery hypoxic mediated vasoconstriction.

- Diagnostic workup involves:
  - PFTs showing **fixed** obstruction
  - VATS lung biopsy
- Management:
  - Macrolide antibiotics
  - Prednisone
- **Combined pulmonary fibrosis and emphysema (CPFE)**
  - Classic imaging features:
    - Emphysematous change (often apical) with fibrosis (basilar)
  - Diagnostic workup involves focusing on the fibrosis component of the disease
  - Management hinges on smoking cessation (and the results of the fibrosis workup)
- **Sarcoidosis (stages II–III), lymphangioleiomyomatosis,** and **pulmonary Langerhans** all may present with obstructive PFTs or an isolated low DLCO (ie, preserved volumes)
  - For imaging, diagnostic workup, and management, see previous specific discussions under restricted PFTs

ACUTE HYPOXEMIC RESPIRATORY FAILURE WITH A DIFFUSE PARENCHYMAL LUNG DISEASE PATTERN SEEN ON CHEST CT IMAGING

- Patients are admitted to the hospital (or ICU) with hypoxemic respiratory failure, associated with a diffuse parenchymal process, demonstrating either **acute on chronic disease** or denovo DPLD, when compared with prior imaging
- **Acute on chronic parenchymal disease:**
  - Differential diagnosis based on CT appearance and clinical features (eg, fever or peripheral edema)
  - **DPLD with superimposed cardiogenic edema** (Fig. 17.14)

53-year-old female with lupus, Sjogren's syndrome, and known lymphocytic interstitial pneumonia (diagnostic resection by video-assisted thoracoscopic surgery lung biopsy) treated with prednisone and Rituximab, admitted with 2 days of SOB, dry cough and chills, found to be hypoxemic. Chest CT with **new ground glass opacities, septal thickening,** and **bilateral pleural effusions.** Echocardiogram showed heart failure with preserved ejection fraction (new/worse from prior). Bronchoalveolar lavage showed edematous airways. Silver stain for pneumocystis jiroveci pneumonia and routine culture were negative. The patient improved rapidly with diuresis.

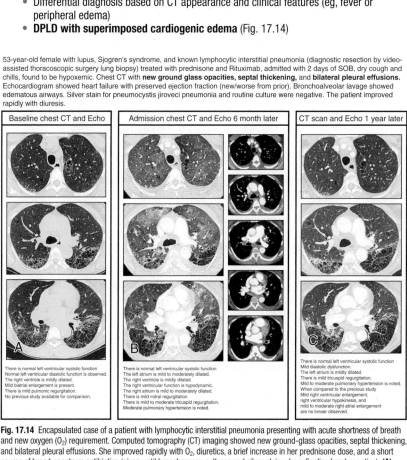

Baseline chest CT and Echo	Admission chest CT and Echo 6 month later	CT scan and Echo 1 year later

There is normal left ventricular systolic function
Normal left ventricular diastolic function is observed.
The right ventricle is mildly dilated.
Mild biatrial enlargement is present.
There is mild pulmonic regurgitation.
No previous study available for comparison.

There is normal left ventricular systolic function
The left atrium is mild to moderately dilated.
The right ventricle is mildly dilated.
The right ventricular function is hypodynamic.
There is mild mitral regurgitation.
There is mild to moderate tricuspid regurgitation.
Moderate pulmonary hypertension is noted.

There is normal left ventricular systolic function
Mild diastolic dysfunction.
The left atrium is mildly dilated.
There is mild tricuspid regurgitation.
Mild to moderate pulmonary hypertension is noted.
When compared to the previous study
Mild right ventricular enlargement,
right ventricular hypokinesis, and
mild to moderate right atrial enlargement
are no longer observed.

Fig. 17.14 Encapsulated case of a patient with lymphocytic interstitial pneumonia presenting with acute shortness of breath and new oxygen (O_2) requirement. Computed tomography (CT) imaging showed new ground-glass opacities, septal thickening, and bilateral pleural effusions. She improved rapidly with O_2, diuretics, a brief increase in her prednisone dose, and a short course of broad-spectrum antibiotics (given until bronchoscopy cultures and silver stain where finalized and negative). **(A)** Baseline CT scan demonstrating a diffuse subpleural reticular pattern with basilar cysts and ground-glass opacities. Baseline echocardiogram shows heart failure with preserved ejection filtration (HFpEF), despite normal diastolic function as evidenced by biatrial enlargement. The left atrial enlargement (and the bilateral pleural effusion) prove that the pulmonary hypertension and right-sided heart failure are caused **not** by her underlying lung disease (and vascular destruction) but rather by HFpEF. Her diastolic filling abnormality may only occur intermittently, during exercise or sleep, leading to sustained HFpEF (despite normal LV diastolic filling during a resting echocardiogram). **(B)** Admission CT scan showing diffuse ground glass with areas of septal thickening (a.k.a. crazy paving) and (small) bilateral pleural effusions (most easily seen on mediastinal windows). No pulmonary embolism is seen. Interestingly the effusion disappears at the right base, presumably because of pleural scarring, effectively pleurodesing much of the right lower lobe. The echocardiogram at admission showed biventricular heart failure with right-ventricular systolic dysfunction (presumably from left-ventricular diastolic dysfunction, which is not commented on), evidenced by worsening left-arterial enlargement (in addition to pleural effusions). The patient improved rapidly with diuresis, leaving the hospital with a prescription for home O_2. This presentation of acute pulmonary edema was likely caused by her underlying lung disease leading to hypoxemia and diastolic dysfunction $\pm$ a viral syndrome. **(C)** Follow-up CT scan one year later, shows slightly worsening fibrosis, most notably in the superior segment of the right lower lobe. Follow-up echo final demonstrates diastolic dysfunction.

- Special features:
  - Diastolic dysfunction and HFpEF occur commonly in individuals with DPLD
    - Hypoxemia provokes diastolic dysfunction, causing and/or worsening HFpEF:
      - Directly, via subendocardial ischemia and LV stiffening, which impairs filling
      - Indirectly, via reflex tachycardia, which shortens diastole (decreasing filling time)
  - Patients may demonstrate or complain of orthopnea, weight gain, and edema
- Classic imaging features:
  - Preexisting DPLD pattern with new pleural effusions, increased ground-glass opacities, and septal thickening
    - Importantly, pleural effusions may be small or absent, as subpleural fibrosis and/or pleural scarring can effectively cause bilateral pleurodesis
- Diagnostic (therapeutic) workup involves:
  - Diuresis (1–2 L net negative fluid balance daily) with loop diuretics to euvolemia (no edema or effusions)
  - Diagnosis is confirmed by a rapid, complete response to diuresis to euvolemia
  - If peripheral edema and pleural effusions resolve but hypoxemia, dyspnea, and ground-glass opacities persist, workup and/or empiric treatment of worsening or relapsed DPLD is warranted
- **DPLD with superimposed TYPICAL pneumonia pattern (new dense consolidation[s])**
  - Special features:
    - Patients with DPLD (especially with bronchiectasis) are at increased risk for bacterial pneumonia
    - Patients may complain of and/or demonstrate acute onset fever, productive cough, elevated WBC count, and rhonchi during examination
  - Classic imaging features:
    - Preexisting DPLD pattern with new area(s) of dense consolidation $\pm$ ground-glass opacity
  - Diagnostic workup:
    - Recovery of a pathogen on sputum (and/or blood culture) or positive urine antigen test for *Streptococcus pneumonia* or legionella
    - Response to antibiotics (albeit slow)
  - Management:
    - Broad-spectrum antibiotics initially covering MRSA, pseudomonas (GNRs), and legionella (atypical bacteria)
- **DPLD with superimposed *atypical* pneumonia pattern (new ground-glass opacity $\pm$ septal thickening)**
  - Special features:
    - More indolent presentation with dry cough or viral syndrome ($\pm$ sick contacts)
    - DDx Differential diagnosis: PJP, lower-respiratory-tract viral infection, mycoplasma, and chlamydia
      - PJP only seen with immunosuppression—typically HIV, prednisone treatment, or hematologic malignancy
  - Classic imaging features:
    - Preexisting DPLD pattern with new ground-glass opacity ($\pm$ septal thickening, a.k.a. crazy paving)
      - Pleural effusions and/or dense consolidation **not** anticipated
  - Diagnostic workup involves:
    - Patients at risk for PJP (even remotely) deserve a BAL with silver stain and/or DFA for PJP
      - Occasionally patients are deemed too sick for BAL ($\pm$ elective intubation), and because of a compelling clinical radiographic picture, PJP is treated empirically
    - Rapid influenza screen
    - Preforming a bronchoscopy solely for a viral respiratory PCR panel (that often does not alter management) in an individual with acute hypoxemic respiratory failure, often is **not** worth the risk

- Acute and convalescent titters can be sent for mycoplasma and chlamydia (but these take time) such that empiric therapy should always be given to cover these organisms
  - Management:
    - Treat proven or strongly suspected PJP with sulfamethoxazole/trimethoprim and prednisone
    - Treat proven influenza pneumonia with oseltamivir
    - Treat noninfluenza lower–respiratory tract viral infections with supportive care $\pm$ prednisone
    - Empirically treat mycoplasma and chlamydia with a macrolide or quinolone
- **Acute exacerbation (or relapse) of previously diagnosed DPLD (not UIP/IPF)**
  - Special features:
    - Individuals have a known diagnosis of DPLD
    - Relapse of COP, CEP, sarcoidosis, and DAH may be obviously associated with weaning of immunosuppression (simplifying the case)
  - Diagnostic workup involves:
    - Failing empiric treatment for superimposed heart failure and PNA
    - Failing empiric therapy may not be required for individuals who present without volume overload or an infectious prodrome, or for those in whom immunosuppression has just been weaned
      - These patients still require aggressive maintenance of euvolemia and often empiric antibiotics while an exacerbation of DPLD is simultaneously treated with steroids
  - Management:
    - Intravenous methylprednisolone is the mainstay of therapy for managing acute exacerbations and/or relapses of steroid-responsive (or possibly responsive) DPLD
    - Steroid dosing should be high enough to ensure that "steroid-responsive" conditions will be affected while also balancing the risks of side effects (mainly hyperglycemia and delirium)
      - For NSIP, HP, COP, and DAH, the methylprednisolone dose typically ranges from 240 mg daily (divided 60 mg IV q 6 hours) to 1 g daily (divided 250 mg IV q 6 hours)
      - For connective tissue disease–associated DPLD, 1 g of methylprednisolone may be given daily (divided 250 mg IV q6)
- **Acute exacerbation of definite UIP/IPF** (Fig. 17.15)
  - Special features:
    - Individuals with a known diagnosis of UIP/IPF, presenting with worsening oxygenation and fibrosis seen by imaging (ie, more honeycombing, volume loss, and ground-glass opacity)
    - These individuals have a high mortality
    - The hope for these patients is that they will stabilize at a new baseline where they are still supportable and functional on ≤ 6 L of oxygen (allowing them to leave the hospital)
    - The concern is that they will have worsening and/or refractory hypoxemia and either be stuck on high-flow oxygen $\pm$ BiPAP (unsustainably poor quality of life) and/or die in the hospital (in days to weeks)
  - Diagnostic workup involves:
    - Failing empiric treatment for superimposed heart failure and PNA
      - Failing empiric therapy may not be required in individuals who present without volume overload or an infectious prodrome
        - These patients still require aggressive maintenance of euvolemia and empiric antibiotics while suffering an exacerbation of UIP/IPF
  - Management:
    - A trial of IV methylprednisolone (hoping that the original diagnosis is wrong) is usually warranted

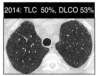

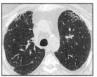

Usual interstitial pneumonia (UIP) pattern found incidentally

2012: TLC 60%, DLCO 49%

- Mr. M suffers a fall and seeks medical attention
- A chest x-ray is obtained suggesting fibrosis
- Follow-up chest CT shows diffuse parenchymal lung disease in a UIP pattern
- Patient endorses occasionally dyspnea on exertion (DOE), but is largely asymptomatic

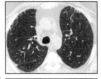

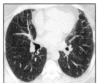

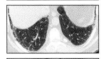

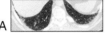

A

First deterioration 2 years later

2014: TLC 50%, DLCO 53%

- Patient does well until 2014 when he is admitted for heart failure and pneumonia
- He improves with diuresis but does not return to baseline
- Post hospitalization pulmonary function tests reveal worsening restriction
- Post hospitilization imaging shows progressive fibrosis (UIP pattern)

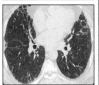

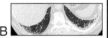

B

Admit for idiopathic pulmonary fibrosis exacerbation

2016: Admitted From PFT LAB For Hypoxemia (O₂sat 75% on RA)

- Patient was again stable, for 2 years, until 2016 when he experienced a subacute worsening of his DOE
- He was referred to pulmonary, and PFTS were ordered
- He was unable to complete PFTs because of severe hypoxemia
- The patient was admitted to the hospital, from the PFT lab, for acute on chronic hypoxemic respiratory failure
- Admission CT scan showed new diffuse ground glass opacities and worsening fibrosis
- Patient denied infectious or heart failure symptoms
- Mr. M was initially diuresed and given empiric broad spectrum antibiotics (with atypical coverage)

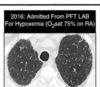

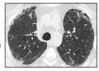

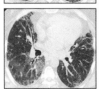

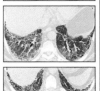

C

Fatal progression

2016: 2 weeks after admission

- When he failed to improve he was started on steroids (240 mg of methylprednisalone daily)
- He completed a 12 day course of antibiotics and maintained a daily even to negative fluid balance throughout his hospital stay
- Despite this Mr. M had progressive worsening of his hypoxemia and dyspnea
- Repeat CT scan showed increased ground glass and fibrosis
- Mr. M was then increased to 1gm of methylprednisalone daily
- At the point of continuous BiPAP dependence, a family meeting was held and goals of care were changed to comfort
- Mr. M died comfortably shortly after

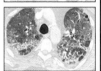

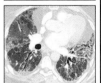

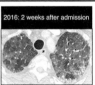

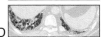

D

Fig. 17.15 See figure legend on opposite page.

- Steroid dosing should be high enough to ensure that "steroid-responsive" conditions will be affected while also balancing the risks of side effects (mainly hyperglycemia and delirium)
  - A typical dose lies somewhere between 240 mg to 1 g a day (in divided doses)
- Do not celebrate a steroid response **too** early
  - Patients (nearly) uniformly report a subjective improvement (or no worsening) with initiation of steroid therapy
  - The daily portable chest x-ray for patients with an acute exacerbation of UIP/IPF is extremely vulnerable to differences in expansion
    - The day after steroids are started, you may see the right heart boarder again, for the first time in days, only to lose it again the next day
  - Premature celebration creates an emotional roller coaster for patients and family
- Lung transplant is often suggested at this point
  - Patients not already listed and admitted to their transplant center cannot be transported, let alone transplanted, during a terminal exacerbation
    - The idea of a lung transplant can create a false sense of hope and should not be entertained unless it is feasible (ie, the patient is lucky enough to be admitted to a lung transplant center)
- BiPAP improves lung expansion and gas exchange and decreases work of breathing
  - Unfortunately, during an exacerbation, patients tend to transition quickly from nocturnal use, to intermittent daytime use, to continuous use, which is uncomfortable and time limited (days)
  - Intubation must be pursued as a last resort, given the concern that patient will either die during intubation or be immediately unsupportable after intubation, from extremely poor compliance and gas exchange
    - These individuals uniformly require paralysis and deep sedation
    - The majority of the time, they will ultimately be forced to pursue compassionate/terminal extubation
    - Because of this, patients must be encouraged to say goodbye to their loved ones and establish parameters for continued care (ie, change to do not actively resuscitate (DNAR) if a pulseless electrical activity (PEA) arrest from refractory hypoxemia becomes imminent) before intubation occurs
- **New** DPLD pattern discovered on imaging (or no prior imaging/history of lung disease) in an individual presenting with acute hypoxemic respiratory failure
  - Initial differential diagnosis is generated by the pattern of disease seen by a chest CT scan, integrated with the clinical presentation:
    - Mimics like cardiogenic edema and atypical pneumonia are more common than true DPLD in patients with no history of lung disease and/or normal prior imaging, who present with acute hypoxemic respiratory failure and a diffuse pattern on imaging
    - Because of this, failing empiric antibiotics and diuresis is often required before concern for DPLD occurs

---

Fig. 17.15 Encapsulated case of UIP/IPF, with death occurring from disease progression in stepwise decrements over a 4-year period after the initial "possible UIP" pattern was incidentally found by computed tomography (CT) imaging of the chest **(A)**. His first deterioration occurred at 2 years, with a hospitalization for heart failure and pneumonia. Despite improving, he did not return to baseline, and his posthospitalization pulmonary function tests (PFTs) and chest CT scan showed worse restriction with increased bibasilar fibrosis **(B)**. He did well for another 2 years until he developed a subacute, dramatic worsening of his dyspnea during exertion, ultimately being admitted to the hospital from the PFT laboratory because of profound hypoxemia. **(C)** His admission CT scan showed new lower-lobe ground-glass opacities and worse basilar "honeycombing." Despite having no definitive evidence of volume overload or infection, diuresis was perused and he was treated for 12 days with antibiotics. Because he did not improve, steroids were also given (ultimately 1 g daily) with no effect. **(D)** Tragically, his CT scan 2 weeks after admission showed rapid progression with diffuse ground-glass opacities and dramatically worsening fibrosis. At this point the patient was transitioned to comfort care, where he experienced a dignified death (within days).

- That said, a diffuse subpleural reticular infiltrate ($\pm$ honeycombing) always raises the concern for (at least) underlying DPLD (especially UIP/NSIP)
  - This concern is heightened in at-risk individuals (ie, patients with rheumatoid arthritis)
- Bronchoscopy with BAL should always be considered in the investigation of a new symptomatic DPLD pattern
  - Patients with marginal oxygenation may be offered elective intubation
    - Elective intubation followed by bronchoscopy is much safer than precipitating respiratory failure and intubating during the procedure
  - Risk of respiratory failure and/or intubation must be weighed against the potential yield from a BAL and the risk of empiric steroids ($\pm$ sulfamethoxazole and trimethoprim for PJP in the appropriate clinical scenario)
    - Bronchoscopy is high yield and/or the gold standard for the diagnosis of eosinophilic pneumonias (acute and chronic), diffuse alveolar hemorrhage, alveolar proteinosis, and PJP pneumonia
  - The risk of short-term, high-dose steroid administration is small and relates to:
    - Hyperglycemia (which causes free water depletion and impaired wound healing)
    - Psychosis and/or manic symptoms
  - Typical and atypical bacterial pneumonia (TB aside) are not anticipated to worsen acutely after steroids
  - A rapid and/or dramatic response to steroids is strongly suggestive of an eosinophilic pneumonia (AEP or CEP) or COP
- Patients with evidence of symptomatic DPLD with a UIP or NSIP/HP/LIP pattern always deserve consideration for a VATS lung biopsy
  - Unfortunately, patients in active, acute hypoxemic respiratory failure are often too sick to safely preform a VATS (need to tolerate one lung ventilation)
- **New UIP, NSIP, LIP, or HP pattern seen by CT scan:**
  - Differential diagnosis:
    - De novo presentation of UIP/NSIP/LIP/HP $\pm$ superimposed cardiogenic edema, typical, or atypical pneumonia
  - Special features:
    - Patients with a de novo presentation of DPLD often:
      - Retrospectively report gradually progressive DOE before their acute presentation
      - Have risk factors for DPLD:
        - Medications (eg, Amiodarone)
        - Underlying connective tissue disease (eg, RA)
        - Or a classic hypersensitivity-related exposure (eg, famer's lung, bird fancier's lung)
  - Classic imaging:
    - Diffuse subpleural reticular infiltrate, ground-glass opacities, traction bronchiectasis:
      - Upper-lobe predominance suggests HP
      - Lower-lobe predominance suggests UIP
      - Even distribution suggests NSIP
      - Predominant ground glass suggests NSIP (Fig. 17.16)
      - Architectural distortion (greater than or equal to two rows of "honeycombing") suggests UIP
      - Nodules and cysts suggest Langerhans (or HP)
      - Diffuse cysts suggest LIP
  - Diagnosis and management:
    - Empiric therapy for heart failure and pneumonia
      - Bronchoscopy is low yield for the diagnosis of DPLD in this setting and is typically reserved for immunosuppressed patients to exclude atypical pathogens

Non-specific Interstitial Pneumonia Pattern

Chest CT scan showing:
- Diffuse subpleural reticular infiltrate
- Diffuse ground glass opacities
- Traction bronchiectasis
- Minimal or no 'honeycombing'
- Disease evenly distributed between upper and lower lobes

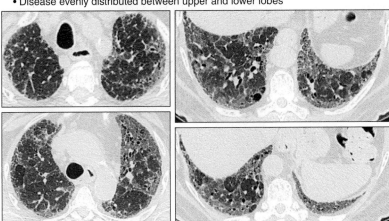

Fig. 17.16 Chest computed tomography (CT) imaging showing an nonspecific interstitial pneumonia pattern, as evidenced by a diffuse subpleural reticular infiltrate (**not** worse at the bases) and predominant ground-glass opacities with traction bronchiectasis (not honeycombing).

- VATS lung biopsy may be helpful if a UIP pattern is present but is usually **not** safe to perform in the setting of acute hypoxemic respiratory failure
  - Definitive UIP diagnosis has important (negative) prognostic value
- Empiric trial of methylprednisolone (240 mg to 1 g) IV daily in divided doses, as outlined under acute exacerbation of UIP/IPF
  - Look for objective improvement within 3–5 days
- Patients who fail to improve have a grave prognosis and few options besides comfort care
- **New ground-glass opacities and dense consolidations** (± septal thickening and scattered reticular changes)
  - These CT findings are not specific, such that the differential diagnosis is based on additional radiographic and/or clinical features:
    - **Dense consolidations *and* ground-glass opacities** (Fig. 17.17), with fever, leukocytosis, and cough, suggest:
      - Severe bacterial pneumonia/acute respiratory distress syndrome
        - Productive cough, respiratory pathogen often recovered (or suggested by urine antigen test)
        - Treat with antibiotics and supportive care with lung-protective ventilation for those requiring mechanical ventilation
      - Acute eosinophilic pneumonia
        - May have peripheral eosinophilia
        - BAL with >25% eosinophils is diagnostic (given the appropriate clinical radiographic scenario)
        - Steroid response is prompt (24–48 hours)

Acute Eosinophilic Pneumonia, Acute Interstitial Pneumonia or Acute Respiratory Distress Syndrome

Acute eosinophilic pneumonia, acute interstitial pneumonia and acute respiratory distress syndrome (from PNA) all share the following, nonspecific constellation of findings on chest CT:
- Diffuse ground glass opacities with areas of dense consolidation
- No significant pleural effusions, septal thickening, subpleural reticular infiltrates or honeycombing

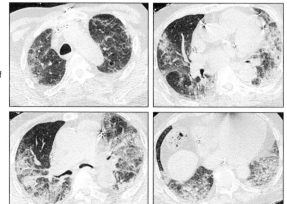

Fig. 17.17 Chest computed tomography (CT) imaging showing diffuse ground-glass opacities with areas of dense consolidation and **no** pleural effusions, septal thickening, subpleural reticular infiltrates, or honeycombing. This nonspecific diffuse parenchymal lung disease pattern can be seen in acute eosinophilic pneumonia, acute interstitial pneumonia, and ARDS (from PNA). This patient had bacterial PNA and devolved ARDS.

- Acutely ill patients should be initially treated with IV steroids at a dose of 240 mg daily
- After unequivocal response (days), transition to 60 mg PO prednisone
  - Taper over weeks
  - Relapse is rare (calls into question the original diagnosis)
- Acute interstitial pneumonia
  - Sputum gram stain 3+ neutrophils, no organisms (also seen in legionella pneumonia)
  - BAL with >25% neutrophils is suggestive
  - May respond to high-dose methylprednisolone (slowly)
    - 1 g daily (250 mg IV q 6 hours), looking for an objective response within 3–5 days
      - If there is a response, taper steroids slowly
      - If there is no response, stop steroid therapy abruptly
- **Ground-glass opacities *alone*** suggest flash pulmonary edema, viral pneumonia, PJP, or DAH
  - DAH is typically seen with anemia, thrombocytopenia, and hypoxemia (Fig. 17.18)
    - Associated with small vessel vasculitis, anti–glomerular basement membrane (anti-GBM) disease (eg, Goodpasture's syndrome), and connective tissue disease
    - Diagnosis made by BAL, showing a progressively bloodier return (macroscopically)
      - When DAH is suspected, a single subsegment should receive three to four BALs
      - Each is collected separately (despite their origin in the same subsegment)
        - A progressively bloodier lavage fluid (in the setting previously outlined) makes the diagnosis
        - Airway trauma from the broncho scope produces the opposite phenomenon (ie, progressively clearer lavage)
    - Treat with high-dose methylprednisolone (500 mg to 1 g in daily in divided doses) until unequivocal response (3–5 days), then transition to prednisone
      - Treat specific underlying disease

Diffuse Alveolar Hemorrhage

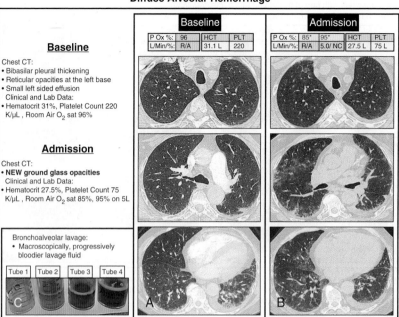

Fig. 17.18 The case of a smoker presenting with shortness of breath, hypoxemia, and acute kidney injury, highlighting the typical pentad presentation of diffuse alveolar hemorrhage (DAH); (1) new ground-glass opacities, (2) hypoxemia, (3) hematocrit drop, (4) thrombocytopenia, and (5) **bronchoalveolar lavage (BAL) with progressively bloodier return** (gold standard for the diagnosis). The patient was ultimately diagnosed with anti-glomerular basement membrane disease by renal biopsy. **(A)** Baseline hematocrit hematopoietic cell transplantation (HCT), platelet count, room air oxygen (O_2) saturation, and chest computed tomography (CT) imaging. Of note, and unrelated to his acute presentation, the patient has baseline bibasilar pleural thickening, left basilar reticular opacities, and a small left-sided effusion. **(B)** Admission data with new hypoxemia, HCT drop, thrombocytopenia, and a chest CT with new ground-glass opacities. The unrelated left basilar process appears improved. **(C)** BAL results demonstrating a visually obvious, progressively bloodier lavage: the gold standard for the diagnosis of DAH.

- Systemic vasculitis may be treated with cyclophosphamide or rituximab
- Anti-GBM disease may require plasmapheresis
- PJP is uniformly seen in the immunosuppressed (for details, see previous discussion under subacute presentation)
  - Treat PJP and acute hypoxemic respiratory failure with po prednisone and IV sulfamethoxazole/trimethoprim
- Viral pneumonia often presents with a viral prodrome and sick contacts (Fig. 17.19)
  - Influenza is diagnosed by nasal swab
    - Bronchoscopy is high yield (via PCR testing) but of very limited utility because specific therapy only exists for influenza
      - Supportive care ± steroids are recommended for those with protracted infiltrates and respiratory failure possibly due to viral pneumonia
- Flash pulmonary edema often has a perihilar distribution with central areas of more dense consolidation (Fig. 17.20)
  - May be obviously associated with myocardial ischemia, acute mitral regurgitation, or hypertensive emergency
  - Supportive care with oxygen, PEEP, diuretics, and specific therapies aimed at improving CO

Crazy Paving Pattern

Chest CT scan from a patient with presumed noninfluenza viral pneumonia, showing diffuse ground glass opacities with septal thickening (a.k.a. crazy paving)
• The opacities cleared and oxygenation returned to normal with supportive care alone

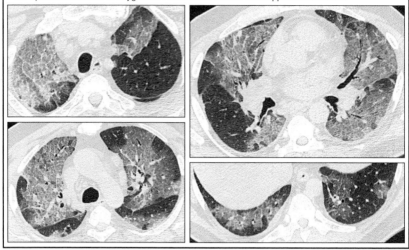

Fig. 17.19 Chest computed tomography (CT) imaging showing a diffuse crazy paving pattern, defined as ground glass combined with septal thickening. This finding is nonspecific and can be seen in cardiogenic pulmonary edema, atypical pneumonia (viral or PJP), lymphangitic spread of tumor, and alveolar proteinosis.

Flash Pulmonary Edema Pattern (Diffuse Parenchymal Lung Disease mimic)

Chest imaging of an individual admitted with a hypertensive emergency causing heart failure with preserved ejection fraction and flash pulmonary edema

Admission chest CT shows:
• Diffuse, perihilar, ground glass opacities
• Coalescing into areas of more dense consolidation (greatest in the superior segment of the right lower lobe)
• With small (evolving) pleural effusions
• Patient has a rapid, complete response to diuresis

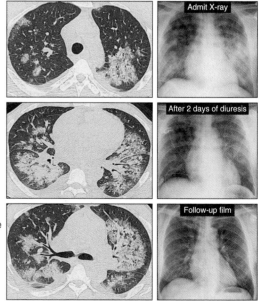

Fig. 17.20 Admission chest computed tomography (CT) imaging and serial chest x-ray films in an individual presenting with flash pulmonary edema from a hypertensive emergency. The initial imaging with diffuse ground-glass opacities and areas of more dense consolidation is compatible with diffuse parenchymal lung disease, yet the clinical scenario, bilateral pleural effusion, and rapid response to diuretics confirm that the parenchymal process is cardiogenic edema.

- **Diffuse cysts'** lower-lobe predominance, with ground-glass opacity and traction bronchiectasis, suggests LIP
- **Bilateral pleural effusion** with ground-glass opacity and respiratory failure strongly suggests cardiogenic edema (or at the very least concomitant volume overload with pulmonary edema)
  - Give threshold-dose loop diuretics to achieve a 1–2 L daily negative fluid balance
  - Only pursue DPLD workup when peripheral edema and pleural effusions resolve and other abnormalities (eg, ground-glass opacity) persist (Fig. 17.21)
- **The "reverse halo sign"** peripheral wedge-shaped, dense consolidations and traction bronchiectasis suggest cryptogenic organizing pneumonia
- **Peripheral distribution** suggests chronic eosinophilic pneumonia
- **Upper-lobe distribution** ± centrilobular nodules suggests hypersensitivity pneumonitis
- **Cavitary centrilobular nodules and/or large cysts** suggests pulmonary Langerhans

Heart Failure with Preserved Ejection Fraction, Volume Overload and Diffuse Parenchymal Lung Disease

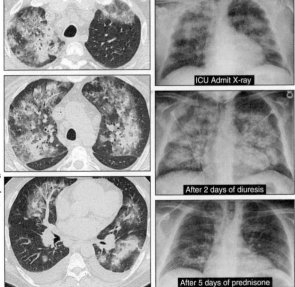

62 year old, admitted with osteomyelitis for IV antibiotic therapy, who was transferred to the ICU on week 3 with sudden hypoxemia and new ground-glass opacities on chest x-ray
- Review of symptoms reveiled weeks of weight gain and orthopnea, with days of cough and fatigue
- His ICU admittance chest CT showed diffuse, perihilar ground-glass opacities, coalescing into areas of more dense consolidation, with small bilateral pleural effusions
- He was treated with diuresis and his peripheral edema and effusions resolved. **BUT his ground glass opacities and hypoxemia persisted**
- Five days after starting steroids the patient was on room air with a dramatically improved ground-glass opacities
- Probable eosinophilic drug reaction to daptomycin

ICU Admit X-ray

After 2 days of diuresis

After 5 days of prednisone

Fig. 17.21 Encapsulated case of an individual transferring from the ward to the intensive care unit complaining of shortness of breath and hypoxemia, with chest imaging compatible with flash pulmonary edema (see Fig. 17.20) and a clinical scenario of volume overload occurring in the setting of weeks of IV antibiotic administration. However, although the patient's peripheral edema and effusions resolved rapidly with diuresis, his ground-glass opacities and hypoxemia persisted, prompting a concern for an additional diffuse parenchymal lung disease process. The patient declined bronchoscopy, opting instead for a brief trial of steroids, which rapidly resolved his infiltrates and hypoxemia. This syndrome was ultimately attributed to a drug reaction to his daptomycin, either pulmonary eosinophilia or cryptogenic organizing pneumonia.

COMMON QUESTIONS GENERATED BY THIS TEACHING

1. When should I pursue VATS lung biopsy in the evaluation of possible DPLD?

    Subacute symptomatic patients (eg, exercise limitation with abnormal PFTs) with imaging suggestive of DPLD deserve consideration for VATS lung biopsy. Biopsy is most likely to alter management when imaging suggests UIP/IPF. Biopsy-proven UIP/IPF mandates antifibrotic medication and consideration for transplant evaluation. Alternatively, a biopsy showing an inflammatory cellular infiltrate warrants a trial of steroids. Patients whose imaging and/or clinical syndrome appears to be inflammatory (ie, predominant ground-glass opacities) or acutely ill patients (too sick for VATS) may be better served by a trial of steroids.

2. When should I perform a bronchoscopy in the evaluation of possible DPLD?

    Bronchoscopy with BAL should be performed to rule out PJP pneumonia in immunosuppressed patients presenting with diffuse ground-glass opacities or in individuals presenting with a radiographic clinical presentation compatible with DAH or eosinophilic pneumonia. Bronchoscopy with endobronchial ultrasound–guided needle aspiration should be performed in individuals with possible sarcoidosis. Bronchoscopy with transbronchial biopsies should be performed when imaging is concerning for lymphangitic spread of tumor.

3. When should I empirically treat DPLD with steroids?

    DPLD should be empirically treated with steroids in symptomatic patients whose imaging and clinical course is suggestive of DPLD if they are too sick (ie, hypoxemic) to tolerate invasive diagnostic workup (ie, BAL or VATS), or in those whose imaging and clinical presentation strongly suggest inflammation/allergy.

4. When should I advise a patient with respiratory failure and DPLD to be DNI because they "will never be able to be extubated"?

    Never, its the wrong way to think and talk about things. Every patient can and may be extubated, even if they will not survive (ie, terminal or compassionate extubation). Patients with definite UIP/IPF experiencing respiratory failure from their underlying disease progression, as determined by failing empiric diuresis, antibiotics, and steroids, should be counseled regarding the futility of intubation, explaining that it will require deep sedation (removing any ability to interact with the outside world) with no benefit (save possible prolongation of life by days). These individuals instead should be encouraged to use medications to reduce dyspnea (ie, narcotics and benzodiazepines), heralding the transition to comfort care.

SHOCK

CHAPTER 18

COMMON MISCONCEPTIONS AND MISTAKES

- Overresuscitating patients with septic shock
- Underresuscitating patients with hemorrhagic shock
- Underresuscitating severe pancreatitis
- Attempting to initially differentiate isolated right-ventricular (RV) cardiogenic shock from left-ventricular (LV) cardiogenic shock by echocardiogram rather than by chest x-ray (looking for pulmonary edema/pleural effusion)
- Missing dependent edema (eg, sacral) during the physical examination
- Failing to consider hemorrhage in inpatients (not admitted for bleeding) who develop shock, instead presuming sepsis

SHOCK

- Pathologically low blood pressure (BP) resulting in end organ hypoperfusion
- Occurs when the normal homeostatic mechanisms protecting organ perfusion (ie, increased sympathetic activity aimed at increasing cardiac output [CO] and systemic vascular resistance [SVR]) fail, leading to systemic tissue hypoxia and organ injury/dysfunction (specifically):
  - Acute kidney injury (often acute tubular necrosis with oliguria)
  - Shock liver (asymptomatic transaminitis or increased international normalized ratio [INR])
  - Decreased mental status (lethargy to obtundation)
  - Lactic acidosis from underperfused skeletal muscle and intestine
- If not reversed, shock will cause death by pulseless electrical activity (PEA) arrest secondary to overwhelming lactic acidosis
- Shock is diagnosed when **end organ hypoperfusion** is proven in the setting of **low BP**
  - Hypoperfusion is evidenced by organ failure and the presence of an elevated serum lactate
- Tachycardia is anticipated in all causes of shock **not** directly related to bradycardia and/or heart block
  - Individuals with baseline conduction system disease may not mount an appropriate tachycardia
    - Shock with "relative bradycardia" may require inotropic/chronotropic support
- There are four distinct pathophysiologic types of shock, with six cardiogenic subtypes (Table 18.1):
  - **Hypovolemic shock**
    - Hypovolemic shock is caused by one of the following:
      - Acute blood loss (hemorrhage)
      - Volume depletion, as seen with gastrointestinal (GI) and renal NaCl loss
      - Third-spacing physiology, as seen in severe pancreatitis or after a large intraabdominal surgery
    - Leads to a decreased central venous pressure (CVP), right ventricular end-diastolic pressure (RVEDP), and left ventricular end-diastolic pressure (LVEDP), reducing stroke volume and thus CO

Table 18.1 Pathophysiologic Types of Shock

TYPE OF SHOCK AND COMMON CAUSES	ANTICIPATED HEMODYNAMICS RED = PRIMARY INSULT BLACK = DIRECT CONSEQUENCE BLUE = COMPENSATORY NEUROHORMONAL RESPONSE	ANTICIPATED EDEMA	ANTICIPATED ECHOCARDIOGRAPHIC FINDING

Hypovolemic
• Blood loss (GI, spontaneous, postprocedure)
• Fluid loss (GI/renal)
• Third spacing
  • Severe pancreatitis
  • Postoperative abdominal surgery
	↓CVP, ↓RVEDP, ↓PAP, ↓ LVEDP, ↓ CO, ↑SVR	No edema	↑RV EF, no PH, nl LA, ↑LV EF

Distributive: • Sepsis without myocardial depression	↓CVP, ↓ RVEDP, ↓ PAP, ↓ LVEDP, ↑CO, ↓SVR	No edema	↑RV EF, No PH, nl LA, ↑LV EF
• Sepsis with myocardial depression	↑CVP, ↑ RVEDP, ↑ PAP, ↑ LVEDP, ↓CO, ↓SVR	Pulmonary edema Peripheral edema	↓RV EF, ↑PAS, ↑ LA, ↓LV EF
• Severe pancreatitis with necrosis • Anaphylaxis • Adrenal insufficiency • Severe acidosis pH <7.2	↓CVP, ↓ RVEDP, ↓ PAP, ↓ LVEDP, ↑ CO, ↓SVR	No edema	↑RV EF, No PH, nl LA, ↑LV EF
LV cardiogenic (systolic dysfunction): • Ischemia, EtOH, viral, tachyarrhythmia (subacute), Takotsubo, idiopathic Long standing: • Aortic or mitral regurgitation, aortic stenosis, HTN	↑CVP, ↑RVEDP, ↑PAP, ↑ LVEDP, ↓ CO, ↑SVR	Pulmonary edema Peripheral edema*	↓RV EF, ↑PAS, ↑ LA, ↓LV EF
LV cardiogenic (diastolic dysfunction): • Tachyarrhythmia (acute) • Hypoxemia (PaO$_2$ < 60 mm Hg) • Volume overload	↑CVP, ↑RVEDP, ↑PAP, ↑ LVEDP, ↓ CO, ↑SVR	Pulmonary edema Peripheral edema*	↓RV EF, ↑PAS, ↑ LA, ↑LV EF

Condition	Hemodynamics	Edema	Echo

LV cardiogenic mechanical failure:
• Mitral regurgitation (acute)
• Aortic regurgitation (acute)
• Outflow tract obstruction
  • Aortic stenosis
  • HOCM
	↑CVP, ↑RVEDP, ↑PAP, **↑ LVEDP, ↓ CO, ↑SVR**	Pulmonary edema
		Peripheral edema*
			Mitral regurgitation
			Aortic regurgitation
			Aortic stenosis
			HOCM

RV cardiogenic, with pulmonary HTN: • Acute PE • CTEPH • IPAH	**↑CVP, ↑RVEDP, ↑PAP, ↓LVEDP, ↓ CO, ↑SVR**	Peripheral edema*	↓RV EF, ↑PAS, nl LA, ↑LV EF
• Mitral stenosis	**↑CVP, ↑RVEDP, ↑PAP, ↓LVEDP, ↓ CO, ↑SVR** (Note: PCWP elevated despite nl LVEDP because of increased LAP and PVP)	Pulmonary edema Peripheral edema*	Mitral stenosis
RV cardiogenic, without pulmonary HTN: • RV infarct	**↑CVP, ↑RVEDP, ↓ PAP, ↓ LVEDP, ↓ CO, ↑SVR**	Peripheral edema*	↓RV EF, no PH, nl LA, ↑LV EF
RV cardiogenic, without pulmonary HTN mechanical failure: • Pericardial effusion with tamponade • Constrictive pericarditis • Restrictive cardiomyopathy	**↑CVP, ↑RVEDP, ↓ PAP, ↓ LVEDP, ↓ CO, ↑SVR**	Peripheral edema*	Echo signs consistent with: • Tamponade physiology • Constrictive pericarditis • Restrictive cardiomyopathy

CO, Cardiac output; CTEPH, chronic thromboembolis pulmonary hypertension; CVP, central venous pressure; EtOH, ethyl acohol; GI, gastrointestinal; HOCM, hypertrophic obstructive cardiomyopathy; HTN, hypertension; IPAH, idiopathic pulmonary arterial hypertension; LAP, left atrial pressure; LVEDP, left ventricular end diastolic pressure; PAP, pulmonary artery pressure; PAS, pulmonary artery systolic; PCWP, pulmonary capillary wedge pressure; PE, pulmonary embolism; PVP, pulmonary venous pressure; RVEDP, right ventricular end-diastolic pressure; SVR, systemic vascular resistance.

↑LV EF = Normal or high LV ejection fraction
↓LV EF = Systolic dysfunction
↑RV EF = Normal or hyperdynamic RV function
↓RV EF = Decreased or hypodynamic RV function and/or RV or RA dilation

*In cases of acute LV and RV cardiogenic shock, peripheral edema takes hours to become appreciable even though right-sided pressures increase instantly.
ᵞPulmonary edema = Interstitial edema, alveolar edema, or pleural effusion

○ Decreased CO triggers an increase in sympathetic activity, leading to tachycardia and a maximally increased SVR (renin–angiotensin system activation)

- **Distributive shock**
  ○ Distributive shock is caused by one of the following:
    - Sepsis (cytokine mediated)
    - Anaphylaxis, as seen in allergic-mediated diffuse mast cell degranulation and histamine release
    - Adrenal crisis, as seen in adrenal insufficiency with provocative stress (eg, bleeding)
    - Severe pancreatitis (cytokine mediated)
    - Neurogenic Shock (central nervous system [CNS] mediated, as in spinal cord injury)
  ○ Leads to inappropriate arteriolar vasodilation **and** increased capillary permeability (capillary leak), which decreases SVR and effective circulating volume, causing hypotension
  ○ Hypotension triggers an increase in sympathetic activity, leading to tachycardia and an increased CO
    - Importantly, distributive shock from sepsis often causes concomitant myocardial depression, decreasing CO
- **LV cardiogenic shock (HFpEF, HFrEF, and mechanical failure)**
  ○ From LV failure, as seen in acute systolic dysfunction from ischemia, acute diastolic dysfunction from arrhythmia or hypoxemia, or mechanical failure (ie, papillary muscle rupture)
  ○ Leads to a decreased CO and an increase in LVEDP, mean pulmonary arterial pressure (mPAP), RVEDP, and CVP
  ○ Decreased CO triggers an increase in sympathetic activity, leading to tachycardia and a maximally increased SVR
- **RV cardiogenic shock (with PH, without PH, and mechanical failure)**
  ○ From isolated RV failure (systolic dysfunction), occurring with pulmonary hypertension (eg, pulmonary embolism), without pulmonary hypertension (eg, RV infarct), or with mechanical failure as in pericardial effusion with tamponade
  ○ Decreased RV stroke volume causes a decrease in RV CO, which leaves the left ventricle underfilled leading to an increased RVEDP and CVP and a decreased LVEDP, LV stroke volume, and LV CO
  ○ The decreased CO triggers an increase in sympathetic activity, leading to tachycardia (unless the conduction system is injured as in inferior wall myocardial infarction with RV infarct) and a maximally increased SVR

INITIAL EVALUATION

- History should focus on screening for symptoms of:
  - Infection (eg, fever, chills, cough, dysuria, abdominal or extremity pain)
  - Bleeding (eg, hematemesis/coffee-ground emesis, bright-red blood per rectum, melena)
  - Left-sided heart failure (eg, paroxysmal nocturnal dyspnea, orthopnea, increased edema, weight gain)
  - Exertional syncope, which is seen in both:
    ○ Isolated right-sided heart failure (eg, pulmonary arterial hypertension [PAH])
    ○ Left-sided heart failure from outflow tract obstruction (ie, hypertrophic obstructive cardiomyopathy [HOCM])
- Physical examination should focus on:
  - Temperature
    ○ Fever and hypotension equal sepsis until proven otherwise
  - Heart rate
    ○ Anticipate sinus tachycardia (relative bradycardia implies conduction system disease or atrioventricular [AV] nodal blockade)

- Blood pressure (BP)
  - Interpret relative to baseline BP:
    - Patients with long-standing, poorly controlled hypertension may experience end organ hypoperfusion despite an mean arterial pressure (MAP) ≥ 60 mm Hg and/or an systolic blood pressure (SBP) ≥ 90 mm Hg
- Mental status
  - Anticipate delirium and/or globally decreased sensorium with septic shock secondary to poor cerebral perfusion and cytokines
  - Anticipate globally decreased sensorium in cardiogenic shock secondary to poor cerebral perfusion from decreased cardiac output
  - Individuals with hemorrhagic shock tend to have a normal mental status despite significant hypotension because cerebral perfusion is maintained by cerebral autoregulation
- Ability to lie flat comfortably (unusual in LV mediated cardiogenic shock)
- Presence or absence of:
  - Oxygen requirement (suggesting LHF, pneumonia, or acute respiratory distress syndrom [ARDS])
  - Heart murmur suggesting valve failure, or a prominent S2 suggesting (pulmonary hypertension [PH]) and/or an S3 suggesting (left-ventricular [LV] dysfunction)
  - Thoracic edema (ie, crackles, decreased breath sounds with dullness) suggesting LHF
  - Peripheral edema suggesting HF
- Markers of cutaneous perfusion may reflect the underlying systemic vascular resistance (ie, poor perfusion implies a high SVR shock state and good perfusion implies a distributive shock state)
  - Skin color (hyperemic or pale)
  - Skin temperature (warm or cool)
- Initial diagnostic labs and imaging include:
  - Complete blood count (CBC) looking for anemia and/or leukocytosis
  - Coagulation studies looking for coagulopathy
  - Chemistries with renal and liver indices and an anion gap calculation
  - Lactate
  - Arterial blood gas (ABG) to check the pH, screen for respiratory failure, and assess gas exchange
    - A pH <7.25 (but typically <7.20) may cause a low SVR state, in and of itself, as intrinsic (and extrinsic) pressors fail in the acidotic milieu
    - Shunt physiology (ie, $PaO_2 < 200$ mm Hg on 100%) is worrisome for either cardiogenic or noncardiogenic pulmonary edema
  - Troponin test looking for evidence of LV or RV ischemia
  - ECG looking for ischemia and/or right heart strain (ie, S I, Q III, flipped T in III)
  - Chest x-ray looking for thoracic fluid and/or pneumonia
  - Urinalysis looking for infection and/or casts consistent with acute tubular necrosis (ATN)
  - Bedside echocardiogram looking at global RV and LV size and function, and screening for a pericardial effusion

DIFFERENTIATING THE TYPES OF SHOCK (FIG. 18.1)

- *First* differentiate **cardiogenic** from **noncardiogenic** etiologies by looking for the **presence or absence** of any peripheral and/or thoracic **edema** (ie, alveolar edema, pulmonary interstitial edema, or pleural effusion)
  - Patients in **hypovolemic** or **distributive** shock will **not** have any **edema** at presentation (unless they had preexisting heart failure and volume overload)
  - Patients with **LV**-mediated **cardiogenic shock** will have **pulmonary edema *and* peripheral edema**
    - Shock from acute LV failure leads to "flash pulmonary edema," a sudden rise in LVEDP, causing dyspnea and gas exchange abnormalities (ie, hypoxemia) with

EVALUATION OF SHOCK

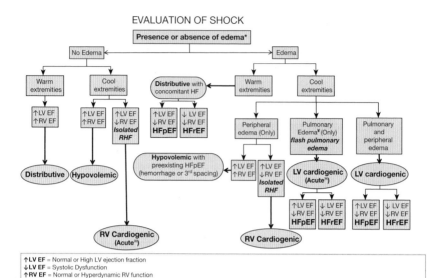

Fig. 18.1 Flow diagram outlining the evaluation of shock by first identifying the presence or absence of **any** edema (peripheral and/or pulmonary). Shock and edema implies either a cardiogenic etiology or preexisting decompensated heart failure with a superimposed distributive or hypovolemic insult. Next, cutaneous perfusion is established by assessing skin temperature (warm vs cool). Shock occurring in an individual with warm extremities implies distributive physiology, whereas shock occurring with cold extremities implies either a cardiogenic or hypovolemic etiology. An echocardiogram is an essential part of the evaluation of an individual with unexplained shock, reliably separating distributive and hypovolemic shock from cardiogenic etiologies. Small, underfilled, hyperdynamic left and right ventricles are seen in cases of distributive and hypovolemic shock. All forms of cardiogenic shock should cause elevated right-sided pressures, evidenced by right-arterial and right-ventricular (RV) dilation and/or RV hypokinesis. RV cardiogenic shock from isolated right-sided heart failure presents with peripheral edema ($\pm$ ascites) alone (no pulmonary edema), unless it happens acutely, in which case patients may have no edema because peripheral edema may take hours to appear. Left-ventricular (LV) cardiogenic shock from biventricular heart failure, both heart failure with preserved ejection fraction (HFpEF) and heart failure with reduced ejection fraction (HFrEF), presents with pulmonary edema and peripheral edema ($\pm$ ascites), unless it happens acutely, in which case pulmonary edema may appear alone (a.k.a. flash pulmonary edema) because peripheral edema may take hours to appear. LV cardiogenic shock can be readily attributed to HFpEF if the LV EF is normal or if HFrEF is reduced. Edematous patients with warm extremities have distributive shock with concomitant heart failure. Edematous patients with cool extremities and small, underfilled, hyperdynamic left and right ventricles have preexisting HFpEF with superimposed hemorrhage (or less likely third spacing). They are not simply volume depleted (ruled out by the presence of peripheral edema).

radiographic evidence of pulmonary edema, often without obvious peripheral edema at presentation
  - Peripheral edema and pleural effusion may take hours to become appreciable (despite an immediate elevation in pulmonary artery pressure [PAP], RVEDP, RA and CVP)
- Patients with **RV**-mediated **cardiogenic shock** (isolated right heart failure) will have peripheral edema **only** (no pulmonary edema)
  - Shock from acute RV failure may present without obvious peripheral edema which may take hours to become appreciable (despite an immediate elevation in RVEDP and CVP)
- *Next* asses cutaneous perfusion (ie, warm vs cool extremities)
  - **Distributive shock** (a low SVR state) produces **warm**, cutaneously well-perfused extremities
  - Both **hypovolemic** and **cardiogenic** shock (high SVR states) produce **cool**, cutaneously poorly perfused extremities

- ***Then*** obtain a cardiac echocardiogram aimed at globally assessing RV and LV function and right- and left-sided pressures (eg, atrial chamber size and estimated pulmonary artery systolic [PAS] pressure) while ruling out tamponade and acute valve failure:
  - The **echocardiogram** is key in **differentiating cardiogenic shock** from **hypovolemic or distributive shock**
  - **Distributive and hypovolemic** shock states cause the right and left ventricles to be underfilled, appearing on an echocardiogram as hyperdynamic (ie, with an increased ejection fraction)
  - **LV-mediated cardiogenic shock** has two possible echocardiographic findings:
    - Decreased systolic function, a.k.a. **HFrEF**
    - Preserved systolic function, a.k.a. **HFpEF**
      - Both HFpEF and HFrEF will cause an increase in LA pressure and mPAP
        - However, echocardiographic evidence of LA enlargement and/or mPAP elevation are not guaranteed
          - The left atrium may not always enlarge under pressure, and echocardiography may underestimate (or miss) pulmonary hypertension
  - **RV-mediated cardiogenic shock** from **mechanical failure** as a result of pericardial effusion with tamponade physiology or LV-mediated cardiogenic shock as a result of aortic or mitral valve failure, can also be readily identified by echocardiogram
  - **RV-mediated cardiogenic shock** (isolated right heart failure) shares the **same** core echocardiographic findings as **LV-mediated cardiogenic shock** caused by HFpEF— namely RV dysfunction with preserved LV function
    - Therefore isolated **RV-mediated cardiogenic shock** is differentiated from **LV-mediated cardiogenic shock due to HFpEF** by the **presence or absence of pulmonary edema** (**not** echocardiographic findings)
      - That said, left atrial enlargement (without mitral valve disease) strongly supports a HFpEF etiology
- **Mixed physiology shock**
  - **Distributive** shock with concomitant **heart failure** occurs relatively commonly, as infection and sepsis can decompensate preexisting heart failure in addition to causing myocardial depression directly (cytokine mediated)
    - Patients will have warm edematous extremities and varying degrees of pulmonary edema
  - **Hypovolemic** shock with preexisting heart failure occurs most commonly when an individual with chronic decompensated heart failure develops hemorrhagic shock or (less commonly) third-spacing physiology
    - Hypovolemic shock causes low CVP, RVEDP, and LVEDP physiology such that:
      - Individuals with preexisting volume overload will have mobilized (resolved) all of their **pulmonary edema** by the time their hypovolemic disease process (eg, GI bleeding) causes shock
      - Long-standing lower extremity edema, however, may persist and be present at presentation in these individuals because this fluid may be slower to mobilize
    - Volume depletion and heart failure **cannot** coexist
      - Volume depletion is a low total-body sodium content state
      - Heart failure is a volume-overloaded, high total body sodium content state

EVALUATION AND MANAGEMENT BY TYPE OF SHOCK

- **Hypovolemia from fluid loss:**
  - Common causes:
    - **Salt and water loss** from the GI tract (vomiting and diarrhea) or kidneys (thiazide diuretic, salt-wasting states)

- **Third-spacing states,** in which fluid weeps into the abdomen, causing sudden, critical intravascular volume depletion, seen in severe pancreatitis and after a large abdominal surgery
- Presentation and evaluation:
  - Patients present hypotensive, tachycardic, and without edema
  - Laboratory results suggest volume depletion (eg, hemoconcentration, elevated blood urea nitrogen (BUN)/creatinine (Cr) >20)
- Support:
  - Aggressive isotonic intravenous fluid resuscitation alone should resolve the shock (ie, not require pressors)
  - Normal saline should be administered in 500–1000 mL boluses (as fast as possible) until heart rate, BP, and urine output normalize (usually 4–6 L)
    - **Third-spacing states** require the highest volume resuscitation because the abdomen may accommodate a large volume of fluid (ie, ascites)
      - **Severe pancreatitis** may require 8–12 L resuscitation in the first 24 hours in an effort to maintain pancreatic perfusion (and prevent necrosis) in the face of third-spacing physiology (Fig. 18.2)
        - Resuscitation should be aggressive enough to cause significant **hemodilution** in the first 6–12 hours
- **Treatment:**
  - GI losses can be treated with antiemetics and antimotility agents (if infectious colitis is **not** a concern)
    - Empiric infectious colitis treatment should be given to those with unexplained profuse and/or bloody diarrhea (including coverage for *Clostridium difficile*)
  - Third spacing improves with time and requires supportive measures only
- **Hypovolemia from blood loss (hemorrhage):**
  - Common causes:
    - **Upper- and lower-GI bleeding** (eg, ulcer, varices, diverticular, arteriovenous malformation [AVM])
    - **Spontaneous bleeding** (eg, retroperitoneal, rectus abdominal sheath, psoas sheath) often occurring in the setting of systemic anticoagulation or coagulopathy
    - Postoperative (eg, partial nephrectomy) or postprocedure (eg, paracentesis) bleeding
  - Presentation and evaluation:
    - Patients present hypotensive, tachycardic, and without edema
    - Physical examination is notable for:
      - **Normal** mental status (despite very low BP)
      - Cutaneous bruising common in retroperitoneal and muscle sheath bleeding
      - Pallor
      - Cold extremities
    - Laboratory and chest x-ray results:
      - In acute hemorrhage, laboratory results are unrevealing (or reveal coagulopathy)
        - Anemia requires time to develop
          - Anemia is seen with acute on chronic hemorrhage (common in cases of GI bleeding)
      - Chest x-ray films show **no** thoracic edema
  - **Support:**
    - Patient's transition from tachycardia and hypotension to PEA arrest with **no warning**
    - Resuscitation must stay ahead of bleeding (administer blood based on estimated loss, **not** last HCT)
      - Persistent or recurrent sinus **tachycardia equals underresuscitation** and/or ongoing bleeding

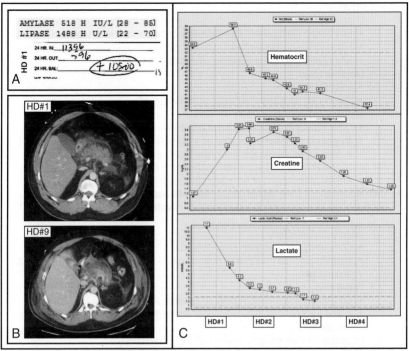

Fig. 18.2 Encapsulated case of an individual admitted with acute pancreatitis secondary to alcohol abuse. **(A)** Elevated amylase and lipase in addition to a ~10 L positive fluid balance in the first 24 hours. **(B)** Computed tomography (CT) imaging of the abdomen with contrast on hospital days 1 and 9. The initial CT scan shows an edematous pancreas without definite necrosis, whereas the follow-up CT scan, 9 days later, reveals necrosis. **(C)** The patient's hematocrit, creatinine, and lactate levels over the first 4 hospital days. The patient presents with hemoconcentration (HCT of 53%), an elevated lactate (11 mmol/L), and oliguria. Despite a 10 L resuscitation attempt, the patient's HCT increased to 58% in the first 24 hours with acute kidney injury (prerenal indices), indicating third-spacing physiology.

- Aggressive IVF resuscitation (0.5–1 L) boluses of LR or NS while waiting for blood
  - With "massive transfusion" (ie, >4 units PRBC in 1 hour or 6 units PRBC in 12 hours), each unit of packed red blood cells (PRBC) should be matched 1-for-1 with platelets and fresh frozen plasma (FFP)
    - Check fibrinogen and consider cryoprecipitate for a fibrinogen <150 mg/dL
- Do **not** worry about overresuscitation (hemorrhage is a low LVEDP state)
- A cordis or two large-bore peripheral IVs are required; pressure bags and rapid infusers are useful
  - A Triple lumen catheter is too long and narrow for effective resuscitation (high resistance)
- Although pressors have no primary role, they are often started for refractory shock while resuscitation is ongoing:
  - Vasopressin promotes vasospasm (helpful in cases of hemorrhage)
  - Beta-agonists are useful if HR is inappropriately low (eg, dopamine, norepinephrine)
- Stress dose steroids should be administered if there is any chance of adrenal insufficiency (hemorrhage demands a maximal cortisol response)

- **Treatment:**
  - Upper-GI Bleed
    - Endoscopic management (band, cautery, or clip) of varices or ulcer by GI
    - Embolization by interventional radiology (IR) and/or resection by general surgery for refractory gastric or duodenal ulcer bleeding
  - Lower-GI Bleed
    - Embolization by IR
    - Surgery for refractory diverticular or AVM bleeding
  - Spontaneous internal bleeding
    - Often venous in origin, associated with anticoagulation
    - May be conservatively managed as anticoagulation is reversed
      - Muscle sheath and retroperitoneal bleeds often develop a local tamponade phenomenon as the pressure in the space increases, promoting hemostasis
    - Arterial bleeding and/or refractory bleeding may require embolization by IR
- **Distributive shock from sepsis (decreased SVR and an increased capillary permeability as a systemic manifestation of infection)**
  - Common inciting infections and organisms:
    - Urinary tract infection
      - Community acquired from *Escherichia coli*
      - Hospital acquired from enteric gram-negative rods (GNRs), staph, enterococcus and candida
    - Pneumonia
      - Community acquired from strep, pneumonia, and staph
      - Hospital acquired from pseudomonas and methicillin-resistant Staphylococcus aureus (MRSA)
    - Hepatobiliary infection from enteric GNRs and enterococcus
    - Cellulitis/necrotizing fasciitis from strep > staph
    - Endocarditis from staph > strep
  - Presentation and evaluation:
    - Patients present hypotensive, tachycardic, and without edema (unless they have preexisting volume overload/heart failure)
      - Often with an obvious infectious prodrome and/or source
    - Physical examination is notable for:
      - Focal pulmonary findings in cases of pneumonia
      - Abdominal and right upper quadrant (RUQ) tenderness in hepatobiliary and intraabdominal infection
      - Redness, warmth, and pain in cases of cellulitis; central anesthesia (ie, pain at the edges only) in cases of necrotizing fasciitis
      - Cutaneous embolic phenomenon in cases of endocarditis
      - Decreased mental status (nonspecific)
  - **Support and treatment** (Fig. 18.3):
    - BP drop and tachycardia tend to occur gradually (over hours), unlike the sudden drop seen in hemorrhagic shock
    - Broad-spectrum IV antibiotics should be administered immediately in patients with possible septic shock
    - Adequate resuscitation is necessary, but **overresuscitation** is **dangerous** and is associated with renal and respiratory failure
    - Patients typically require between 2 and 6 L of IVF
      - If they have peripheral edema (ie, volume overload) when they become septic, closer to 2 L
        - Target circulating volume
        - Give in 500 mL boluses
        - Screen for pulmonary edema between boluses

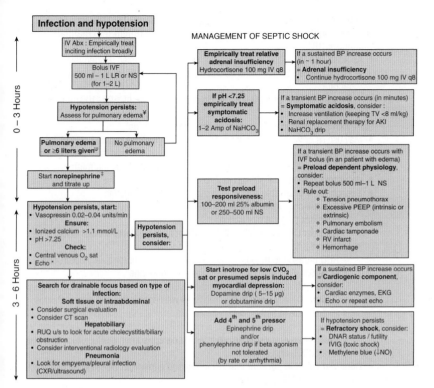

Fig. 18.3 Flow diagram outlining the management of septic shock, starting with empiric broad-spectrum antibiotics and IV fluids. Fluid resuscitation continues until a patient develops edema or >6 L of IV fluid is given. At that point, patients should be considered volume overloaded or fluid unresponsive (respectively), and norepinephrine should be started and titrated up. If hypotension persists, one should simultaneously start vasopressin, rule out hypocalcemia and symptomatic acidosis, and check an echocardiogram (if not already done) and a central venous oxygen (CVO₂) saturation to screen for a significant concomitant cardiogenic component (and surprises like a pericardial effusion with tamponade). Additionally, one should search for a drainable, or surgically intervenable, focus (eg, necrotizing fasciitis, appendicitis, diverticular abscess) with ultrasound and possible computed tomography (CT) scan and/or surgical consultation. Relative adrenal insufficiency should be empirically treated with hydrocortisone 100 mg IV every 8 hours. If oxygenation is adequate, preload responsiveness should be tested with colloid or fluid. If these measures fail (and/or the CVO₂ saturation is low), an inotrope (eg, beta-agonist dose dopamine or dobutamine) should be started for presumed myocardial depression. If shock persists, an epinephrine drip (and/or phenylephrine if epinephrine is not tolerated by rate or arrhythmia) should be started. At this point the patient should be considered moribund, and a change to DNAR status (given futility) should be pursued. Last-ditch efforts may include IVIG (if toxic shock syndrome possible) or methylene blue infusion to scavenge nitric oxide.

- If they are outpatients with a "poor PO" prodrome, closer to 6 L
  - The first 3–4 L fill the interstitium, and the next 2 L restore circulating volume
  - Give in 500 mL to 1 L boluses
  - Screen for pulmonary edema after each liter
- Stop resuscitation at 6 L or at the first sign of pulmonary edema, pleural effusion, or generalized edema

- If hypotension persists, patients should be considered fluid unresponsive, and pressors should be initiated and titrated up as required to maintain an "adequate BP"
  - An adequate BP is one in which systemic tissue perfusion is adequate
    - Evidenced by normal urine output (assuming no AKI) and/or a falling or normal lactate
    - Typically a MAP of $\geq$60–70 mm Hg or a systolic BP of $\geq$90–100 mm Hg will be adequate
- Start with a mixed alpha/beta-agonist (eg, norepinephrine)
  - May use α_1 or v_1 receptor agonist alone (ie, phenylephrine or vasopressin) if the patient is excessively tachycardic (ST >130 bpm) or suffering from a tachyarrhythmia
- If hypotension persists despite maximum norepinephrine (20 mcg/min):
  - Vasopressin should be started (0.2–0.4 units/min)
  - **Search for a drainable focus** based on the type of infection
    - Soft tissue or intraabdominal:
      - Consider surgical evaluation
      - Consider CT imaging (though the patient must be stable enough to leave the unit)
    - Hepatobiliary:
      - RUQ ultrasound to look for acute cholecystitis and/or biliary obstruction
      - Consider IR evaluation for percutaneous drainage
        - Patients with shock from cholecystitis should be evaluated by surgery **but** typically need to be stabilized with antibiotics and percutaneous drainage initially
    - Pneumonia:
      - Look for an empyema (ie, an infected parapneumonic effusion) with a chest x-ray (CXR) and ultrasound
  - **Consider relative adrenal insufficiency** and administer stress dose steroids (ie, hydrocortisone 100 mg IV q 8)
    - A sustained increase in BP occurring 40–60 minutes after steroid administration strongly supports adrenal insufficiency
  - Ensure ionized calcium is >1.1 mmol/L
    - Hypocalcemia can occur in the setting of resuscitation and impair vascular tone
  - Check pH to rule out symptomatic acidosis
    - A pH <7.25 (but typically <7.20) may impair vascular tone by preventing catecholamine-mediated vasoconstriction
    - Symptomatic acidosis can be tested for by administering an ampule of sodium bicarbonate ($NaHCO_3$)
      - A rapid, significant, and transient increase in BP suggests that the refractory shock may be mediated by the low pH
        - This can be treated by:
          - Renal replacement therapy for patients with AKI
          - Increasing minute ventilation (while keeping TV <8 mL/kg) in those receiving mechanical ventilation
          - $NaHCO_3$ drip (3 amps of $NaHCO_3$ mixed in 1 L of D_5W run at 150–333 mL/hr)
            - 333 ml/hr $\approx$ 1 amp/hr
            - Sodium bicarbonate will significantly worsen volume overload
  - **Screen for a cardiogenic component** of the shock by checking an echocardiogram and a central venous O_2 saturation (normal is >65%)
    - Sepsis may cause significant myocardial depression, leading to global LV systolic dysfunction
      - Low central venous O_2 saturation and/or LV dysfunction seen by echocardiogram should prompt consideration for inotropic support with isolated beta-agonists (dopamine in the 5–15 μg range or dobutamine)

- A high or relatively high central venous O_2 saturation suggests distributive physiology (eg, sepsis)
- **Check for preload-dependent physiology** (ie, fluid responsiveness despite total body volume overload)
  - Use 100–200 mL boluses of colloid (eg, 25% albumin) or 250–500 mL of lactated Ringer's (LR) or normal saline (NS), and observe the hemodynamic effect
    - A transient increase in BP after fluid administration (despite edema) suggests preload-dependent physiology
  - Edematous patients who respond to preload should be evaluated for superimposed RV-mediated cardiogenic shock (ie, isolated right-sided heart failure) or superimposed hemorrhagic shock
    - Obtain echocardiogram
      - Rule out pericardial effusion with tamponade
      - If RV function is impaired and LV function is preserved, consider pulmonary embolism (PE) and RV infarct
      - If RV function and LV function are preserved, consider hemorrhage, tension pneumothorax, and excessive PEEP (intrinsic or extrinsic)
        - If extrinsic, attempt to wean PEEP as tolerated by gas exchange
        - Intrinsic PEEP (see Breath stacking auto peep and impaired venous return under special situations below)
  - Isolated RV systolic dysfunction with shock should be supported with inotropes (eg, dopamine)
- **If hypotension persists** despite norepinephrine, vasopressin, dopamine/dobutamine, phenylephrine, and stress dose steroids, and if no drainable focus of infection exists and an echocardiogram is unrevealing, the patient has refractory septic shock and a grave prognosis
- **Refractory septic shock, consider:**
  - A change of code status to DNAR, given potential futility of resuscitation efforts (eg, refractory acidosis despite renal replacement therapy and NaHCO$_3$ infusion)
  - Epinephrine drip
  - Intravenous immunoglubulin (IVIG) infusion for toxic shock syndrome seen with:
    - Group A strep infection as a complication of pharyngitis or cellulitis/soft tissue infection
    - Staph infection associated with nasal packing or tampons
  - Methylene blue infusion as nitric oxide scavenger, though most anecdotes involve cirrhotics
- **Distributive shock from severe pancreatitis with necrosis:**
  - Common causes:
    - Alcohol and gallstones
  - Presentation and evaluation:
    - Patients present hypotensive, tachycardic without edema, complaining of severe abdominal pain
    - Physical examination reveals midepigastric tenderness (occasionally with Cullen's sign, a.k.a. periumbilical bruising)
    - Laboratory results show hemoconcentration, prerenal azotemia, and an elevated serum amylase and lipase
    - CT of abdomen with contrast shows an edematous pancreas ± necrosis
  - Support:
    - Aggressive resuscitation (8–12 L in 24 hours) to stay ahead of third spacing, attempting hemodilution until significant (tense) ascites develops, then use vasopressors
    - Screen for abdominal compartment syndrome, caused by tense ascites, with bladder pressures (should be <25–30 cm H$_2$O)
    - Avoid anticoagulation to prevent conversion to hemorrhagic necrosis

- Treatment:
  - Bowel rest
  - Consider empirically treating infected pancreatic necrosis
    - Use carbapenem to achieve adequate pancreatic penetration
- **Distributive shock from anaphylaxis:**
  - Common causes:
    - Food or drug allergy
  - Presentation and evaluation:
    - Patients present hypotensive, tachycardic, and without edema
    - Physical examination reveals large areas of confluent erythema $\pm$ wheezing
    - Labs demonstrate an elevated tryptase level (transiently)
  - Support:
    - Epinephrine 0.1 mL of 1:1000 IV push (may be repeated; rarely requires IV drip)
    - IV fluid resuscitation
  - Treatment:
    - Identification and avoidance of allergen
    - Histamine receptor blockade, both H_1 and H_2 (ie, diphenhydramine and cimetidine)
    - Steroids to mitigate late-phase anaphylaxis (which is based on inflammatory cell recruitment)
- **Distributive shock from relative and absolute adrenal insufficiency:**
  - Causes of absolute adrenal insufficiency:
    - Addison's disease (autoimmune adrenal insufficiency), hemorrhagic adrenal injury (eg, Sheehan syndrome, a.k.a. postpartum hemorrhage), and granulomatous replacement of the adrenals (eg, TB)
  - Causes of relative adrenal insufficiency:
    - Steroid administration and poor adrenal reserve (idiopathic)
  - Presentation and evaluation:
    - Shock associated with adrenal insufficiency (relative or absolute) occurs when individuals experience a sympathetic stressor (eg, hemorrhage)
    - Inadequate (or absent) cortisol secretion impairs the sympathetic nervous system's ability to increase vascular tone
    - Absolute adrenal insufficiency can be diagnosed by a cortisol value of $<5\,\mu g/dL$ in the setting of shock
    - Symptomatic relative adrenal insufficiency is difficult to test for and instead is empirically treated in those with fluid and pressor refractory shock
  - Treatment:
    - Hypotension associated with adrenal insufficiency should respond dramatically and promptly to IV steroid administration (within 40–60 minutes)
      - All glucocorticoid preparations will work, but hydrocortisone is the fastest
- **Left ventricular cardiogenic shock from systolic dysfunction:**
  - Common causes of systolic dysfunction:
    - Ischemia, ethyl alcohol abuse, viral myocarditis, tachyarrhythmia (subacute), Takotsubo (catecholamine surge), idiopathic cardiomyopathy, or cardiomyopathy secondary to long-standing aortic or mitral regurgitation, aortic stenosis, or hypertension (HTN)
  - Presentation and evaluation:
    - Patients present hypotensive and tachycardic (unless conduction system injured), with pulmonary edema
    - Laboratory results show a brain natriuretic peptide (BNP) >100 pg/mL
    - Elevated BUN/Cr ratio >20 (cardiorenal)
  - Support:
    - Inotropic support with dopamine or dobutamine
    - Diuresis
    - Noninvasive positive pressure ventilation (or intubation)

- Treatment:
  - Euvolemia
  - Revascularization and/or valve repair when appropriate
- **Left ventricular cardiogenic shock from HFpEF:**
  - LV diastolic dysfunction decreases LV CO and increases LVEDP
  - Increased LVEDP triggers a reflexive increase in mPAP and RVEDP
  - RV volume/pressure overload further decreases RV CO, leading to shock (as the RV falls off of its starling curve)
  - Common causes of acute diastolic dysfunction (HFpEF) are:
    - Volume overload
    - Hypoxemia (PaO$_2$ < 60 mm Hg)
    - Tachyarrhythmia
  - Presentation and evaluation:
    - Patients present hypotensive and tachycardic, with pulmonary edema
    - BNP may not be elevated because LV is not dilated
    - Elevated BUN/Cr ratio >20 (cardiorenal)
  - Support:
    - Diuresis
    - Noninvasive positive pressure ventilation (or intubation)
    - Inotropic support with dopamine or dobutamine
  - Treatment:
    - Euvolemia, oxygen support, BP, and heart-rate control
- **Left ventricular cardiogenic shock from mechanical failure:**
  - Common causes:
    - Mitral regurgitation (acute), aortic regurgitation (acute), left ventricular outflow track obstruction (eg, aortic stenosis and HOCM)
  - Presentation:
    - Decompensated biventricular heart failure (ie, peripheral and pulmonary edema)
    - Outflow tract obstruction may present with exertional syncope (or cardiac arrest)
    - Acute valve failure often presents with flash pulmonary edema
      - May be asymmetric in the case of a flail mitral valve leaflet giving focal edema associated with the regurgitant jet trajectory
  - Support:
    - Inotropic support
    - Mechanical ventilation
  - Treatment:
    - Percutaneous or surgical intervention (ie, valve replacement)
- **Right ventricular cardiogenic shock with pulmonary HTN:**
  - Common causes:
    - Acute PE
    - Mitral stenosis
    - Chronic thromboembolic pulmonary hypertension (CTEPH)
    - Idiopathic pulmonary arterial hypertension (IPAH)
  - Presentation, support, and treatment (by specific disease entity):
    - Acute PE
      - Presents with:
        - Isolated right-sided heart failure with right-sided heart strain (right-axis deviation seen by ECG)
        - Often obvious DVT during examination
        - PA filling defects seen on CT angiography
      - Support and treat with:
        - Inotropic support and adequate (but not excessive) preload
        - Thrombolytics and possible inferior vena cava (IVC) filter placement

- CTEPH
  - Presents with:
    - Exercise limitation with exertional syncope (presyncope)
    - Peripheral edema without pulmonary edema
    - Often patients have a history of DVT/PE
    - Chronic (eg, laminar) proximal clot, RV hypertrophy, and mosaicism on lung windows (reflecting areas of decreased perfusion juxtaposed to areas with increased perfusion) possibly seen on CT angiography
  - Support and treat with:
    - Inotropic support and diuresis to euvolemia
    - Anticoagulation, IVC filter placement, and urgent pulmonary thromboendarterectomy
- IPAH
  - Presents with:
    - Exercise limitation with exertional syncope (presyncope)
    - Peripheral edema without pulmonary edema
    - Pulmonary hypertension and isolated RV failure (with a small, underfilled LA and LV) seen during echocardiography
  - Support and treat with:
    - Inotropes (ie, dopamine) and direct pulmonary vasodilators (eg, prostacyclin)
    - Diuresis to euvolemia
    - Anticoagulation
- Mitral stenosis
  - Presents with:
    - Shortness of breath and exercise limitation
    - Pulmonary and peripheral edema
    - Mitral valve stenosis, LA enlargement, pulmonary hypertension, and varying degrees of RV dysfunction seen during echocardiography
  - Support and treat with:
    - Diuresis to euvolemia
    - Inotropes (aimed at RV failure [ie, dopamine])
    - Mitral valve replacement
- **RV cardiogenic shock without pulmonary HTN:**
  - Common cause:
    - RV infarct
      - Presents with:
        - Hypotension, often with bradycardia or heart block (as occurs with inferior wall ischemia)
        - Right-sided ECG leads (a.k.a. Lewis leads) showing ST segment elevation in II, III, and aVF
        - Depressed RV systolic function **without** pulmonary hypertension, LA enlargement, or LV dysfunction seen during echocardiography
      - Support and treat with:
        - Inotropic support and adequate (but not excessive) preload
        - Cardiac catheterization
- **RV cardiogenic shock without pulmonary HTN from mechanical failure:**
  - Common causes:
    - Pericardial effusion with tamponade
    - Constrictive pericarditis
    - Restrictive cardiomyopathy
  - Presents with:
    - Exercise limitation and exertional syncope
    - Peripheral edema without pulmonary edema
    - In cases of pericardial effusion with tamponade, a CXR possibly showing a large, globular "water bottle" heart

- Support and treatment (by specific disease entity):
  - Pericardial effusion with tamponade
    - Emergent pericardiocentesis ± pericardial drain placement
  - Constrictive pericarditis and restrictive cardiomyopathy
    - NSAIDs and TB treatment if appropriate
    - Pericardiectomy

GENERAL PRINCIPLES OF SHOCK MANAGEMENT

- Management of shock requires a continual **clinical** reassessment of the essential hemodynamic parameters—namely **filling pressures, cardiac output, and SVR**
- Clinical assessment is **more** important and useful than CVP and/or right-sided heart catheterization data, both of which are prone to error and often misleading (Fig. 18.4)

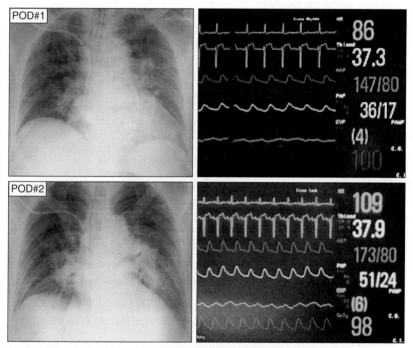

- Postoperative patient given intravenous fluid boluses targeting a CVP ≥ 10 mm Hg as part of "Triple H therapy" protocol (Induced hypertension, hypervolemia, and hemodilution)
- Achieves a 2.2 L positive fluid balance on POD #2 and becomes edematous
- Develops perihilar 'bat-wing' pulmonary edema with left > right pleural effusions (and impaired oxygenation)
- Heart rate, blood pressure and pulmonary artery pressures pressure all increased significantly demonstrating the worsening volume overload
- Central venous pressure, however, starts unbelievably low (given the chest x-ray) at 4 mm Hg and barely increases to 6 mm Hg

Fig. 18.4 Encapsulated case showing the chest x-ray (CXR) film and monitor screen grab of an intensive care unit (ICU) patient with a right-sided heart catheter (not wedged) on POD #1 and POD #2, after a 2.2 L positive fluid balance. The patient was receiving "triple-H therapy" and induced hypertension, hypervolemia, and hemodilution aimed at maintaining adequate cerebral perfusion in the setting of impaired cerebrovascular autoregulation after a complicated aneurism repair. On POD #1, his CXR shows perihilar edema (indicating an elevated left-ventricular end-diastolic pressure). His right-heart catheter shows a pulmonary artery systolic (PAS)/pulmonary artery distial (PAD) of 36/17 mm Hg, with a central venous pressure (CVP) of 4 mm Hg. After being net positive ~2 L overnight, his CXR develops a classic "bat wing" pulmonary edema pattern with left > right pleural effusion. Additionally, the patient develops hypertension and tachycardia, and his RHC shows that his PAS and PAD have increased significantly to 51/24 mm Hg, all indicating worsening left-sided heart failure and volume overload. His central venous pressure, however, barely budges, topping out at 6 mm Hg.

- Filling pressures should be presumed to be adequate when patients develop fluid overload (effusions and edema)
  - In the absence of fluid overload, fluid responsiveness should be repeatedly tested with IVF boluses (to a maximum based on the clinical scenario, eg, 6 L for septic shock, 10 L for pancreatitis)
- When patients develop fluid overload during resuscitation pressors should be started
  - The initial pressor should be a mixed alpha and beta agonist (eg, norepinephrine), unless the patient is excessvily tachycardic, in which case it should be an alpha agonist alone (eg, neosynephrine)
- Cardiac output can be assessed by end organ perfusion (urine output), lactate, and central venous O_2 saturation
  - Useful when adjusting vasopressors to ensure improvement rather than worsening
    - A low central venous O_2 saturation should prompt inotropic support with a beta agonist (eg, dopamine)
  - Urine output is very sensitive to renal perfusion and in turn cardiac output if intrinsic renal injury (ie, ATN) is not present
  - When urine output drops while weaning pressors, consider increasing the MAP goal (eg, from 65 mm Hg to 70 mm Hg)

SPECIAL SITUATIONS

- **Shock that is out of proportion to the clinical scenario:**
  - Consider adrenal insufficiency
  - Consider toxic shock syndrome (rule out nasal packing or tampon, pharyngitis, and/or skin/soft issue infection)
- **Urosepsis:**
  - Patients get better quickly (often despite documented bacteremia)
- **_C. difficile_ infection:**
  - Patients with _C. difficile_ colitis often have significant septic physiology from poor bowel wall integrity (without bacteremia), before toxic dilation and perforation
- **Splenectomy:**
  - Splenectomized patients are vulnerable to high-grade bacteremia from encapsulated organisms and extremely rapid deterioration and death
  - Prompt empiric antibiotic administration and supportive care are critical
- **Rash and shock:**
  - Consider endocarditis, toxic shock syndrome, meningococcemia and erlichosis
- **Isolated diastolic hypotension:**
  - Patients who can not be weaned off of vasopressors because of low MAPs from isolated diastolic hypotension, despite resolution of all other signs of shock (often sitting in a chair at the bedside)
    - Commonly (but not exclusively) seen when noninvasive BP measurements are being used
    - Treat by changing vasopressor titration goal from an MAP $\geq$60 mm Hg to an SBP $\geq$90 mm Hg
      - Occasionally you must sit in the room (providing reassurance to nursing), chatting with the patient, as the vasopressor drip is finally stopped
      - Tough out a few asymptomatic low BP readings (as endogenous catecholamines return)
- **Sedation related low SVR:**
  - SVR is often low, or inappropriately low, secondary to pain medication and sedation
  - Sedation-related reductions in SVR are easily treated with low-dose alpha-agonists (eg, 50–100 mcg/kg/min of phenylephrine)
- **Breath stacking auto peep and impaired venous return:**
  - Consider in intubated patients who develop sudden tachycardia, hypotension, and an inability to ventilate

- Rule out impaired venous due to high intrinsic peep by disconnecting the patient from the ventilator, allowing a complete exhalation
- A rapid reduction in HR, and an increase in BP after disconnection from the ventilator, confirms the diagnosis
  - To prevent reassurance, the respiratory rate on the ventilator must be reduced, or the patient must be sedated (or paralyzed) if he or she is overbreathing the set rate

CIRRHOSIS

- Cirrhotic patients have a low SVR and an increased cardiac output at baseline (from pathologic vasodilatation)
- They are prone to AKI, with only minor decreases in renal blood flow
  - Additionally, decreased renal blood flow is capable of triggering hepatorenal syndrome
- Cirrhosis is a sodium-avid state such that decompensated cirrhotics are often volume overloaded at the time they develop their hemorrhagic or distributive shock
- Hemorrhagic shock, secondary to portal-hypertensive–associated bleeding (eg, variceal), is the most common cause of shock in this population
  - Mysterious shock in a cirrhotic patient equals UGIB until proven otherwise
  - Bleeding is often accompanied by worsening hepatic encephalopathy and an elevated BUN secondary to ammonia generation from ingested/digested blood
  - Bleeding (as always) requires aggressive resuscitation
- Septic shock, often related to spontaneous bacterial peritonitis, is also common
  - Sepsis occurring in an edematous cirrhotic patient should involve minimal NaCl resuscitation (1–2 L maximum), with early pressor administration
- Lactic acid levels are often very high in cirrhotic patients with shock, and prognosis hinges on the rapidity of clearance (rather than absolute magnitude)

COMMON QUESTIONS GENERATED BY THIS TEACHING

1. Is pulmonary HTN with RV systolic dysfunction, in the setting of normal LV systolic function, pathognomonic for PAH and, if associated with shock, virtually diagnostic of acute pulmonary embolism?
   No. The most common cause of RV systolic dysfunction is an elevated mPAP and LVEDP from the biventricular heart failure reflex (HFpEF or HFrEF). The most common cause of RV systolic dysfunction occurring with pulmonary hypertension and preserved LV systolic function is HFpEF. The presence of pulmonary edema and/or left atrial enlargement (in the absence of mitral valve disease) clinches the diagnosis.
2. Is GI always the "first call" for a patient with massive lower-GI bleeding?
   No. Unlike upper-GI bleeding, in which endoscopic hemostasis is the primary therapeutic approach, endoscopy has little or no role in the management of hemorrhagic shock secondary to lower-GI bleeding. Interventional radiology (via angiography and embolization) and general surgery (via resection) are the services that achieve hemostasis in massive lower-GI bleeding.
3. Is CVP useful in guiding resuscitation?
   No. CVP values are unreliable, and optimal CVP pressures are not known. Many patients suffer iatrogenic HFpEF when resuscitation targets a CVP greater than some number (typically 6–12 L). Applying reasonable limits to resuscitation (ie, 2–6 L) and carefully reassessing patients for the development of edema during resuscitation is a much better approach.
4. Do steroids improve blood pressure in patients with adrenal insufficiency (relative or absolute) by increasing sodium reabsorption in the kidney (ie, mineralocorticoid effect)?
   No. It is the glucocorticoid effect on vascular smooth muscle cells and sympathetic receptors that is required for normal vascular tone and/or intrinsic/extrinsic pressor response. Any glucocorticoid should work in 40–60 minutes.

CHAPTER 19

INVASIVE MECHANICAL VENTILATION

COMMON MISCONCEPTIONS AND MISTAKES

- Believing that patients with acute respiratory distress syndrome (ARDS) require advanced modes of mechanical ventilation (eg, airway pressure release ventilation [APRV])

- Changing the ventilator mode from volume control to pressure control because of high peak airway pressures, without urgently working up the change in pulmonary mechanics

- Attempting lung-protective ventilation while allowing patients to have tidal volumes (TVs) >6 mg/kg by ignoring "double triggering" of the ventilator

- Missing breath stacking and severe intrinsic positive end-expiratory pressure (PEEP)

- Missing the tell-tale warning signs of endotracheal tube (ET) tube occlusion with biofilm—namely, increasing peak inspiratory pressures; unchanged plateau pressures and reports of intermittent difficulty passing the suction catheter

INVASIVE MECHANICAL VENTILATION

- The **goal** of **invasive mechanical ventilation** is **always the same** (in every patient):
  - to provide **adequate** respiratory support **without causing** ventilator-associated **lung injury**

- This requires a **lung-protective ventilation** strategy where **low lung volumes** (6–8 mg/kg) are prioritized
  - Low lung volumes have been proven to improve survival in individuals with ARDS (Ventilation with Lower Tidal Volumes as Compared with Traditional Tidal Volumes for Acute Lung Injury and the Acute Respiratory Distress Syndrome, ARDSNET, N Engl J Med 2000; 342:1301–1308, May 4, 2000)

- Mechanical ventilation is capable of causing life-threatening injury by causing either (or both):
  - Noncardiogenic pulmonary edema/ARDS (by alveolar overdistension and trauma)
  - Pneumothorax (PTX)
  - Most likely to occur when:
    - Lung volumes are high (>8 mg/kg)
    - Peak airway pressures are high (>40 cm H_2O)
    - Plateau pressures (P_{plat}) are high (>30 cm H_2O)

- **Adequate** as opposed to **full** support; prioritizes **low lung volumes** over **normal pH and pco_2**

- In patients with abnormal lung mechanics, this often requires permitting a respiratory acidosis (a.k.a. permissive hypercapnia) to maintain a **safe** TV of ~6 mg/kg, **ideal body weight (IBW)** (Table 19.1)

Table 19.1 Safe Tidal Volumes Based on Height (Ideal Body Weight)

HEIGHT (FT)	INCHES	CENTIMETERS	FEMALE TIDAL VOLUME (ML) 6 MG/KG	FEMALE TIDAL VOLUME (ML) 8 MG/KG	MALE TIDAL VOLUME (ML) 6 MG/KG	MALE TIDAL VOLUME (ML) 8 MG/KG
5′	60	152	270	360	300	400
5′3	63	160	310	420	340	455
5′6	66	168	350	480	380	510
5′9	69	175	400	530	420	560
6′	72	182	430	580	460	610
6′6	78	198	520	690	550	730
6′10	82	208	575	770	600	800

- Males: IBW = 50 kg + 2.3 kg for each inch over 5 feet
- Females: IBW = 45.5 kg + 2.3 kg for each inch over 5 feet

- Permissive hypercapnia requires tolerating hemodynamically asymptomatic pH decreases (often in the low 7.1–7.2 range)

- Prioritizing low lung volumes means that increasing the minute ventilation is done by increasing the rate, **not** the TV
  - Maximum respiratory rate is determined by exhalation time and varies widely based on the pulmonary mechanics (ie, 15 breaths/min for obstructive disease vs 35 breaths/min for restrictive disease)
  - Practically speaking, maximum respiratory rate is determined by examining the expiratory flow waveform and ensuring that flow returns to zero before the next breath is delivered (Fig. 19.1A)
    - The rate is then slowly increased to the point just before breath stacking (delivery of the next breath before complete exhalation of the last one) (Fig. 19.1B)

- In patients with severely abnormal lung mechanics, lung-protective ventilation typically requires deep sedation and paralysis to avoid dyssynchrony, which can:
  - Prevent effective ventilation (via high pressures generated by patient struggling/misplaced effort)
  - Cause breath stacking (previously described)
  - Cause double triggering, where acidosis and air hunger cause the patient to trigger a breath immediately after the last breath terminates (before complete exhalation), leading to the delivery of nearly twice the set TV (Fig. 19.1C)

CHOOSING A MODE OF VENTILATION (VOLUME CONTROLLED VS PRESSURE CONTROLLED)

- All individuals requiring mechanical ventilation can be appropriately managed with either volume-controlled (VC) or pressure-controlled (PC) ventilation
  - There is no disease state that requires exotic modes of ventilation

- Volume controlled
  - TV is **set** and fixed
  - Airway pressures vary based on airway resistance and lung compliance

Basic Ventilator Wave Form Analysis

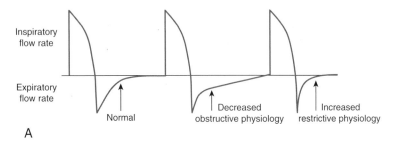

A

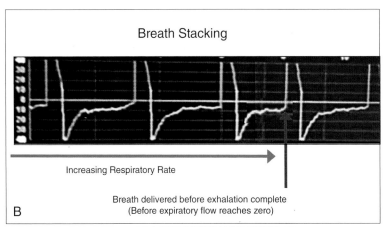

B

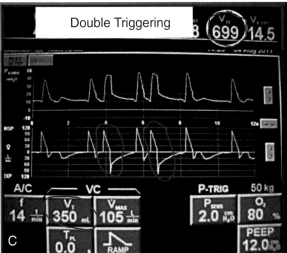

C

Fig. 19.1 See figure legend on opposite page.

- Pressure controlled
  - Peak airway pressure is **set** and fixed
  - TV varies based on airway resistance and lung compliance

- **Volume-controlled ventilation** is the **preferred** mode of ventilation for individuals with **normal to moderately abnormal** pulmonary mechanics, because:
  - It prioritizes control of tidal volume, which is the hallmark of a lung-protective ventilatory strategy
  - It is the most commonly used mode, making it the safest
    - Staff familiarity (specifically with high airway pressure alarms) makes this the easiest mode to troubleshoot
  - It is more comfortable than pressure control, requiring less sedation
  - Volume-controlled ventilation is only problematic when patients have severely abnormal pulmonary mechanics (ie, extremely increased airway resistance or low compliance)
    - In these situations it can take time to find the minimally acceptable TV (based on airway pressure alarming), delaying adequate support and placing the individual **at risk for barotrauma**

- **Pressure-controlled ventilation** is the **preferred** mode of ventilation for individuals with **severely abnormal pulmonary mechanics**
  - Pressure control can protect patients with severe obstruction or poor compliance from barotrauma, while rapidly establishing the minimally effective/safe TV
  - However, this protection from barotrauma puts them **at risk for underventilation**, as TV is sacrificed to avoid high airway pressures
    - PIPs are fixed; therefore TV drops when mechanics worsen
  - In pressure control mode **the low exhaled TV alarm** (used to detect circuit disconnect in VC mode) becomes the **most important** alarm, signaling a change in mechanics (akin to the peak airway alarm in VC mode)
    - Ensure that it is set high enough, reflecting the lowest TV you would be comfortable with (eg, 350 mL in a patient with a TV target of 450 mL)
  - The low minute ventilation alarm is also important in pressure control, screening for underventilation

VOLUME CONTROL: INITIAL VENTILATOR SETTINGS AND ADJUSTMENTS FOR PATIENTS WITH NORMAL TO MODERATELY ABNORMAL MECHANICS (FIG. 19.2)

- Normal lung mechanics:
  - TV: 8 mL/kg IBW
  - Rate: 15 breaths/min
  - FiO_2: start with 50% FiO_2
  - PEEP: 5 cm H_2O

Fig. 19.1 (A) Representative tracing of a flow vs time ventilator waveform, showing three mechanical breaths delivered under three hypothetical situations; normal pulmonary physiology, obstructive physiology, and restrictive physiology, highlighting the difference in expiratory flow rate and thus expiratory time. Obstructive physiology is evidenced by a decreased expiratory flow rate and a long exhalation time, where restrictive physiology is evidenced by a supranormal expiratory flow rate, and a shortened exhalation time. **(B)** Flow vs time tracing of a patient with obstructive physiology demonstrating breath stacking, occurring after an increase in respiratory rate. This is evidenced by the delivery of a breath before the complete exhalation of the last one. **(C)** Pressure vs time and a flow vs time tracing illustrating "double triggering," a phenomenon where the patient triggers a mechanical breath before exhalation of the last one, leading to the delivery of nearly twice the set tidal volume (TV). This is evident by comparing the set TV in the lower left of the figure with the actual exhaled TV in the upper right portion of the figure. Double triggering must be avoided during lung-protective ventilation.

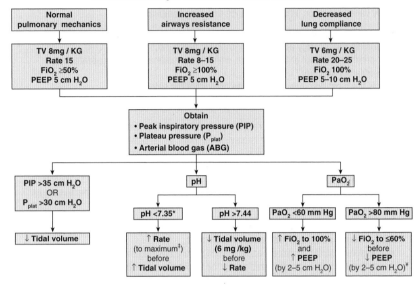

NORMAL to MODERATELY IMPAIRED RESISTENCE or COMPLIANCE:
Initial Ventilator Settings, Preferred Mode = **VOLUME CONTROL**

* Avoid acidosis to avoid dyspnea, patient discomfort, and increased sedation needs

‡ **Maximum rate** = as fast as possible without breath stacking (typically 12–15 b/m for obstructive disease, 25–35 b/m for ARDS)

¥ In ARDS **wean PEEP slowly** (ie, decrease by 2–5 cm H_2O q 12–24 hrs) to avoid derecruitment, In cardiogenic edema PEEP may be weaned more quickly

Fig. 19.2 Flow diagram showing initial ventilator settings and adjustments for individuals with normal to moderately impaired pulmonary mechanics. Patients with normal lungs, like those intubated for a surgical procedure, will generally tolerate a tidal volume (TV) of 8 mg/kg better than 6 mg/kg (less air hunger/sedation needs). Ventilating patients with increased airway resistance requires a low enough respiratory rate to allow complete exhalation before breath delivery. Ventilating patients with restrictive physiology requires low lung volumes (6 mg/kg) and faster respiratory rates. Regardless of the pulmonary mechanics, ventilator adjustments, aimed at achieving safe airway pressure and adequate ventilation and oxygenation, are the same. High airway pressures require a decrease in TV. A symptomatic respiratory acidosis requires an increase in rate (just to the point before breath stacking), before an increase in TV. A respiratory alkalosis requires a decrease in TV to 6 mg/kg (safest TV) before a decrease in rate. A $PaO_2 < 60$ mm Hg on 60% mandates a FiO_2 of 100% and an increase in PEEP. When PaO_2 improves, first wean FiO_2 to 60% and then wean PEEP (watching closely for intolerance/derecruitment).

- **Mild to moderate increase in airway resistance:**
  - TV: 8 mL/kg IBW
  - Rate: 8–15 breaths/min
  - FiO_2: start with ≥100% FiO_2
  - PEEP: 5 cm H_2O

- **Mild to moderate decrease in lung compliance:**
  - TV: 6 ml/kg IBW
  - Rate: 20–25 breaths/min
  - FiO_2: start with 100% FiO_2
  - PEEP: 5–10 cm H_2O

- **Adjusting the ventilator in volume control mode based on safe airway pressures and adequate arterial blood gas (ABG) values:**
  - Obtain the PIP, the P_{plat} and ABG values
    - If the PIP is >35 cm H_2O or the P_{plat} is >30 cm H_2O, decrease the TV
    - If the pH is <7.35, increase the rate (to the maximum tolerated before breath stacking), then consider increasing the TV, watching airway pressures closely

- If the pH is >7.44, decrease the TV to 6 mg/kg before decreasing the rate
- If the Pao_2 is <60 mm Hg, increase the Fio_2 to 100% and increase the PEEP by 2–5 cm H_2O
- If the Pao_2 is >80 mm Hg, decrease the Fio_2 to ≤60% before decreasing PEEP by 2–5 cm H_2O

- Things to remember about volume control:
  - Patient always gets full TV with every breath; PIP and P_{plat} vary
  - Breath stacking (where the next breath is triggered before complete exhalation) is a major problem when ventilating patients with obstructive lung disease in acute respiratory failure because of both:
    - Prolonged exhalation and a rapid intrinsic respiratory rate (increased drive from acidosis)
    - Flow vs time waveform reveals that the next breath is delivered before flow returns to zero (ie, before exhalation is complete)
      - This can lead to dynamic hyperinflation, high intrinsic PEEP, and ultimately an increase in intrathoracic pressure high enough to impair venous return
      - This causes shock and failure to ventilate
        - Physical examination reveals tachycardia, hypotension, and failure to ventilate secondary to "high pressure" limits, with no air movement despite connection to the ventilator
        - Temporarily disconnecting the patient from the ventilator, allowing complete exhalation, provides instantaneous resolution to the acute ventilatory failure and hemodynamic instability
        - Rate must be decreased and/or the patient must be sedated (± paralyzed) to prevent rapid recurrence

PRESSURE CONTROL: INITIAL SETTINGS AND ADJUSTMENTS FOR PATIENTS WITH SEVERELY ABNORMAL LUNG MECHANICS

- **Severely increased airway resistance:** (Fig. 19.3)
  - Driving pressure: 25–35 cm H_2O
  - PEEP: 5 cm H_2O
  - Rate: 8–15 breaths/min
  - Fio_2: 100%
  - Low exhaled TV alarm: 300–400 mL

- **Severely decreased lung compliance:** (Fig. 19.4)
  - Driving pressure: 20 cm H_2O
  - PEEP: 10–20 cm H_2O
  - Rate: 20–30 breaths/min
  - Fio_2: 100%
  - Low exhaled TV alarm: 300–400 mL

- Adjust the ventilator in pressure control mode based on safe TVs and adequate ABG values
  - Obtain the TV, the P_{plat}, and an ABG
  - If the TV is too high (>8 mg/kg in increased airway resistance, or >6 mg/kg in decreased lung compliance) or the P_{plat} is >30 cm H_2O, decrease the driving pressure
  - If pH is <7.20 (and affecting hemodynamics), increase the rate to maximum (ensuring adequate exhalation time/avoid breath stacking), then increase driving pressure unless TV ≥8 mg/kg
    - In this situation sodium bicarbonate may be administered, but this comes with obligatory volume that must be diuresed

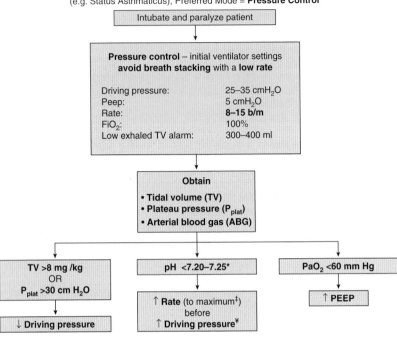

EXTREMELY HIGH AIRWAYS RESISTANCE:
Initial Ventilator Settings for Difficult to Ventilate Patients
(e.g. Status Asthmaticus), Preferred Mode = **Pressure Control**

Intubate and paralyze patient

Pressure control – initial ventilator settings
avoid breath stacking with a **low rate**

Driving pressure:	25–35 cmH$_2$O
Peep:	5 cmH$_2$O
Rate:	**8–15 b/m**
FiO$_2$:	100%
Low exhaled TV alarm:	300–400 ml

Obtain
• Tidal volume (TV)
• Plateau pressure (P$_{plat}$)
• Arterial blood gas (ABG)

TV >8 mg /kg
OR
P$_{plat}$ >30 cm H$_2$O
→ ↓ **Driving pressure**

pH <7.20–7.25*
→ ↑ **Rate** (to maximum‡)
before
↑ **Driving pressure**¥

PaO$_2$ <60 mm Hg
→ ↑ **PEEP**

* **Tolerate a lower pH (a.k.a. permissive hypercapnia) if no symptoms** (ie, no supraventricular tachycardia or refectory hypotension)
‡ **Maximum rate** = as fast as possible without breath stacking (typically 12–15 b/m)
¥ **Keep peek air way pressure** (driving pressure + PEEP) **<40–50 cm H$_2$O**
(to avoid pneumothorax)

Fig. 19.3 Flow diagram showing the initial approach to the mechanical ventilation of a patient with extremely high airway resistance. Paralysis is necessary to avoid breath stacking. Driving pressure is set to achieve a tidal volume (TV) of 6 to 8 mg/kg. Rate is set slow enough to avoid breath stacking, determined by examination of the flow vs time plot on the ventilator, ensuring expiratory flow returns to zero before the next breath is initiated. Positive end-expiratory pressure (PEEP) sensitive shunt physiology is uncommon in obstructive disease such that a PEEP of 5 cm H$_2$O is typically adequate. Matching auto PEEP is of no benefit in a paralyzed/sedated patient with extremely high airway resistance. High TVs require a decrease in driving pressure. A hemodynamically symptomatic respiratory acidosis requires an increase in rate (just to the point before breath stacking), before an increase in driving pressure. A respiratory alkalosis requires a decrease in driving pressure to achieve a TV of 6 mg/kg (safest TV) before a decrease in rate. A PaO$_2$ < 60 mm Hg on a FiO$_2$ of 100% requires an increase in PEEP. When PaO$_2$ improves, first wean FiO$_2$ to 60% and then wean PEEP (watching closely for intolerance/derecruitment). In pressure control mode, the most important alarm is the low exhaled TV. It must be set high enough to alert you of a meaningful change in airway resistance.

- If the patient also has renal failure, renal replacement therapy should be considered to help with the renal compensation (metabolic alkalosis) component
- If PaO$_2$ < 60 mm Hg, increase PEEP by 2–5 cm H$_2$O
  - Shunt physiology is not a common problem in patients with increased airway resistance (ie, obstructive disease) such that an FiO$_2$ ≥ 60% and a physiologic PEEP of 5 cm H$_2$O will usually attain a PaO$_2$ > 60 mm Hg
  - Although matching intrinsic PEEP with expiratory postive airway pressure (EPAP) in patients with obstructive disease on bilevel positive airway pressure (BiPAP) can decrease the work of breathing and prevent intubation, matching intrinsic PEEP in mechanically ventilated patients is not as helpful and increases PIPs

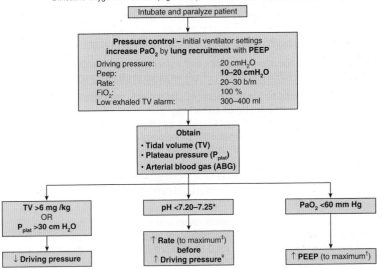

EXTREMELY LOW COMPLIANCE:
Initial Ventilator Settings for
Difficult to Oxygenate Patients (e.g. ARDS), Preferred Mode = **Pressure Control**

Intubate and paralyze patient

Pressure control – initial ventilator settings
increase PaO$_2$ by **lung recruitment** with **PEEP**

Driving pressure:	20 cmH$_2$O
Peep:	**10–20 cmH$_2$O**
Rate:	20–30 b/m
FiO$_2$:	100 %
Low exhaled TV alarm:	300–400 ml

Obtain
- **Tidal volume (TV)**
- **Plateau pressure (P$_{plat}$)**
- **Arterial blood gas (ABG)**

TV >6 mg /kg
OR
P$_{plat}$ >30 cm H$_2$O → ↓ **Driving pressure**

pH <7.20–7.25* → ↑ **Rate** (to maximum[†])
before
↑ **Driving pressure**[¥]

PaO$_2$ <60 mm Hg → ↑ **PEEP** (to maximum[†])

[‡] **Maximum rate** = as fast as possible without breath stacking (typically 25–35 b/m)
[*] **Tolerate a lower pH if no symptoms** (ie, no supraventricular tachycardia or refectory hypotension)
[†] **Maximum PEEP** = as high a PEEP as possible without hypotension (impaired venous return), typically 15–25 cm H$_2$O
[¥] **Keep peek air way pressure** (driving pressure + PEEP) **<40–50 cm H$_2$O** (to avoid pneumothorax)

Fig. 19.4 Flow diagram showing the initial approach to the mechanical ventilation of a patient with extremely low compliance. Paralysis is necessary because of the need for synchrony with the ventilator (despite uncomfortable ventilator settings). Driving pressure is set to 20 cm H$_2$O to allow for high positive end-expiratory pressure (PEEP) while maintaining a peak inspiratory pressure ≤40 cm H$_2$O. PEEP is set to 10 to 20 cm H$_2$O based on the severity/refractory nature of the hypoxemia. FiO$_2$ is set to 100%. Rate is set to fast (20–30 breaths/min) to maintain an adequate minute ventilation (MV). High TVs and/or a high P$_{plat}$ require a decrease in driving pressure. A hemodynamically symptomatic respiratory acidosis requires an increase in rate (just to the point before breath stacking), before an increase in driving pressure (remembering that PIPs in the 40–50 cm H$_2$O range often result in pneumothoraces). A respiratory alkalosis requires a decrease in driving pressure to achieve a TV of 6 mg/kg (safest TV) before a decrease in rate. A Pao$_2$ < 60 mm Hg on a FiO$_2$ of 100% requires an increase in PEEP. When Pao$_2$ improves, first wean FiO$_2$ to 60% and then wean PEEP (watching closely for intolerance/derecruitment). In pressure control mode, the most important alarm is the low exhaled TV. It must be set high enough to alert you of a meaningful change in compliance.

- Things to remember about pressure control:
  - Pressure is fixed; therefore worsening respiratory mechanics lead to a decreased TV
  - Double triggering is a major problem in patients with noncardiogenic edema because these individuals are at the highest risk for ongoing alveolar injury based on high TVs and alveolar overdistension
    - Double triggering can be seen by examining the ventilator waveform and the (actual) exhaled TV
      - When patients trigger the next breath immediately after the last, they often achieve a TV nearly twice the set value (see Fig. 19.1C)
  - Indicates a need for more sedation and likely paralysis

IMPROVING OXYGENATION

- Oxygenation is increased by increasing Fio$_2$ and end expiratory pressure:
  - Increasing Fio$_2$ to 100% can improve hypoxemia, even with extremely low V/Q physiology
  - Increasing (positive) end expiratory pressure (ie, PEEP):

- At the level of the alveolus, it recruits uninjured alveoli and protects injured alveoli from atelectasis while also forcing intraalveolar fluid to the edges of the air sac, improving diffusion and thus oxygenation
- At the level of the lung segment, it prevents and resolves atelectasis (as seen in individuals with obesity, whose bases are subject to the collapsing force of their abdomen, often unmasked by sedation/paralysis and loss of abdominal wall muscular tone)

- Shunt physiology is the norm in patients with extremely poor compliance (eg, ARDS), and often an Fio_2 of 100% and high PEEP are required to attain a $Pao_2 > 60$ mm Hg

- Increasing PEEP should be the first maneuver for patients demonstrating shunt physiology (ie, $Pao_2 < 200$ mm Hg on 100% Fio_2)
  - Optimal PEEP, the PEEP at which most lung units are inflated but none are overdistended, is different in every patient and changes within an individual over the course of his or her illness
  - Increasing PEEP will increase PIP variably based on the stiffness of the lung and the degree of lung inflation
    - When PIP increases 1 to 1 with PEEP, it is concerning for overdistension
    - When PIP stays the same despite increased PEEP, it is reassuring for recruitment
      - This may take time (24–48 hours)

- PEEP >12 cm H_2O may decrease venous return and cardiac output, causing hypotension (worse in patients with abnormal RV function and hypovolemia)
  - This hemodynamic consequence must be balanced against the significant cost of a $Pao_2 < 60$ mm Hg (ie, heart failure, renal failure, and central nervous system [CNS] dysfunction)
  - This type of preload-dependent physiology should only be treated with normal saline in the nonedematous (no pleural effusions) patient
    - Volume overload significantly worsens pulmonary mechanics and **must** be avoided
  - Volume overloaded patients suffering hypotension possibly related to high levels of PEEP (required to maintain a $Pao_2 > 60$ mm Hg) should have a trial of inotropes to improve RV functioning (preventing the need for excessive preload/volume)

- Increasing inspiratory time:
  - A normal inspiratory/expiratory ratio is 1:3–1:4
  - Increasing the inspiratory time will increase mean airway pressure, improving oxygenation, (a.k.a. inverse ratio ventilation), but
  - The longer the inspiratory time, the shorter the expiratory time, leading to underventilation
    - Often not tolerated in a lung-protective ventilation strategy in which ventilation is already minimal (based on low lung volumes)

- Aggressive diuresis:
  - The FACTT trial (Comparison of Two Fluid-Management Strategies in Acute Lung Injury, ARDSNET, N Engl J Med 2006) showed that targeting a low **central venous pressure (CVP) <4 cm H20**, with **aggressive diuresis** decreased ventilator days and had a trend toward improved survival in patients with lung injury
    - Because decreased ventilator days decrease the risk of ventilator acquired pneumonia (VAP) and thus ICU mortality, the trend toward improved survival (in these dry patients) is most certainly real

PEEP RESPONSE IN CARDIOGENIC AND NONCARDIOGENIC EDEMA (AVOIDING ALVEOLAR DERECRUITMENT)

- Pao_2 may respond to PEEP in hours or days, depending on the disease state
  - Cardiogenic edema responds quickly to PEEP (eg, $Pao_2 > 200$ mm Hg on 100% Fio_2 in hours)
    - Here PEEP works mainly by redistributing fluid in the alveolus and by decreasing preload (more than by alveolar recruitment)

- PEEP weaning generally occurs fast, with desaturation expected to respond quickly to PEEP increase
- Noncardiogenic edema (ie, ARDS) responds more slowly to PEEP (eg, $PaO_2 > 60$ mm Hg on 100% FiO_2 12 hours later)
  - Here PEEP works by alveolar recruitment
  - PEEP weaning must occur slowly because patients are vulnerable to **derecruitment**, where **desaturation** responds **slowly** to PEEP increase and recovery may take 12–24 hours

- Avoid derecruitment by weaning PEEP slowly and **not** disconnecting patient from the ventilator circuit
  - Bronchoscopy, or even transporting a patient (disconnecting, manual bagging), can lead to 24–48 hours of lost progress

- When mechanics appear to have improved wean PEEP **very** slowly
  - Decreasing PEEP by no more than 2 cm H_2O, q12 hours (until demonstrated tolerance)
    - If PaO_2 drops significantly after PEEP reduction, **immediately** go back up on the PEEP (in addition to the FiO_2 if the $PaO_2 < 60$ mm Hg)

TROUBLESHOOTING A SUDDEN CHANGE IN RESPIRATORY MECHANICS (FIG. 19.5)

- Examine the patient (check for dyssynchrony, agitation, breath stacking)
  - Mechanically ventilated patients who experience a change in pulmonary mechanics associated with dyssynchrony despite sedation, deserve a trial of paralysis
  - This either returns pulmonary mechanics back to baseline, or removes dyssynchrony as the etiology

- Obtain PIP and P_{plat} for patients on volume control
  - The peak inspiratory pressure (PIP) reflects the airway pressure in the trachea (normal <25 cm H_2O)
  - The plateau pressure (P_{plat}) represents the pressure in the alveolus (normal <13 cm H_2O)
  - The normal PIP – P_{plat} delta (or difference) is <12 cm H_2O
    - A PIP – P_{plat} difference >15 cm H_2O = obstructive pulmonary physiology
    - A PIP – P_{plat} difference <10 cm H_2O = restrictive pulmonary physiology
  - When peak inspiratory pressure rises in isolation relative to the plateau pressure (ie, PIP – P_{plat} >15 cm H_2O) airways resistance has increased due to partial obstruction somewhere between the ET tube and the alveolus:
    - Anything from a partially occluded ET tube or airway (eg, biting, mucus plug, blood clot, biofilm), to bronchospasm
  - When peak inspiratory pressure rises with the plateau pressure (ie, PIP – P_{plat} <10 cm H_2O) compliance has worsened as may be see with:
    - Dyssynchrony, extremely high auto PEEP (a.k.a. breath stacked), edema (HF or ARDS), collapse, pneumothorax or intrusive abdominal physiology (eg, ileus, ascites)

- Obtain an ABG and a CXR

- Changing modes from volume control to pressure control will **not fix** abnormal pulmonary mechanics, and will instead delay the diagnosis of the real problem
  - Although changing to pressure control may be necessary to prevent barotrauma, this is done in conjunction with troubleshooting as previously outlined

- Worsening respiratory mechanics and respiratory failure, despite mechanical ventilation, are medical emergencies requiring subspecialty attending level input

TROUBLESHOOTING CHANGES IN PULMONARY MECHANICS OCCURRING ON MECHANICAL VENTILATION

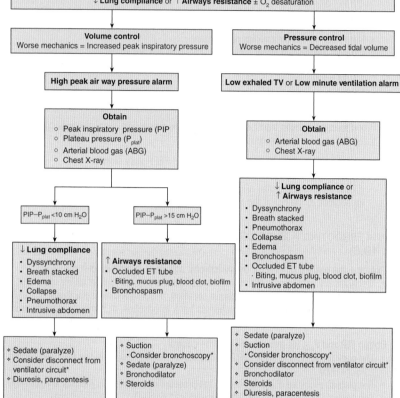

* Disconnection from the ventilator and bronchoscopy causes PEEP loss and possible derecruitment

Fig. 19.5 Flow diagram depicting the approach to trouble shooting a change in pulmonary mechanics based on the mode of ventilation (ie, pressure control vs volume control). In volume control, worsening mechanics are signaled by persistent high peak airway pressure alarms. Evaluation involves obtaining a plateau pressure to establish whether the problem is increased airway resistance (PIP − P_{plat} >15 cm H_2O), or lower compliance (PIP − P_{plat} <10 cm H_2O) followed by an arterial blood gas (ABG) and a chest x-ray (CXR). In pressure control mode, worsening mechanics are signaled by persistently low exhaled tidal volume alarms. Evaluation is limited to physical examination, ABG, and CXR. ABG is helpful in assessing the severity of the situation (ie, how low the pH is and how high the Pco_2 is), whereas the CXR and physical examination often reveal the problem (ie, cardiogenic edema or lobar collapse).
PIP, peak inspiratory pressures; *P_{plat}*, plateau pressures

SPECIAL SITUATIONS

- Respiratory therapy reports "the ET tube cuff is leaking, requiring higher than normal pressures to stay inflated and to prevent an air leak"
  - This typically means that the ET tube has migrated up (and nearly out of the trachea), resting in the subglottic space (much wider than the trachea), explaining the balloon behavior
  - First check the ET tube **position** at the bedside, via physical examination (urgently, to avoid self-extubation), obtain a **stat** CXR

- If the ET tube is in good position, trouble shoot the cuff system
  - Occasionally the pilot balloon valve fails (and can be replaced with a repair kit)
    - Having the cuff actually develop a leak like a bicycle tire is **very** unusual
      - If this occurs the ET tube should be exchanged over a tube changer
- Respiratory therapy and/or nursing report intermittent difficulty passing the suction catheter
  - This should prompt an evaluation of ET tube patency
    - ET tubes may accumulate a thick, rubbery, adherent film (a.k.a. biofilm) that is made worse by absent or inadequate humidification
    - The ventilator flowsheet should be reviewed looking for a trend of increasing peak airway pressure (often unnoticed and unreported when rising from the mid-twenties to the mid-thirties)
    - ET tube occlusion with biofilm often presents suddenly, where a circumferentially narrowed lumen suffers complete occlusion from mucus or biofilm debris
    - Urgent bronchoscopy may be able to clear the lumen, however if the ET remains occluded the patient must be extubated and reintubated (last resort)
- Shunt physiology occurring with mechanical ventilation in morbidly obese patients without significant parenchymal findings (often in the postoperative setting, see CH1 fig 1.5)
  - These patients should be screened for a patent foramen ovale (PFO) with an agitated saline contrast echocardiogram
    - In these cases the PFO is open because of elevated right-sided pressure relative to left, usually a temporary consequence of intubation, sedation and volume overload
    - Treatment hinges on lowering right-sided pressure (diuresis, improved oxygenation) and increasing left-sided pressure (by increasing afterload with deceased sedation or use of pressors)
    - These patients should be screened for pulmonary embolism (as an explanation for increased right atrial pressure and new shunting through a PFO)
  - When a PFO and/or pulmonary embolism is not present, patients should be evaluated for bilateral lower lobe atelectasis, often subtle on the frontal/portable CXR, appearing as low lung volumes only
    - Loss of abdominal muscular tone with sedation, combined with abdominal obesity and supine positioning, leads to lower lobe atelectasis
    - PaO_2 improves with lightened sedation/arousal, sitting upright and spontaneous breathing
  - May perform a spontaneous breathing trial (SBT), despite high FiO_2 and PEEP needs before trial, anticipating improvement as abdominal muscles participate in stenting open the lower thorax, and negative inspiration helps stent open lower lobes
    - One can then rapidly wean PEEP and FiO_2 and extubate if PaO_2 remains >60 mm Hg

Salvage Therapies for Acute Respiratory Distress Syndrome

- Patients with ARDS who do not attain a $PaO_2 > 60$ mm Hg with pressure control and a high PEEP strategy, despite paralysis, increased inspiratory time and diuresis ($\pm$ steroids), deserve consideration for salvage therapies:
  - Prone positioning (rotation) may improve oxygenation by decreasing dependent atelectasis and improving ventilation/perfusion (V/Q) matching temporarily
  - Inhaled NO can be used on the theory that intrinsic V/Q is so deranged; a trial of indiscriminant pulmonary artery vasodilation is warranted (and may produce better V/Q matching)
    - May worsen oxygenation rapidly if left ventricle end-diastolic pressure (LVEDP) is high (cardiogenic edema), or because intrinsic V/Q matching was better
  - In centers with experience, extracorporeal membrane oxygenation (ECMO) should be employed early in patients unresponsive to traditional aggressive support

COMMON QUESTIONS GENERATED BY THIS TEACHING

1. **What does increasing the inspiratory flow rate do? RT suggested I do this this based on the flow volume waveform.**
   In patients with air hunger and normal mechanics (eg, overwhelming metabolic acidosis) increasing the inspiratory flow rate can better match patient desire (decreasing sedation needs). This increases peak inspiratory pressure and is not tolerated when mechanics are abnormal, in which case sedation may be increased.

2. **I had a patient have a pulseless electrical activity arrest secondary to acidosis from ventilatory failure despite mechanical ventilation in VC+ mode. No ventilator alarms went off before the cardiac arrest. How can that happen?**
   VC+ (volume targeted pressure control) is a pressure control mode. As in all pressure control modes, worsening respiratory mechanics cause decreased TVs and underventilation. If the low exhaled TV and/or the low MV alarms are set too low, patients may become critically acidotic from underventilation, without the ventilator alarming.

3. **When should I "permit" hypercapnia?**
   Whenever eucapnia would require high lung volumes or airway pressures.

4. **What is a normal lung compliance?**
   Lung compliance quantifies the pressure–volume relationship for the lung. Normal lung compliance is 50 to 80 mL/cm H_2O. This means that if you apply 1 cm H_2O pressure to a lung, you should increase its volume by 50 to 80 mL. Said differently, a driving pressure of 20 cm H_2O should yield a TV of 1000 to 1600 mL. Poor compliance (a.k.a. stiff lungs) will yield a much lower tidal volume for the same driving pressure.

CHAPTER 20

NONINVASIVE VENTILATORY SUPPORT WITH BILEVEL POSITIVE PRESSURE VENTILATION

COMMON MISCONCEPTIONS AND MISTAKES

- Believing that somnolence makes a trial of bilevel positive pressure ventilation (BiPAP) unsafe
- Believing that any hemoptysis, regardless of the volume or context, makes a trial of BiPAP unsafe
- Starting BiPAP for respiratory failure using inadequate pressure settings (ie, 12/4)
- Ordering BiPAP like a nebulizer treatment (ie, **not** being at the bedside when initiating BiPAP for respiratory failure)
- Sedating a patient for anxiety/agitation related respiratory failure while using BiPAP

NONINVASIVE VENTILATORY SUPPORT

- Patients in need of ventilatory assistance can be managed either noninvasively with positive pressure applied to the nose and mouth via face mask, or invasively with positive pressure applied directly to the lungs via an endotracheal tube (gold standard)
- Most arousable patients in need of ventilatory support, or improved oxygenation despite 100% FiO_2, deserve a trial of noninvasive BiPAP before intubation, assuming:
  - They have the ability to wear a mask (ie, no preclusive facial or scalp wounds) and
  - Do not require continual oral clearance (ie, emesis, copious pulmonary secretions, massive hemoptysis)
- BiPAP:
  - Allows for differential setting of inspiratory positive airway pressure (IPAP) and expiratory positive airway pressure (EPAP), a.k.a. positive end expiratory pressure (PEEP)
    - The driving pressure for ventilation comes from the difference between the IPAP and the EPAP
      - Minimum driving pressure (IPAP − EPAP) appropriate for acute respiratory failure = 10 cm H_2O
      - **Isolated increases in** IPAP will increase driving pressure and may further decrease the work of breathing
    - Minimum EPAP (PEEP) = 5 cm H_2O (physiologic)
      - **Increasing** EPAP (a.k.a. PEEP) may provide additional support in two settings:
        - Patients with obstructive lung disease, suffering dynamic hyperinflation (ie, breath stacking) and significant intrinsic PEEP (a.k.a. auto-PEEP), typically "tripoding" on the edge of the with and pursed-lip breathing
          - Increasing EPAP can match intrinsic PEEP, making the initiation of inhalation easier, decreasing the work of breathing

- Patients with cardiogenic pulmonary edema and hypoxemia
  - Increasing EPAP can redistribute fluid in the alveolar space and improve oxygenation
- A high EPAP is uncomfortable for patients
  - EPAP should be increased slowly (increments of 2 cm H_2O) to avoid precipitating intolerance
  - Feedback regarding comfort must be solicited
    - Successfully matching intrinsic PEEP should provide the patient instantaneous improvement

INITIATION OF BILEVEL POSITIVE AIRWAY PRESSURE (FIG. 20.1)

- Respiratory failure represents an unstable situation requiring immediate action to avoid respiratory arrest

- The definitive therapy for respiratory failure is invasive endotracheal intubation and mechanical ventilation

- In the absence of contraindications, use of BiPAP to prevent intubation is appropriate, but requires care and vigilance to ensure that respiratory arrest **does not** ensue if BiPAP fails (or is **not** tolerated)

- Initiation of BiPAP for acute respiratory failure **requires** a physician to be at the bedside to ensure initial tolerance and efficacy
  - Intolerance of the mask and/or sudden worsening of respiratory status should prompt immediate rapid sequence intubation (RSI)

- BiPAP has its greatest efficacy in assisting ventilation (unloading the diaphragm and decreasing the work of breathing), but it may also improve oxygenation in hypoxemic respiratory failure, by increasing mean airway pressure, which:
  - Facilitates recruitment
  - Redistributes fluid to the edge of the alveolus
  - Decreases preload (helpful in cardiogenic edema)

- The contraindications to BiPAP are:
  - Obtundation (unarousable)
    - BiPAP requires that a patient have sufficient oral-pharyngeal reflexes to clear oral secretions and protect their airway from aspiration (generally absent in the obtunded)
  - Facial or scalp wounds (eg, surgical flap) precluding the use of a mask and securing straps
  - The need for continual oral clearance (not possible with a mask strapped to your face), as seen with:
    - Copious respiratory secretions (phlegm)
    - Ongoing emesis
    - Massive hemoptysis

INITIAL SETUP, SETTINGS, AND ADJUSTMENTS (TO BE PERFORMED BY THE PHYSICIAN AT THE BEDSIDE)

- Mask fit is crucial for patient tolerance and efficacy
  - Assist respiratory therapy (RT) in mask placement
  - Focus on creating the facial seal while the RT fixes the straps
  - Dentures will **assist** in mask fit, but need to be removed if RSI is required

INITIATION OF BIPAP FOR ACUTE HYPERCAPNIC OR HYPOXEMIC RESPIRATORY FAILURE

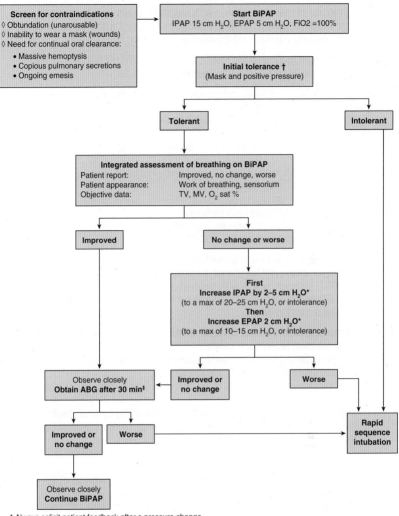

* Always solicit patient feedback after a pressure change

‡ May be able to leave the bedside at this point while awaiting ABG (but don't go far)

† Patients who fight (pulling off the mask), or whose respiratory failure worsens precipitously, should be intubated

Fig. 20.1 Flow diagram showing the approach to initiating bilevel positive pressure (BiPAP) ventilation. Initiating BiPAP (instead of electively intubating a patient) must be done carefully to avoid respiratory arrest. If this occurs, it makes the decision to use BiPAP look flawed. Some patients will demonstrate an immediate intolerance to BiPAP, typically because their respiratory failure is too advanced (and they are in extremis, unable to cooperate) or because of claustrophobia and mask intolerance. These individuals should be immediately intubated (respiratory arrest imminent). Once a patient demonstrates initial tolerance, improvement is usually obvious. Individuals who look about the same (or worse) deserve a trial of more support by increasing inspiratory positive airway pressure (IPAP) to the maximum tolerated by comfort and then doing the same for expiratory positive airway pressure (EPAP; again as tolerated). Worsening at this point necessitates intubation. Stability or improvement should prompt continued observation. It is important to objectively document the success of BiPAP by demonstrating stability, improvement, or resolution of the initial respiratory acidosis or hypoxemeia (presumably present).

- Standard initial settings: IPAP 15 cm H_2O, EPAP 5 cm H_2O, and FiO_2 100%

- Although Haldol can be used in those with hospital delirium (constantly picking and pulling at things), in general, patients in **respiratory failure with significant agitation require intubation**, sedation, and mechanical ventilation

- Patients who fight (pulling off the mask), or whose respiratory failure worsens precipitously, should emergently undergo RSI

- After initial tolerance is established, an integrated assessment of the patient's breathing on BiPAP is undertaken
  - Illicit a subjective assessment of the BiPAP mask and pressure from the patient (ie, "Does this feel better?")
    - Though in respiratory failure, patients are typically able to indicate via nod or thumb gesture
  - Assess the patient's work of breathing and level of consciousness (ie, improved, no change, worse)
  - Ensure that:
    - Tidal volume is adequate (ie, >6 mg/kg)
    - Minute ventilation is adequate (ie, >5 L/min)
    - O_2 saturations are adequate (ie, >94%)

- If the patient appears to have improved, then close clinical observation is warranted for 30 minutes, at which point an arterial blood gas (ABG) should be obtained
  - If the ABG is improved or stable (ie, resolved or stable respiratory acidosis and/or $PaO2 > 60$ mm Hg), then BiPAP should be continued and the patient closely observed for worsening respiratory status

- If the patient appears the same or worse, BiPAP pressures should be adjusted in an attempt to increase support and comfort
  - Unless the patient specifically communicates the sense that the pressure is too high, decreasing IPAP initially is usually **not** helpful
  - Instead increasing support should be the first maneuver to make the patient more comfortable:
    - Adjusting BiPAP pressures should be done while eliciting continual feedback on comfort by the patient (ie, "I'm going to increase the pressure in the mask, tell me if this feels better, worse or the same")
    - First increase IPAP in small increments (2–5 cm H_2O*) to a maximum of 20–25 cm H_2O, based on patient tolerance
    - Then increase EPAP in small increments (2 cm H_2O*) to a maximum of 10–15 cm H_2O, based on patient tolerance
    - May increase EPAP earlier if the patient has obstructive disease with presumed high intrinsic PEEP
  - Maximum settings typically achievable (based on tolerance and comfort):
    - IPAP 20–25 cm H_2O, EPAP 10–15 cmH_2O, and FiO_2 100%

- If the BiPAP adjustments yield improvement or stability then observe for 30 minutes and obtain an ABG

- Worsening clinical status and/or ABG values signal a failure of BiPAP and should prompt intubation

- BiPAP is only a support device, such that simultaneous attempts must be made to decrease airway resistance and improve compliance, depending on the clinical scenario (ie, nebulized β-agonist, IV steroids, IV loop diuretics)

- Patients who are inappropriate for, or who fail BiPAP require urgent intubation

TRIALING PATIENTS OFF OF BILEVEL POSITIVE AIRWAY PRESSURE

- Most often BiPAP is a rescue device for patients who have suffered a sudden increase in the work of breathing as a result of a change in pulmonary mechanics
- Resolving respiratory failure with initiation of BiPAP is usually clinically obvious
  - Visible decrease in work of breathing, improved mental status, improved respiratory acidosis, and/or oxygenation
- Consider a trial off BiPAP when:
  - Work of breathing returns to normal
  - Respiratory acidosis resolves and/or oxygenation improves
  - Mechanics improve (ie, after diuresis or steroids)
    - Patients should be included in the decision (ie, asked if they feel ready)

COMMON QUESTIONS GENERATED BY THIS TEACHING

1. I had a patient that I thought was obtunded so I didn't want to try BiPAP. My resident did a sternal rub and got the patient to transiently open his eyes. How awake does an individual have to be to make BiPAP safe?
   Clinical judgment is required, but if a significant portion of the patient's somnolence is as a result of CO_2 narcosis, one can anticipate rapid progress with improved ventilation (ie, 15–30 minutes on BiPAP). The danger posed to the obtunded patient on BiPAP is twofold: 1) emesis and 2) completion of hypoventilation (ie, a quiet respiratory arrest). If the patient is not experiencing emesis, then BiPAP may be safe, even in the initially barely arousable patient, assuming they are actively watched, at their bedside, for worsening hypoventilation.

2. Why can't I give a patient in acute respiratory failure, on BiPAP, a benzodiazepine to help them relax and become more comfortable?
   Respiratory failure causes appropriate anxiety, which must be treated by adequate respiratory support. Sedating patients in respiratory failure may precipitate BiPAP failure, necessitating intubation. Instead, attempt to increase patient comfort by adjusting the pressure settings and perhaps the mask.

CHAPTER 21

HEMOPTYSIS

COMMON MISCONCEPTIONS AND MISTAKES

- Believing that a double-lumen tube is the preferred airway in a patient with massive hemoptysis

- Failing to treat patients with bronchiectasis and hemoptysis with antibiotics (Abx) because there is no fever or elevated white blood cell (WBC) count

- Believing that intubation should be done, preemptively for airway protection, to prevent respiratory failure in patients with massive hemoptysis

- Focusing risk stratification on the amount of blood reported to have been coughed up in the 24 hours before presentation

- Believing that the priority positioning in a patient with massive hemoptysis is "good lung up"

- Being reassured by a stable hematocrit in a patient reporting an episode of massive hemoptysis

- Believing that bronchoscopy is the preferred (gold standard) way to localize bleeding in a patient with massive hemoptysis

INITIAL ASSESSMENT/RISK STRATIFICATION

- Hemoptysis is a very common complaint that encompasses a wide spectrum, from reports of blood-tinged oral secretions that "may have been" coughed up to presentations of voluminous, bright-red blood being expelled from the airway

- Risk stratification: **massive**, **at risk for massive**, and **non–life-threatening** hemoptysis (Fig. 21.1)
  - Massive hemoptysis
    - Individuals who actively cough up voluminous, bright-red blood and clot at the time of evaluation are suffering from massive hemoptysis
    - These patients need localization via a chest CT (typically with arterial-phase contrast looking for bronchial arteries) and definitive intervention via embolization (interventional radiology) or resection (CT surgery)
  - At risk for massive hemoptysis
    - Individuals who report (or demonstrate) **hemoptysis *and*** who have a known history of **bronchiectasis** (the most common cause of massive hemoptysis) are **at risk for massive hemoptysis**
      - These individuals should:
        - Be admitted for observation
        - Be given IV antibiotics with Gram-positive cocci (GPC) and Gram-negative rod (GNR) coverage
        - Have their bleeding localized via a chest CT scan

EVALUATION AND MANAGEMENT OF HEMOPTYSIS

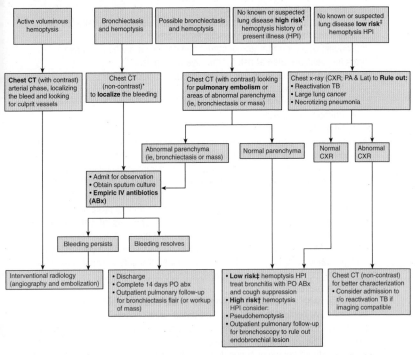

* Contrast (arterial phase) may be used if embolization is likely (i.e. **high risk** hemoptysis HPI) but is unnecessary with a **low risk** hemoptysis HPI
† **High risk** hemoptysis HPI = no cough, phlegm, or respiratory illness
‡ **Low risk** hemoptysis HPI = productive cough, blood tinged sputum, respiratory illness

Fig. 21.1 Schematic showing the evaluation and management of hemoptysis. Patients presenting with active voluminous hemoptysis require urgent evaluation by interventional radiology (IR) and possibly CT surgery. Either way, an arterial-phase computed tomography (CT) scan of the chest should be the first step in attempting to localize active hemoptysis (and survey for culprit vessels). Patients with known bronchiectasis typically have recurrent exacerbations or flairs where sputum becomes more purulent and blood clots and streaks appear with phlegm. This is a "low-risk" presentation for an individual with known, symptomatic bronchiectasis and should be evaluated with a noncontrast CT scan (for localization) as part of admission for antibiotics and observation. Patients with known bronchiectasis who have a "high-risk" presentation (ie, no change in cough or phlegm, just sudden hemoptysis) probably deserve a contrast CT scan (arterial phase) and an urgent IR evaluation. Patients with known parenchymal lung disease (ie, pulmonary fibrosis) but no history of clinical bronchiectasis (ie, recurrent lung infections and chronic sputum purulence) should be treated like individuals with no known lung disease (ie, pulmonary embolism should be excluded with a contrast CT timed for pulmonary artery [PA] opacification). If the CT scan demonstrates bronchiectasis or a mass, the patient should be admitted for observation. Patients with bronchiectasis and hemoptysis deserve intravenous antibiotics (even if they deny a change in cough or phlegm). When a new parenchymal mass is discovered, antibiotics should be considered for postobstructive pneumonia or imaging suggestive of a lung abscess (ie, necrosis with an air-fluid level). Individuals reporting hemoptysis who have normal Chest CT angiography (CTA) are **not** at risk of death by massive hemoptysis (or pulmonary embolism) and can be discharged from the emergency room with outpatient follow-up. Individuals who have a "high-risk" presentation (ie, no cough, phlegm, or respiratory illness) should be followed up in pulmonary clinic to have bronchoscopy considered to exclude an airway mucosal source of bleeding (ie, early squamous cell cancer). Patients without lung disease and with "low-risk" presentation (ie, cough, phlegm, blood-tinged sputum) should be screened for tuberculosis and necrotic pneumonia with a PA and lateral chest x-ray (CXR). A clear CXR confirms the diagnosis of bronchitis, which should be treated with antibiotics and cough suppression (and smoking cessation attempts if applicable). An abnormal CXR in an otherwise healthy person presenting with hemoptysis in the clinical setting of "bronchitis" (ie, cough and phlegm) but not "fever and shaking chills" (ie, pneumonia) warrants a CT scan for better characterization of the abnormality.

- The majority of the time, bleeding (and sputum) will improve with antibiotics (requiring no further intervention)
- Those with ongoing bleeding, despite antibiotics, should be evaluated by interventional radiology for possible embolization
- Individuals who report (or demonstrate) hemoptysis **and** who may have bronchiectasis are **also** at risk for massive hemoptysis
  - Common bronchiectasis risk factors in adults include:
    - Nontuberculous mycobacterial infection
    - Thoracic radiation therapy (ie, external beam radiation therapy for lung cancer)
    - Pulmonary fibrosis
    - Fibrocavitary tuberculosis
  - Less common causes include immunodeficiency (and recurrent lung infection), poorly treated bacterial pneumonia in youth, ciliary dyskinesia syndromes, and partial cystic fibrosis (CF) gene mutations, and immunoglobulin deficiencies
  - Patients at risk for massive hemoptysis deserve a chest CT (typically noncontrast) looking for a focal parenchymal explanation for their bleeding (ie, lung cancer, arteriovenous malformation, necrotic pneumonia, or area of bronchiectasis)
- Individuals without known or suspected lung disease who present with a **high-risk hemoptysis story** (ie, significant hemoptysis without cough, phlegm production, and/or an antecedent respiratory illness) deserve a chest CT scan with contrast (pulmonary arterial phase) looking for pulmonary embolism and/or a parenchymal source to explain their bleeding (ie, lung cancer, arteriovenous malformation, necrotic pneumonia, or an area of bronchiectasis)
  - Individuals with a **normal CT angiogram of the chest** are **not** at risk of dying from massive hemoptysis and may be treated more conservatively (ie, outpatient pulmonary follow-up and possibly bronchoscopy to look for an endobronchial explanation [ie, early squamous cell cancer])
- Individuals without known or suspected lung disease who present with a **low-risk hemoptysis story** (ie, blood tinged sputum or clots mixed with phlegm in the setting of a respiratory illness) deserve a PA and lateral CXR looking for reactivation TB, lung cancer, and/or necrotic pneumonia
  - Individuals with a low-risk story and a clear CXR should have bronchitis treated with PO antibiotics and cough suppression

PATHOPHYSIOLOGY AND MANAGEMENT OF MASSIVE HEMOPTYSIS

- Massive hemoptysis kills by **large airway obstruction** with clot
  - Not by hemorrhagic shock or alveolar filling of blood with subsequent hypoxemia

- Massive hemoptysis most commonly occurs when large, ectatic **bronchial** and **intercostal arteries** (arising from the aorta) rupture, often in the setting of an **acute on chronic bronchiectasis** infection or exacerbation
  - Bronchiectasis produces abnormal bronchial and intercostal arteries via:
    - Poor secretion clearance, leading to chronic lung infection and inflammation, leading to pathologic angiogenesis

- Other common causes of massive hemoptysis include:
  - Large proximal lung cancers (especially squamous cell carcinoma)
  - Invasive fungal infection
  - Pulmonary artery bleeding (as in Rasmussen's aneurysm [ie, calcified granulomatous lymphoid tissue eroding into the pulmonary artery])
  - Diffuse alveolar hemorrhage (<30% of the time)

- Pulmonary venous bleeding from pulmonary vein stenosis (eg, after ablation for atrial fibrillation [AFIB])
- May require definitive intervention (ie, IR embolization vs CT surgical resection)
- When definitive therapy is required, the pulmonologist localize the bleeding to a region of the lung (eg, right vs left, upper lung zone vs lower lung zone)
  - Subsegmental resolution is **not** required (culprit vessels arise directly from the aorta)
  - CXR and CT scan typically show an area of parenchymal abnormality
    - If multiple abnormalities exist, the area of most change compared with the prior is presumed to be the area of activity, either the bleeding lesion itself or an area of aspirated blood (close to the bleeding lesion)
  - Patients are good at localizing their own bleeding source and should be asked, "Do you have any idea where the bleeding is coming from? Have you had any strange sensations in an area of your chest—popping, bubbling, or gurgling sensations?"
    - Often they will point with one finger to the abnormal area identified by imaging (high pretest probability sign)
  - Upper lobe fibrocavitary change should prompt consideration of reactivation of TB or chronic fibrosing pulmonary aspergillosis
- Bronchoscopic localization is **extraordinarily difficult** during active bleeding (Fig. 21.2)
  - Blood quickly coats all of the airways during active bleeding and coughing
    - Blood always appears to be dripping from the upper lobes and pooling in the lower lobes
  - Should be reserved for patients who are in respiratory failure, already intubated, or too unstable for CT imaging

INTUBATION IN MASSIVE HEMOPTYSIS (WHEN, WHY, AND WITH WHAT)

- An awake patient with a strong cough and respiratory reserve will prevent large airway occlusion **better** than you and your ET tube and bronchoscope (Fig. 21.3)
- Optimal patient positioning (in the nonintubated) is whatever position the patient finds most comfortable (expectorating blood)
  - Typically this is upright positioning, often on the side of the bed (with a basin)
- Intubate only when a patient has developed respiratory failure (**not** preemptively)
  - After intubation, only small bits of clot can be removed (via bronchoscopic suctioning), increasing the likelihood of fatal airway obstruction
- It is safer for awake patients with a strong cough, who are adequately clearing their airways, to undergo interventional radiology (IR) embolization with oral suctioning and close observation for respiratory compromise
- When intubation is required for respiratory failure, the **preferred airway** is a **large, single-lumen ET tube** (ie, number 8 or number 10) combined with a therapeutic bronchoscope
  - Double-lumen tubes are easily mispositioned (and more easily clogged)
    - They are too small to suction through (will only accept a pediatric bronchoscope)
  - A bronchial blocker can be used with a large single-lumen ET tube and a therapeutic bronchoscope, but they are also easily and frequently dislodged
- Continued suctioning via a therapeutic bronchoscope (in the IR suite as necessary) is the most reliable way to maintain airway patency in an intubated patient with massive hemoptysis

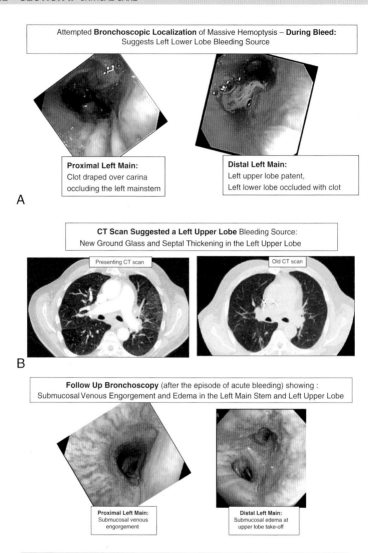

Attempted **Bronchoscopic Localization** of Massive Hemoptysis – **During Bleed:**
Suggests Left Lower Lobe Bleeding Source

Proximal Left Main:
Clot draped over carina
occluding the left mainstem

Distal Left Main:
Left upper lobe patent,
Left lower lobe occluded with clot

A

CT Scan Suggested a Left Upper Lobe Bleeding Source:
New Ground Glass and Septal Thickening in the Left Upper Lobe

Presenting CT scan

Old CT scan

B

Follow Up Bronchoscopy (after the episode of acute bleeding) showing :
Submucosal Venous Engorgement and Edema in the Left Main Stem and Left Upper Lobe

Proximal Left Main:
Submucosal venous
engorgement

Distal Left Main:
Submucosal edema at
upper lobe take-off

Final Diagnosis: Left Main and LUL bleeding from **left anterior pulmonary vein stenosis,**
occurring after an ablation procedure for atrial fibrillation

C

Fig. 21.2 (A) Bronchoscopic images obtained during the attempted localization of bleeding in a patient with massive hemoptysis. Left-sided bleeding is suggested by the presence of an occlusive left mainstem clot. After the proximal clot was removed (bit by bit) the distal left main was inspected and revealed a patent upper lobe takeoff with a completely occluded lower lobe, suggesting a left lower lobe bleeding source. (B) Computed tomography (CT) scan obtained before bronchoscopy revealing new ground glass and septal thickening in the left upper lobe. The rest of the CT scan, including the lower lobe, was unchanged from the prior and therefore the CT scan suggested a left upper lobe bleeding source. The bronchoscopy was pursued to confirm the CT scan localization because the upper lobe changes did not suggest a bleeding source (ie, there was no bronchiectasis or mass). (C) Bronchoscopic images obtained during repeat bronchoscopy after the bleeding had stopped, revealing the cause of the patient's hemoptysis—namely varix-like submucosal venous engorgement in the left main and left upper lobe, secondary to left anterior pulmonary vein stenosis (occurring as a complication of an ablation procedure for atrial fibrillation). The patient ultimately underwent angioplasty of his left anterior pulmonary vein with stent placement, leading to resolution of his hemoptysis and improvement in his submucosal edema and venous engorgement pattern.

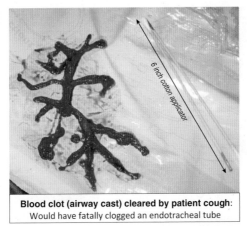

Blood clot (airway cast) cleared by patient cough:
Would have fatally clogged an endotracheal tube

Fig. 21.3 Photograph of an expectorated clot from an individual suffering massive hemoptysis. The patient suffered a desaturation, coughed forcefully, and cleared this nearly 6-inch-long, mainstem occluding clot. This same bleeding event would have led to fatal airway/endotracheal tube obstruction had the patient been "preemptively" intubated.

INTERVENTIONAL RADIOLOGY VS CARDIOTHORACIC SURGERY

- The first-line therapeutic intervention for massive hemoptysis involves embolization of a culprit vessel by IR

- Unfortunately IR embolization may be complicated by **spinal cord infarction** (just under 5% of the time), often leading to permanent paralysis (Fig. 21.4)
  - The spinal arteries arise from the aorta, as do the bronchial and intercostal arteries (the major targets of IR embolization in massive hemoptysis)
    - Thus erroneous embolization of a spinal artery can occur
    - And even worse, the **artery of Adamkiewicz** is a vascular variation in which the left posterior intercostal artery (T8 to L1) supplies the anterior spinal artery
      - In this situation the successful embolization of a culprit vessel may still lead to spinal cord infarction
  - Patients with diabetes, specifically diabetic myelopathy, may have aorta and spinal artery atherosclerotic disease such that instrumentation alone causes embolization of debris and spinal cord ischemia
  - Occasionally the embolization catheter slips out of the vessel orifice as the embolization beads are being deployed, leading to systemic embolization capable of infarcting **any** systemic arterial bed

- Individuals with good pulmonary reserve and an obvious parenchymal focus for massive hemoptysis should be evaluated by CT surgery for resection
  - Practically speaking, most individuals with bronchiectasis have diffuse lung disease with poor pulmonary reserve such that anatomic lung resection to obtain hemostasis is not a good first-line option
  - That said, focal areas of bronchiectasis occurring in the young, with otherwise normal lung parenchyma (as seen in fibrocavitary TB), may be amenable to surgical resection (providing definitive therapy without the risk of spinal cord injury)

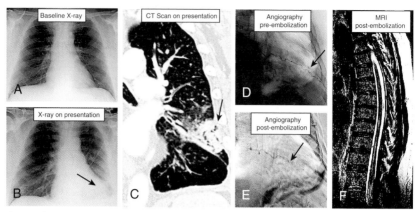

Fig. 21.4 (A) Baseline chest x-ray of an individual presenting with massive hemoptysis. (B) The presenting film with an obvious new left basilar opacity *(black arrow).* (C) Subsequent computed tomography scan, which better defines the lesion as a rounded, bronchiectatic (dilated airways visible) consolidation *(black arrow).* The patient went straight from the emergency room to the interventional radiology suite, where he underwent angiography. (D) The initial angiogram identifying a left basilar intercostal artery with abnormal caliber and tortuosity in the area of the bronchiectatic consolidation *(black arrow).* (E) Postembolization angiogram demonstrating embolization of the distal third of the vessel with an immediate result (hemoptysis stopped). Unfortunately the patient was unable to move his legs after the procedure. (F) Magnetic resonance image demonstrating a linear high attenuation band in the center of the spinal cord consistent with infarction *(red arrow).* Despite the location, no artery of Adamkiewicz was found during close review of the angiography. The patient was a diabetic with diabetic myelopathy and may have had preexisting aorta and spinal artery atherosclerotic disease such that instrumentation alone was to blame.

NONMASSIVE HEMOPTYSIS

- Pseudohemoptysis
  - The nasopharyngeal passages are **very** common sources of bleeding because the upper airway mucosa is prone to inflammation (much more so than the lungs)
  - It is very common for epistaxis or dental bleeding to be aspirated, expectorated, and thought to be hemoptysis
    - "Hemoptysis" occurring with epistaxis is typically pseudohemoptysis

- **Small-volume hemoptysis with a productive cough** (eg, blood-tinged sputum or blood clots with phlegm) occurs most commonly in the setting of bronchitis
  - In this situation the bleeding is from large airway mucosal irritation and inflammation
    - The most common presenting scenario goes something like "Doc, I've been coughing for 5 days. The cough is so bad, the last 2 nights I have been unable to sleep and this morning there was blood mixed in with the phlegm."
  - Treat with antibiotics and cough suppression
  - Very low threshold to obtain a CXR for unusual features (eg, chest pain and/or shortness of breath [not anticipated with bronchitis])

- If the clinical scenario **does not support bronchitis** (ie, no cough, phlegm production, or antecedent respiratory illness) **consider:**
  - Pulmonary embolism
    - Rule out with a contrast CT scan timed for pulmonary artery opacification
  - Reactivation TB
    - Rule out with a CXR/CT scan showing normal lung apices
  - Early endobronchial malignancy (especially squamous cell carcinoma)
    - 90% of malignant hemoptysis is caused by large, central tumors made obvious on chest imaging

- Consider bronchoscopy for individuals with unexplained hemoptysis and risk factors to rule out an early endobronchial malignancy
- Diffuse alveolar hemorrhage (DAH)
  - Only a minority of patients with DAH will experience hemoptysis
    - Patients with hemoptysis, thrombocytopenia, anemia, and ground glass infiltrates should be evaluated for DAH
      - The diagnosis of DAH is made bronchoscopically by the demonstration of a progressively bloodier bronchial alveolar lavage
- Pulmonary edema
  - Patients with alveolar edema often report pink, frothy sputum and frank, blood-tinged sputum
  - In this situation the bleeding is from hydrostatic capillary injury and does not require specific treatment (beyond reducing left ventricle end-diastolic pressure [LVEDP])

COMMON QUESTIONS GENERATED BY THIS TEACHING

1. **When should you perform a bronchoscopy on a patient with massive hemoptysis?**
   When he or she is too unstable for the CT scanner (often immediately after intubation) to maintain airway patency and to localize the bleeding

2. **When should I use a double-lumen ET tube?**
   Never (for massive hemoptysis). The preferred airway is the patient's trachea, and failing that, a number 8 (or greater) ET tube.

3. **How much blood does somebody need to report coughing up to warrant admission for observation?**
   Individuals are notoriously unreliable when reporting the volume of their hemoptysis. Those who are concerned and want you to be concerned overreport (ie, young, anxious smokers), and those who are not concerned (individuals with longstanding bronchiectasis and recurrent hemoptysis) underreport. Risk stratification for massive hemoptysis is best done based on the anatomy of the thorax and the likelihood that it may contain abnormal/ ectatic bronchial or intercostal arteries or a large, central necrotic lung cancer (the most common causes of life-threatening massive hemoptysis).

4. **Should patients with massive hemoptysis be positioned with their "good" nonbleeding lung up?**
   Nonintubated patients should be positioned to optimize their comfort, while they cough and clear blood and clots. Typically this involves sitting upright, often on the side of the bed, with a basin to cough into. Intubated patients are better served supine, with a bronchoscopist responsible for keeping the nonbleeding segments from occlusion.

5. **I had a patient who reported coughing up 200 mL of blood, but his hematocrit (HCT) was at baseline. Why is this not this reassuring?**
   Massive hemoptysis kills by airway obstruction with clot, **not** by blood loss or anemia. The HCT is **not** a part of the risk stratification for hemoptysis.

6. **I admitted a patient with bronchiectasis and hemoptysis. Pulmonary was upset that I did not give antibiotics, but the patient had a normal WBC count and was afebrile. Why should I have given Abx?**
   Hemoptysis is very common in patients with bronchiectasis. It typically occurs when they transition from chronic low-level infection to more acute infection. This manifests as increased cough, change in sputum, and hemoptysis, not fever or an elevated WBC count. All patients with bronchiectasis admitted for hemoptysis and observation require Abx (typically IV) aimed at GPCs and GNRs.

CHAPTER 22

SALT AND WATER: THE PHYSIOLOGY AND REGULATION OF VOLUME AND TONICITY

COMMON MISCONCEPTIONS AND MISTAKES

- Behaving as if humans are "brittle" with regard to volume status—namely that they transition quickly from total body volume overload to volume depletion (in a dangerous way)
- Not resuscitating hypovolemic individuals for fear that the sodium correction will be too rapid
- Treating hyponatremia based on the calculated Na^+ deficit and desired rate of increase
- Treating hypernatremia based on the calculated free water deficit, giving half back in the first 24 hours and the remaining half over the next 24–48 hours

VOLUME STATUS AND TONICITY

- Life evolved in saltwater; thus humans need constant access to water and salt
- Normal euvolemic (nonedematous) humans store ~10 L of saltwater in the interstitium of their bodies, with ~3–4 L in the interstitium of their extremities (lower extremity > upper extremity in the upright position)
  - This provides at least a 48-hour buffer against dehydration and volume depletion if water is scarce
- The kidneys **regulate volume status** by adjusting glomerular filtration rate (GFR) and sodium balance, manipulating the **amount of NaCl** in the urine
- The hypothalamus, pituitary (via anti-diuretic hormone [ADH] secretion and thirst), and the kidneys (by adjusting water reabsorption, responding to ADH) **regulate tonicity** by manipulating the **amount of water** or **concentration** of the urine
- Maintenance of adequate circulating **volume** (sodium balance) is the body's ultimate **priority**
  - **Therefore tonicity** is **sacrificed** to maintain adequate volume (resulting in Hyper- and hyponatremia presentations)
- **Tonicity** (practically speaking, **cell size**) is dictated by water balance
  - Dehydration is a state of inadequate body water, increased tonicity, and shrunken cells, ultimately causing central nervous system (CNS) dysfunction
- **Total body volume status** is dictated by **sodium balance**
  - **hypovolemia equals total body sodium depeltion, implying =** no reserve saltwater in the interstitium, no edema anticipated
  - **euvolemia equals normal sodium balance**, implying > 5 L of reserve saltwater in the interstitium, no edema anticipated

- **hypervolemia equals total body sodium overload**, implying excessive saltwater in the interstitium, manifesting as peripheral edema
- Volume overload is a problem of NaCl intake, **not** water intake
  - To illustrate, if a human eats 10 g of NaCl in a day he or she will:
    - Drink, responding to thirst as tonicity threatens to increase
    - Experience a pressure natriuresis in an attempt to prevent volume overload
    - Gain 1–2 lbs as he or she expands his or her interstitial fluid volume to the 10+ L maximum of interstitial reserve (often manifesting as sock edema)
  - Alternatively, if a human drinks 10 L of water in a day he or she will:
    - Urinate 9.5 L of a dilute urine to prevent decreased tonicity
    - Not gain weight (or manifest edema)

THE NORMAL HOMEOSTASIS OF VOLUME STATUS AND SODIUM BALANCE

- Hypovolemia leads to a decreased circulating volume, perceived by the kidney as a decreased renal blood flow
  - Decreased renal blood flow causes a decreased GFR with subsequent activation of the renin–angiotensin–aldosterone system, leading to:
    - Decreased urine output
    - **Increased sodium reabsorption** to conserve salt (urine Na^+ <10 mmol/L)
    - **Increased ADH** secretion concentrating the urine to conserve water (>300 mOsm/kg)
- Hypervolemia leads to an increased circulating volume perceived by the kidney as increased renal blood flow
  - Increased renal blood flow leads to an increased GFR leading to **sodium spillage** "a.k.a. pressure natriuresis"
    - Increased urine output
    - **Sodium spillage** to return volume status to normal (urine Na^+ >20 mmol/L)
    - **Decreased ADH** secretion diluting the urine to remove water (<100 mOsm/kg)

THE NORMAL HOMEOSTASIS OF TONICITY AND WATER BALANCE

- The hypothalamus, pituitary, and the kidney attempt to maintain tonicity homeostasis by manipulating ADH
  - Increased tonicity (ie, hypernatremia) causes increased ADH secretion, concentrating the urine
  - Decreased tonicity (ie, hyponatremia) causes decreased ADH secretion, diluting the urine
- **Inadequate water** intake leads to an increased serum sodium and thus **increased tonicity**
  - Increased tonicity is perceived by the hypothalamus, which creates thirst and activates ADH secretion from the pituitary, leading to:
    - Increased water intake
    - Increased water reabsorption in the collecting tubule
    - Concentrated urine (>300 mOsm/kg)
- **Water excess** leads to decreased serum sodium and thus **decreased tonicity**
  - Decreased tonicity inhibits thirst (hypothalamus) and suppresses pituitary ADH secretion, leading to:
    - Decreased water intake
    - Decreased water reabsorption in the collecting tubule, Increasing urine output
    - Dilute urine (<100 mOsm/kg)

THE PATHOPHYSIOLOGY AND EVALUATION OF HYPONATREMIA

- **Hyponatremia** represents a state of excessive plasma water
  - This is either a result of volume depletion (in an attempt to maintain circulating volume), impaired water excretion (syndrome of inappropriate antidiuretic hormone secretion [SIADH]), or excessive water intake (overcoming the body's ability to excrete water)
  - The most common causes of hyponatremia are:
    - Hypovolemic (gastrointestinal [GI] losses) > dilutional (occurring as a complication of volume overload) > SIADH > low sodium intake > excessive water ingestion

- Symptoms of hyponatremia are caused by decreased tonicity
  - Decreased extracellular tonicity creates an osmotic gradient, causing water to shift into cells (intracellular tonicity, which is based on potassium, remains normal)
  - This shift of water into cells makes them swell (poorly tolerated by central neurons)
    - Causing headache, confusion, seizure, coma, and even herniation (water intoxication)
    - An **acute** drop in serum sodium causes:
      - Confusion ($Na^+ \leq 125$)
      - Seizure, coma, and herniation ($Na^+ \leq 115$)
    - A **chronic** drop in serum sodium is often asymptomatic until the $Na^+ \leq 115\,mEq/L$
      - When Na^+ drops gradually, brain cells compensate (over days or weeks) by reducing intracellular osmolality
        - This poses a danger if chronic hyponatremia is rapidly corrected
        - The previous compensatory decreased intracellular osmolality in the neurons causes them to shrink rapidly as extracellular tonicity normalizes
          - This is associated with the devastating osmotic demyelination syndrome (the disease formerly known as "central pontine myelinolysis")

- The **first step** in evaluating a **low**-serum sodium is establishing **total body volume status** (ie, edema vs no edema) (Fig. 22.1)
  - The next step is obtaining a urine Na^+ and a urine osmolality (obtain **before** IVF is given or expect some Na^+ spillage)
  - Finally, observe the urine output

- *Edematous* patients are **volume overloaded** from either heart failure, cirrhosis, or renal failure
  - Hyponatremia occurring with volume overload is **dilutional**:
    - Heart failure or cirrhosis lead to decreased renal blood flow and decreased GFR (which directly impairs water excretion)
    - Decreased renal blood flow is **erroneously** perceived by the kidneys as hypovolemia, causing activation of the renin–angiotensin–aldosterone system (which causes sodium retention)
    - Angiotensin II leads to **nonosmolar**-mediated ADH secretion, sacrificing tonicity in an erroneous attempt to increase circulating volume
    - Together this signaling causes:
      - Low urine output from the "cardio-renal" physiology previously described
      - Concentered urine (>300 mOsm kg) with a low Na^+ (<10 mEq/L)
        - A low urine osmolality implies concomitant psychogenic polydipsia
        - A high urine Na^+ implies loop diuretic use or acute tubular necrosis (ATN)
    - Treat with diuresis (loop diuretics) and water restriction
  - Renal failure may impair free water excretion directly
    - Treat with loop diuretics, water restriction, and consider renal replacement therapy

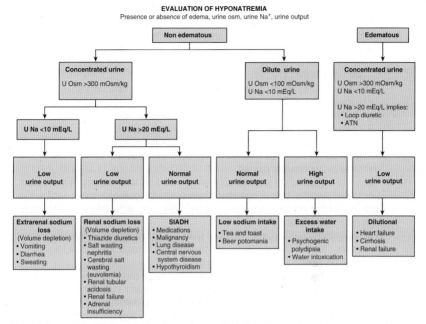

EVALUATION OF HYPONATREMIA
Presence or absence of edema, urine osm, urine Na⁺, urine output

Fig. 22.1 Flowchart showing the evaluation of hyponatremia, which initially hinges on the presence or absence of edema. The most common cause of hyponatremia is volume depletion (no edema), and the second most common cause is dilutional (generalized edema). Edematous patients with hyponatremia need no additional studies or workup (just diuresis and fluid restriction). The next aspect of the evaluation is establishing whether the urine is concentrated or dilute, distinguishing volume depletion and syndrome of inappropriate antidiuretic hormone secretion (SIADH) (concentrated urine) from very low sodium or excessive water intake (dilute urine). The next step in the evaluation of the nonedematous hyponatremic individual with a concentrated urine is ruling out volume depletion with an assessment of urine sodium. Volume-depleted individuals will have a low urine sodium. A concentrated urine with a high urine sodium suggests SIADH. Hyponatremic individuals with a dilute urine have either a very low sodium diet or excessive water intake. Individuals who have excessively consumed water will have a high urine output as anti-diuretic hormone is appropriately inhibited and their kidneys attempt to excrete the excess water.

- **Nonedematous patients with hyponatremia** are suffering from **volume depletion, impaired water excretion, very low Na⁺ intake,** or **very high water intake**
  - **Volume depletion** (suggested by hypotension, tachycardia, and low urine output)
    - Volume depletion (insufficient Na⁺) leads to decreased renal blood flow
      - This is correctly perceived by the kidneys as hypovolemia, resulting in the activation of the renin–angiotensin system and leading to:
        - **Nonosmolar**-mediated ADH secretion, sacrificing tonicity in an appropriate attempt to increase circulating volume
        - Concentered urine (>300 mOsm/kg)
        - Low urine output
  - **Hypovolemic hyponatremia** is caused by **NaCl loss** (either renal or extrarenal)
    - Extrarenal NaCl loss is seen with vomiting, diarrhea, and profound sweating
      - Concentrated urine, **low urine sodium**, and low urine output
    - Renal NaCl loss is seen with **thiazide diuretics**, salt-wasting syndromes, adrenal insufficiency, and distal renal tubular acidosis (RTA)
  - **Euvolemic patients** with **hyponatremia either** have **impaired water excretion** from inappropriate ADH secretion (ie, **SIADH**) **or** engage in such voluminous water intake (ie, nonosmotic polydipsia) that they overcome their ability to excrete it (typically >15 L a day)

- Inappropriately secreted ADH causes water reabsorption from the collecting tubules, leading to:
  - An inappropriately concentrated urine (>300 mOsm/kg)
  - A decreased serum sodium (and tonicity)
  - An increased circulating volume, increasing renal blood flow and GFR leading to sodium spillage (ie, a high urine Na$^+$ [>20 mEq/L])
  - **SIADH** is common and is caused by myriad medications (eg, selective serotonin reuptake inhibitors [SSRIs]) and conditions, from pulmonary, CNS or thyroid disease to pain
- **Very low Na$^+$ intake** (a.k.a. "tea and toast" or "beer potomania")
  - **Very low sodium intake** causes decreased tonicity, leading to:
    - Inhibition of ADH secretion and a dilute urine (<100 mOsm/kg)
    - Urine Na$^+$ remains low because of total body Na$^+$ depletion
    - Urine output remains normal
  - Very low sodium intake is a phenomenon of individuals who eat only "tea and toast" (ie, a diet devoid of salt) or who consume only alcohol (beer potomania)
- **Excessive water intake exists** in a spectrum, from acute water intoxication to chronic psychogenic polydipsia
  - An acute ingestion of a large volume of water (5–10 L) in an hour or two, or a chronic ingestion (10–15 L day), can overcome the body's maximum water excreting ability, causing decreased tonicity and leading to:
    - Osmotic-mediated inhibition of ADH secretion and a dilute urine (<100 mOsm/kg)
    - Urine Na$^+$ that remains low (<10 mEq/L) because plasma volume does not expand when ADH is inhibited (as almost all ingested water is excreted)
    - **High** urine output (500–1000 mL/hr) because ADH is appropriately inhibited
  - An acute, massive water ingestion is typically seen in "water-drinking contests" or psychiatric illness
  - Chronic, daily ingestion of large volumes of water (>10 L every 24 hours) is a psychiatric illness known as psychogenic polydipsia

- Assessment of **urine output** is critical to the evaluation of both volume and ADH status (Fig. 22.2)
  - **Hypovolemic** patients have **low** urine output
  - The transition from hypovolemia to euvolemia is demonstrated by the resolution of oliguria (ie, resuscitation is over when the individual starts to urinate)
  - **Volume-overloaded** patients with cardiorenal or cirrhotic physiology will also have **low** urine output
  - When **ADH is inhibited**, urine volume is **high**, and dilute

TREATMENT OF HYPONATREMIA (FIG. 22.3)

- Treatment of hypovolemic hyponatremia
  - **Resuscitate to euvolemia** with normal saline (NS) in 500 mL bolus (typically 1–2 L)
    - Normalize heart rate (HR), blood pressure (BP), and **urine output**
  - Resolution of hypovolemia (the nonosmotic stimulus for ADH secretion) allows for osmotic-mediated ADH inhibition and thus water excretion
    - **Excess water excretion cannot occur until volume is restored**
  - **After resuscitation,** correct **tonicity,** taking into account **chronicity** and **symptomology**
    - Correct hyponatremia **slowly** such that serum Na$^+$ changes by ≤12 mEq/L in a 24-hour period
      - **Acute hyponatremia** should be corrected to ≥120 mEq/L within 24 hours
      - **Chronic hyponatremia** should be corrected to ≥115 mEq/L within hours
    - Asymptomatic:
      - Encourage oral sodium intake
      - Recheck serum Na$^+$ q 6 hours

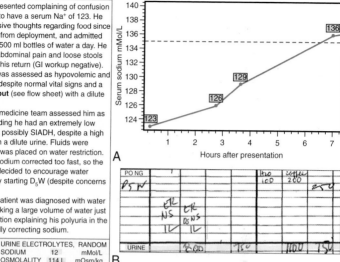

Water intoxication

- 29 year old presented complaining of confusion and was found to have a serum Na⁺ of 123. He reported obsessive thoughts regarding food since returning home from deployment, and admitted to drinking four 500 ml bottles of water a day. He complained of abdominal pain and loose stools occurring since his return (GI workup negative).
- In the ED he was assessed as hypovolemic and given 2L of NS despite normal vital signs and a **high urine output** (see flow sheet) with a dilute urine.
- The admitting medicine team assessed him as euvolemic, deciding he had an extremely low sodium diet and possibly SIADH, despite a high urine output with a dilute urine. Fluids were stopped and he was placed on water restriction.
- The patient's sodium corrected too fast, so the medicine team decided to encourage water intake, ultimately starting D₅W (despite concerns of SIADH)
- Untimely, the patient was diagnosed with water intoxication, drinking a large volume of water just prior to presentation explaining his polyuria in the setting of a rapidly correcting sodium.

URINE ELECTROLYTES, RANDOM		
SODIUM	12	mMol/L
OSMOLALITY	114 L	mOsm/kg

Fig. 22.2 Encapsulated case of water intoxication initially mischaracterized as hypovolemic hyponatremia despite normal vital signs and an elevated urine output (not compatible with volume depletion). The patient was given a total of 2L normal saline over 2 hours, made 0.8 L of urine, and his serum sodium went from 123 mmol/L to 126 mmol/L. He was then admitted to medicine, reassessed by the admitting medical team as euvolemic, and placed on fluid restriction. The next hour he urinated another 0.75 L and his sodium increased another 3 mEq/L to 129 mEq/L. He was then encouraged to drink. He drank 300 mL, was given D₅W at 250 mL/hr, and urinated 1.85 L, correcting his sodium to normal. This was his third admission to the intensive care unit in 2 months with the same presentation; each time he was discharged with instructions to eat more salt and drink less water. Hyponatremia that corrects in the setting of polyuria with a dilute urine is caused by water excess. During this admission he was confronted with the fact that his presentation could only be explained by drinking liters of water in the hours just before his presentation. He was also warned about the real danger of herniation. He never admitted to excessive water intake, but he did not get angry or upset (as one would expect if he actually felt that he had a mysterious disease and his doctors did not trust him). After confrontation his sodium remained normal and he had no more episodes of hyponatremia. He continues to obtain routine primary care in our institution.

- Confusion or lethargy:
  - Give 1–2 L of normal saline at 250 mL/hr and recheck serum Na⁺ q 2–4 hours
  - Repeat normal saline (NS) infusions as necessary to meet the previously outlined goals (based on chronicity)
  - Encourage PO NaCl intake
- Seizure or coma:
  - Give 3% saline 50 mL/hr for 1–2 hours, then recheck serum Na⁺
  - Give 1–2 L of normal saline at 250 mL/hr, then recheck serum Na⁺ q 2–4 hours
  - Repeat NS infusions as necessary to meet the previously outlined goals (based on chronicity)

- **Treatment of Euvolemic Hyponatremia (low sodium intake, SIADH, and excessive water intake)**
  - Low sodium intake:
    - Asymptomatic:
      - Encourage PO sodium intake
      - Recheck serum Na⁺ q 6 hours
    - Confusion or lethargy:
      - Give 1–2 L NS at 250 mL/hr, then recheck serum Na⁺ q 2–4 hours
      - Repeat NS infusions as necessary to meet the previously outlined goals (based on chronicity)

TREATMENT OF HYPONATREMIA

Correct **SLOWLY** and never overcorrect

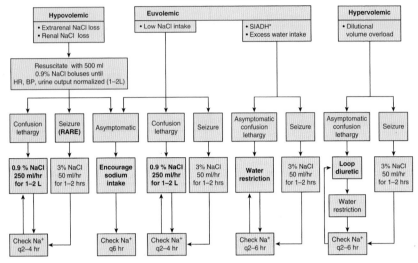

Correct **ACUTE** Hyponatremia ≥120 mEq /L by 24 hr
Correct **CHRONIC** Hyponatremia ≥115 mEq /L by 24 hr

* Uncommonly, severely symptomatic syndrome of inappropriate antidiuretic hormone secretion (SIADH) may be treated with loop diuretic or aquaretic (see figure legend)

Fig. 22.3 Flowchart showing the treatment algorithm for hyponatremia. Correcting hyponatremia is much more dangerous than correcting hypernatremia with regard to seizure, herniation, and death. To avoid complications, sodium should be corrected slowly, focusing on getting the patient to a safe range within 24 hours (115 mEq/L for chronic and 120 mEq/L for acute). Intravenous saline should be discontinued as soon as symptoms resolve. Further sodium administration, if required, by sodium defect, can be given by mouth via food or salt tabs. Hypovolemic patients are often lethargic but rarely have complications and do well with 1–2 L of normal saline. Individuals with a low-sodium diet do well with oral sodium alone. Individuals with excessive water intake do well with water restriction, correcting themselves as they urinate a voluminous dilute urine. Attempts to avoid rapid autocorrection with D_5W at rates approaching urine output (ie, 750 mL/hr) are met with increased urination, barely deflecting the rate of correction. Some advocate attempting to avoid rapid autocorrection by using desmopressin (DDAVP). This may be used in high-risk individuals (ie, chronic psychogenic polydipsia presenting with a very low sodium) who are undergoing correction over hours. Individuals with syndrome of inappropriate antidiuretic hormone secretion (SIADH) may be unable to excrete any free water such that isotonic fluid (ie, normal saline) may worsen their hyponatremia. Hypotonic fluid may cause seizure and/or death. Very symptomatic patients with SIADH may be given 1–2 doses of a loop diuretic to assist with water removal (at the cost of Na^+ and volume). More recently V_2 receptor antagonist aquaretics have been developed that compete with arginine vasopressin at the collecting tubule, allowing for water excretion. These drugs may cause rapid correction so they must be used cautiously and only when significant symptoms are present. Hypervolemic patients rarely need anything more than fluid restriction and diuresis (despite the urging of V_2 receptor antagonist drug representatives).

- Seizure or coma:
  - Give 3% saline 50 mL/hr for 1–2 hours, then recheck serum Na^+
  - Give 1–2 L of normal saline at 250 mL/hr, then recheck serum Na^+ q 2–4 hours
  - Repeat NS infusions as necessary to meet the previously outlined goals (based on chronicity)
- **SIADH and** excessive water intake are treated with **fluid restriction**
  - Asymptomatic:
    - Recheck serum Na^+ q 6 hours
  - Confusion or lethargy:
    - Recheck serum Na^+ q 2–4 hours
  - Seizure or coma:
    - Give 3% saline 50 mL/hr for 1–2 hours, then recheck serum Na^+
    - Continue fluid restriction

- Patients with **SIADH must not** receive hypotonic fluid because this may lead to a rapid drop in sodium
  - Decreasing serum Na^+ in response to isotonic fluid (ie, normal saline) is diagnostic of SIADH

THE PATHOPHYSIOLOGY AND EVALUATION OF HYPERNATREMIA

- Hypernatremia represents a state of decreased plasma water occurring when water loss is greater than water intake
  - The major mechanism protecting against hypernatremia (increased tonicity) is thirst
    - Thirst is one of the most profound drives in humans
      - A serum Na^+ of 146 mEq/L should cause obsessive thirst
  - Increased tonicity stimulates thirst and ADH secretion, increasing water intake and decreasing renal water loss, thereby preventing hypernatremia
    - Therefore, in addition to water loss, hypernatremia requires impaired access to, ingestion of, or absorption of water
      - Impaired or absent thirst is very rare and is associated with inherited (adipsia) or acquired hypothalamic injury
    - The most common causes of hypernatremia are:
      - GI losses (vomiting and diarrhea) > Osmotic diuresis (ie hyperglycemia) > Iatrogenic (ie failure to provide water) > Diabetes insipidus (nephrogenic > central) without access to water
- Symptoms of hypernatremia are caused by increased tonicity
  - Hypertonicity shrinks cells most significantly in the CNS, causing symptoms on a spectrum ranging from lethargy to coma
  - Neurons attempt to balance the increased tonicity of the extracellular fluid by creating idiogenic osmoles (poorly understood)
    - Rapidly correcting hypernatremia may cause cerebral edema (very rare)
      - Gradual correction allows for the idiogenic osmoles to be removed from the cell
    - Overall, treating hypernatremia is much less dangerous than hyponatremia with regard to permanent CNS injury (osmotic demyelination)
- The first step in evaluating hypernatremia is establishing volume status (Fig. 22.4)
  - First surveying for edema, and then, in its absence
    - Assessing intravascular volume via ancillary signs (ie, HR, BP, urine output)
- **Hypovolemic hypernatremia** occurs as a consequence of extrarenal or renal hypotonic fluid loss (ie, water loss > salt)
  - The sodium loss explains the volume depletion, whereas the water loss, in excess of salt, is responsible for the hypernatremia
  - Occurs most commonly from **extrarenal water loss** as seen in vomiting, diarrhea, and profuse sweating
    - Urine Na^+ is low (<10 mEq/L) to conserve sodium
    - Urine is maximally concentrated (>500 mOsm/kg) to conserve water
    - Urine output is low (because of the previously mentioned facts)
  - **Renal (water > sodium) loss** occurs as a consequence of osmotic diuresis, most commonly glycosuria (but also mannitol infusion and urea)
    - Urine Na^+ is high (>20 mEq/L) because salt follows water
    - Urine is dilute (<100 mOsm/kg) because of the osmotically mediated water loss
    - Urine output is low on presentation because of volume depletion
- **Euvolemic hypernatremia** occurs in states of pure water loss
  - **Extrarenal water loss** consists of insensible losses (ie, water vapor lost from skin or the respiratory tract)

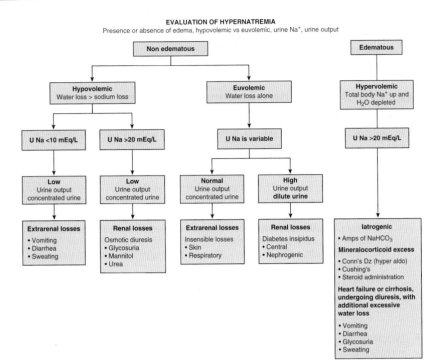

EVALUATION OF HYPERNATREMIA
Presence or absence of edema, hypovolemic vs euvolemic, urine Na⁺, urine output

Fig. 22.4 Flowchart showing the evaluation of hypernatremia. Although the initial step in evaluating hypernatremia also hinges on the presence or absence of edema, unlike hyponatremia, edema is very uncommon. The vast majority of hypernatremic individuals are volume depleted from gastrointestinal illness or glycosuria. Euvolemic hypernatremia from insensible loss typically occurs in demented individuals who are unable to express thirst or ask for water. Hypernatremia with a high urine output suggests diabetes insipidus (DI) with either impaired access to water, as seen in nephrogenic DI (associated with lithium therapy), or impaired thirst, as seen in central DI. Edematous patients with hypernatremia come in three distinct variates: (1) iatrogenic, (2) mineralocorticoid excess, and (3) diuresis with additional excessive water loss. Iatrogenic hypernatremia occurs when individuals receive hypertonic fluid—typically amps of sodium bicarbonate for symptomatic metabolic acidosis. Patients with mineralocorticoid excess may develop hypertension, edema, and hypernatremia (eg, Cushing's syndrome, from ectopic adrenocorticotropic hormone production, or primary hyperaldosteronism). The most common cause of hypervolemic hypernatremia occurs when a hospitalized patient with total body volume overload, undergoing daily diuresis, develops additional water loss from diarrhea, vomiting, glycosuria, or fever.

- This occurs when individuals are not provided adequate water
  - Urine Na⁺ is variable based on sodium intake
  - Urine is maximally concentrated (>500 mOsm/kg) to conserve water
  - Urine output is normal
- **Renal water loss** occurs either when ADH is absent (central diabetes insipidus) or when the kidneys are unable to respond to it (nephrogenic diabetes insipidus)
- Central diabetes insipidus is caused by pituitary disease and nephrogenic diabetes insipidus by renal disease (most commonly as a complication of lithium therapy)
  - Urine Na⁺ is variable based on sodium intake
  - Urine is dilute (<100 mOsm/kg) because of the absent or ineffective ADH
  - Urine output is high because of the absent or ineffective ADH and subsequent water loss

- **Hypervolemic hypernatremia** is most often iatrogenic but may also be seen in primary hyperaldosteronism and Cushing's syndrome
  - **Iatrogenic** hypernatremia occurs commonly:
    - After aggressive resuscitation with ampules of NaHCO₃
    - With exogenous mineralocorticoid excess (eg, florinef, high-dose hydrocortisone)

- During diuresis of volume-overloaded individuals when additional water loss occurs (eg, diarrhea, glycosuria, fever)
  - Urine Na$^+$ is high (>20 mEq/L), reflecting total body sodium overload (and loop diuretics)
  - Urine is maximally concentrated (>500 mOsm/kg) to conserve water

TREATMENT OF HYPERNATREMIA (FIG. 22.5)

- **Estimating the free water deficit does not affect therapy but is easy to do and helps define the magnitude of the derangement**
  - Serum Na$^+$ 146 mEq/L = ~2-L water deficit
  - Serum Na$^+$ 150 mEq/L = ~3-L water deficit
  - Serum Na$^+$ 160 mEq/L = ~6-L water deficit
  - Serum Na$^+$ 170 mEq/L = ~9-L water deficit

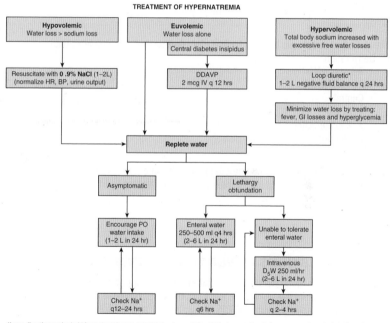

Fig. 22.5 Flowchart showing the treatment algorithm for hypernatremia. Correcting hypernatremia (rehydrating humans) is much safer than correcting hyponatremia. Enteral water consumed in accordance with thirst is the best way to treat hypernatremia. Lethargic individuals unable to drink volumes of water should have an nasogastric (NG) tube placed to facilitate enteral water administration. As soon as they awaken the NG tube can be removed and the patient can be encouraged to drink. Only individuals intolerant to enteral water (ie, ileus, diarrhea) require D$_5$W. Hypovolemic patients should be resuscitated with normal saline (despite the traditional teaching arguing for hypotonic fluid). Isotonic fluid is required to restore vascular volume in a timely manner. Hypervolemic patients can usually tolerate continued diuresis while they have their water repleted (acknowledging that loop diuretics will increase their water loss). Diuretics should be held to hasten water repletion if the hypernatremia is symptomatic, either by decreased mental status or thick, tenacious (endotracheal tube–clogging), pulmonary secretions. Central diabetes insipidus patients refractory to water intake may receive desmopressin (DDAVP) 2 mcg intravenously every 12 hours and via nasal inhaler for outpatient use.

- The general rule of water repletion is, replete half of the deficit in the first 24 hours and the remaining deficit over the next 24 to 48 hours
- Replete water based on symptoms and ability to tolerate enteral water (the preferred route)
  - Asymptomatic:
    - Encourage 1–2 L of water intake in 24 hours
      - Check Na^+ q 12–24 hours
  - Symptomatic (lethargy to coma):
    - Enteral water 250–500 mL q 4 hours for a total of 2–6 L in 24 hours
      - Check Na^+ q 6 hours
    - If unable to tolerate enteral water, use intravenous (IV) D_5W 250 mL/hr for a total of 2–6 L in 24 hours
      - Check Na^+ q 2–4 hours while administering IV water (highest risk for rapid swings)
- Symptoms should always be reassessed, and water repletion slowed, as symptoms improve
- Treatment of hypovolemic hypernatremia
  - Resuscitate to euvolemia with **normal saline** in 500-mL boluses (typically 1–2 L)
    - Normalize HR, BP, and **urine output**
  - Replete water
- Treatment of **euvolemic hypernatremia** (dehydration and diabetes insipidus)
  - Dehydration
    - Replete water
  - Diabetes insipidus
    - Central
      - DDAVP 2 mcg IV q 12
      - Replete water
    - Nephrogenic
      - Replete water
- Treatment of hypervolemic (edematous) hypernatremia
  - Attempts should be made to minimize additional water loss by treating fever, hyperglycemia, or diarrhea
  - Replete water
  - Diuresis

COMMON QUESTIONS GENERATED BY THIS TEACHING

1. **Does renal failure alone (without heart failure) lead to volume overload?**
   Although renal failure causes volume overload, the development of edema occurs after left ventricle end-diastolic pressure (LVEDP) is elevated (a.k.a. heart failure)

2. **I thought calculating the sodium deficit was the most important aspect of hyponatremia treatment (establishing IV fluid rate and volume to infuse)?**
   The most important aspect of treating hyponatremia is to go slow and never overcorrect (highest risk of osmotic demyelination). This is best achieved with frequent monitoring (q 2-hour sodium checks) and oral sodium intake vs 0.9% normal saline IV infusion. Three-percent saline should be reserved for patients with life-threatening neurologic complications like seizure and herniation, and they should only be infused for a short time.

3. **I thought calculating the free water defect was the most important aspect of hypernatremia treatment (establishing the water goal for the first 24 hours)?**
Replacing water in dehydrated individuals is much safer than replacing sodium in hyponatremic individuals. The free water deficit may be estimated based on the serum sodium (ie, 2 L for 146 mEq/L, 3 L for 150 mEq/L, 6 L for 160 mEq/L, 9 L for 170 mEq/L) but does not affect management much. Practically speaking, enteral water is given until patients wake up, at which point thirst and access to water correct the rest of the deficit. Neurologic complications are almost theoretical/exceedingly rare when rehydrating people.

CHAPTER 23

DIABETIC EMERGENCIES

COMMON MISCONCEPTIONS AND MISTAKES

- Extreme hyperglycemia **always** implies profound dehydration and is pathognomonic for a hyperosmolar-type presentation

- Diabetic ketoacidosis (DKA) **always** requires aggressive fluid resuscitation

- Attributing ketoacidosis to starvation

- Attributing obtundation to hyperosmolarity when the calculated serum osmolality (without the blood urea nitrogen [BUN]) is <360 mOsm/kg

- Failing to administer potassium to a DKA patient on presentation because his or her potassium was **normal** (ie, 3.5 mmol/L)

ACUTE DIABETIC PRESENTATIONS

- Diabetics in crisis present on a spectrum from DKA to the hyperglycemic hyperosmolar nonketotic syndrome (HHNKS)

- Management decisions should be made based on the **specific derangements** occurring at the time of presentation and not on the type of diabetes (ie, type 1 or 2) or a single feature of the presentation (eg, extreme hyperglycemia) (Fig. 23.1)

- **Do not** attempt to **treat** via **algorithm**
  - Manage each derangement independently; for example:
    - Ketoacidosis is treated with insulin and prompts a search for a possible sympathetic stressor (ie, **infection** or myocardial **infarction**), even if **indiscretion** (medication/insulin noncompliance) is likely
    - Extreme hyperglycemia occurs as a consequence of renal failure (most often prerenal azotemia); therefore it is treated with insulin, resuscitation (ie, IVF), and possibly a workup of acute kidney injury (AKI)
    - Hypernatremia occurs as a consequence of profound water depletion (often >10 L) caused by weeks of severe hyperglycemia and glycosuria; therefore it is treated with enteral free water replacement and improved glucose control

KETOACIDOSIS

- Respect ketosis:
  - Measurable serum ketones causing a significant metabolic acidosis is **never** normal physiology
    - **Do not** attribute to starvation
  - Ketoacidosis occurs in (only) three clinical situations:
    - DKA, the hyperglycemic hyperosmolar state with ketoacidosis, or alcoholic ketoacidosis (AKA)

Important Points	HHNKS Hyperglycemic Hyperosmolar (Hypernatremic) Nonketotic Syndrome	DKA Diabetic ketoacidosis

• **Extreme Blood Glucose Elevation (ie, BG > 600 mg/dL) implies Anuria**
  •GFR approaches zero and glycosuria stops allowing BG to skyrocket
  • *Not the Hyperosmolar State*
  • *Not Profound Dehydration*
• **High Corrected Na$^+$ = Hyperosmolar state**, from profound dehydration
• **Absence of urine ketones** argues against DKA positive urine ketones only prove fasting (ketones concentrated in urine)
• **Hyperkalemia** occurs secondary to potassium's **Acidotic Shift** out of cells
• Blood urea nitrogen (BUN) included in calc Osm to check for an osmolar gap (ie, to compare to measured Osms), **NOT** to assess for **symptomatic hyperosmolarity** (ie, Osm ≥ 360 mOsm/kg)
  • BUN does not draw water out of cells
  • This mistake can lead to **erroneously attributing obtundation to the hyperosmolar state** (delaying workup eg, ABG, head CT)
	• 57 yo ALS patient, no h/o DM
	• Started on Tube Feeds 2 mo prior c/o 2 wks polyuria, increased thirst and
	• **Decreased mental status**
		• 50 yo Type I DM, CKD 3, blindness, presents c/o 2 days of n/v, ↓PO intake
		• Held insulin the last 24 hrs
		• **Normal mental status**

HHNKS values:
Glucose Level	865 mg/dL	
Sodium	154 mmol/L	
Potassium	3.8 mmol/L	
Chloride	115 mmol/L	
CO2	29 mmol/L	
BUN	57 mg/dL	
Creatinine	0.82 mg/dL	
uKetones Negative	(Cr↑ from 0.3)	

DKA values:
	1297 H*	
	124 L	
	6.7 H*	
	83 L	
	4 L	
	74 H	
	3.72 H	
Specimen KET / Serum ** POS	(Cr ↑ from 1.7)	

	HHNKS	DKA
• Anion Gap:	10	• Anion Gap: 37
• Corrected Sodium:	166 mMol / L	• Corrected Sodium: 143 mMol / L
• Free H$_2$O Deficit:	7–8 L	• Free H$_2$O Deficit: None
• Calc Osm with BUN:	384 mOsm/kg	• Calc Osm with BUN: 360 mOsm/kg
• Calc Osm without BUN:	364 mOsm/kg	• Calc Osm without BUN: 346 mOsm/kg

Fig. 23.1 Comparison of the presenting chemistries and calculated values regarding tonicity and water deficit for a patient with hyperglycemic hyperosmolar nonketotic syndrome (HHNK) and a patient with diabetic ketoacidosis (DKA), highlighting that the important difference between the presentations is not the magnitude of the hyperglycemia but rather the sodium and the bicarbonate. The bicarbonate signifies the presence (or absence) of a severe metabolic acidosis and the sodium reflects the duration of the illness, as water depletion takes time (days to weeks). Both patients have an extremely elevated glucose because both are in renal failure. The HHNKS patient's renal failure is likely a result of volume depletion. His corrected sodium is 166 mmol/L, proving he has suffered weeks of glycosuria and is profoundly volume depleted. The DKA patient, however, sick for only 24–48 hours deserves more thought. In this case the DKA patient had significant baseline disease (chronic kidney disease [CKD] III) and was on an angiotensin-converting-enzyme (ACE) inhibitor. The HHNKS patient was lethargic. His tonicity, or calculated serum osms without the blood urea nigrogen (BUN), were 364 mOsm/kg—a satisfying explanation for lethargy. Interestingly, the DKA patient's calculated osms, including the BUN, were 360 mOsm/kg. If he had been lethargic, he would have been vulnerable to the common mistake of misattributing obtundation to hyperosmolarity based on an ineffective osm, namely BUN. His tonicity, or relevant calculated osmolality, is only 346 mOsm/kg, meaning that lethargy should be worked up.

- The common feature of all three is **absolute** or **relative lack of insulin** (ie, **insulinopenia**)
- Insulinopenia (absolute vs relative)
  - Absolute lack of insulin occurs in type 1 diabetics who abstain from taking their insulin or in end-stage pancreatitis where >90% of the pancreas has been destroyed
  - Relative lack of insulin occurs in type 1 or type 2 diabetics when faced with a significant sympathetic stimulus:
    - Increased sympathetic activity overwhelms the ability of insulin to signal fat storage, resulting in unchecked fatty lipolysis
    - This leads to increased free fatty acid (FFA) release and massive unregulated hepatic ketone generation
    - Sympathetic stimulation also **directly** suppresses beta cell insulin secretion (further promoting ketosis)
- Ketoacidosis should prompt a search for hypersympathetic disease states
  - **Myocardial infarction** and **infection** are classic and **common** triggers and should **always** be screened for no matter how likely a lack of insulin administration is to blame
  - Methamphetamine (and other sympathomimetics) are capable of direct pancreatic insulin suppression, triggering hyperglycemia and ketoacidosis in type 2 diabetics (and vulnerable prediabetics)

DIABETIC KETOACIDOSIS CLASSIC PRESENTATION AND PATHOPHYSIOLOGY

- Insulin is held either to avoid hypoglycemia during an illness with poor per os (PO) intake (ie, vomiting) or when *significant* illness leads to catecholamine excess relative to administered insulin:
  - For example, an individual takes 10 U of insulin but needs 30 U because of an unanticipated myocardial infarction and the increased sympathetic activity that ensues

- Absolute (or relative) lack of insulin destabilizes adipose tissue, leading to massive fatty lipolysis, which releases free fatty acid (FFA) into the circulation
  - Unregulated hepatic FFA metabolism generates an excess of acetyl CoA, which is converted to acetoacetate and beta-hydroxybutyrate and then released into the blood; this lowers pH to a critical level, thereby threatening:
    - Hypercarbic respiratory failure secondary to diaphragmatic fatigue in the face of overwhelming metabolic acidosis
    - Hemodynamic collapse, arrhythmia, or pulseless electrical activity (PEA) arrest secondary to severe metabolic acidosis

- Ketoacidosis is a poorly tolerated condition, and thus it always represents a short-duration illness with patients presenting 24–48 hrs after the onset (eg, last insulin dose or onset of extreme stressor)
  - Often the history reveals an obvious illness that led to cessation of insulin or inadequate administration

- Patients present with a normal mental status, **extreme dyspnea**, and an obvious **maximum** ventilatory effort (ie, Kussmaul's respirations), attempting to compensate for the severe acidosis

- Abdominal pain, nausea, and vomiting are common symptoms that are caused by ketoacidosis itself and are often misattributed to a superimposed viral gastroenteritis
  - May be complicated by preexisting diabetic gastroparesis

- A large, anion gap metabolic acidosis, as a result of ketones, is the central feature of the syndrome
  - Serum ketones positive (at some dilution, magnitude **not** helpful) is the gold standard for the diagnosis
  - Usually a small amount of lactic acid also detected (2–4 mmol/L)
  - If serum ketones cannot be measured in a timely fashion (laboratory limitation), ketoacidosis can be reasonably inferred in the appropriate clinical setting by demonstrating:
    - A large anion gap acidosis (>25 mEq/L) with a lactate <5 mmol/L
    - Positive urine ketones
    - No significant osmolar gap (to suggest ethylene or isopropyl alcohol ingestion)

- Blood glucose is typically elevated in the 200–500 mg/dL range, **not** extremely high (ie, >600 mg/dL)
  - Extreme hyperglycemia is only seen if concomitant renal failure is present
    - In straightforward DKA presentations, volume depletion is not usually significant enough to cause renal failure alone
    - Acute renal failure in this setting commonly represents acute or chronic renal disease often complicated by angiotensin-converting-enzyme (ACE) or angiotensin receptor blocker (ARB) therapy

- Significant hyperkalemia (K^+ >5.5 mmol/L) is **expected** and related to the magnitude of the acidosis (from acidotic shift of potassium out of cells)
  - If the potassium is normal or low on admission, it will drop to <3 mmol/L (often <2 mmol/L) when the acidosis resolves, possibly causing ventricular tachycardia and cardiac arrest

- Hypokalemia, at a normal pH, implies total body potassium depletion as seen in the malnourished and in alcoholics (more common in AKA)
  - Hypokalemia should trigger the monitoring of phosphate (also vulnerable to total body depletion in alcoholism and malnutrition)
- **Serum sodium is normal**
  - Blood glucose is usually not high enough to cause significant dilution
  - There is no protracted period of hyperglycemia and water diuresis to cause hypovolemic hypernatremia
- **Fluid-unresponsive hypotension is ominous and is likely related to the triggering event (eg, sepsis) or symptomatic acidosis (much less likely)**
  - Patients with pure DKA are typically only mildly volume depleted (ie, 2–4 L down), given the short duration of their illness

HYPERGLYCEMIC HYPEROSMOLAR NONKETOTIC SYNDROME (HHNK): CLASSIC PRESENTATION AND PATHOPHYSIOLOGY

- HHNK is most commonly seen in patients with poorly controlled type 2 diabetes who experience a subacute presentation, starting with poor glucose control and persistent hyperglycemia
  - This may occur as the de novo presentation of type 2 diabetes, or it may complicate known disease
    - In established type 2 diabetics, the poor glucose control is usually a result of medication and/or diet noncompliance, infection, or steroid administration for an unrelated problem
- The syndrome starts within 2–3 weeks of polyuria and polydipsia from hyperglycemia and glycosuria, which lead to profound water depletion (5–10 L) and extreme hypovolemic hypernatremia, the central feature of the syndrome
  - The hypernatremia increases osmolality, drawing water out of cells, shrinking central neurons, and causing a decreased mental status (lethargy to obtundation) when serum osms rises above 360 mOsm/kg
  - The uncorrected presenting sodium is often only mildly elevated in the setting of extreme hyperglycemia (because of the dilutional effect this causes)
- Symptomatic hypovolemia is caused by the sodium loss incurred by the osmotic diuresis (because salt follows water), manifesting as:
  - Orthostatic hypotension
  - Renal failure from decreased renal blood flow (RBF)
    - Often complicated by acute tubular necrosis (ATN) if the patient was taking an angiotensin blocker, ace inhibitor or nonsteroidal anti-inflammatory drug (NSAID)
- Extreme hyperglycemia, glucose in the 600–1600 mg/dL range, occurs when glomerular filtration rate (GFR) approaches zero and glycosuria stops, allowing blood glucose values to soar
  - Extreme hyperglycemia (itself) causes few or no symptoms (ie, blurry vision) and is significant only in that it indicates oliguric renal failure
- Patients present with decreased mental status (obtundation), profound volume depletion, and dehydration
  - Patients with pure HHNK are profoundly dehydrated (ie, >5 L free water deficit), and volume depleted (ie, >5L down), given the long duration of their illness

OVERLAP SYNDROMES

- Mixed presentations are more common than pure DKA or HHNK presentations alone
- Over 50% of type 2 diabetics presenting with hyperglycemia and hypernatremia will also have ketoacidosis
  - This implies a transition from a hyperinsulinemic state (occurring during the weeks of hyperglycemia) to an insulinopenic state (occurring in the last 24–48 hours before presentation)
  - Often the onset of ketosis can be pinpointed in the history, coinciding with the development of nausea, vomiting, and abdominal pain
- Explained by pancreatic beta cell suppression, or failure from (either or both):
  1. Increased sympathetic activity, which suppresses pancreatic insulin secretion
     - This is often from critical volume depletion but should prompt a search for other sympathetic stressors, such as infection or myocardial infarction
  2. Pancreatic exhaustion
     - Pancreatic exhaustion describes a potentially transient beta cell dysfunction occurring after weeks of hyperglycemia and overstimulation (beta cells may recover function in weeks to months)
     - Type 2 diabetics with ketoacidosis and a normal sodium level (ie, short duration of illness) do not have volume depletion or pancreatic exhaustion to explain their sudden (relative) lack of insulin
       - These individuals should be scrutinized for a sympathetic stimulus (eg, toxicology screen, cardiac markers, blood cultures)
     - Type 1 diabetics presenting with ketoacidosis and extreme elevations of blood glucose (BG) are suffering from acute renal failure which is **not** obviously explained by profound volume depletion (short duration illness); therefore a workup is warranted in the absence of significant baseline renal dysfunction

TYPICAL DERANGEMENTS, CAUSES, AND INITIAL TREATMENTS OF DIABETIC EMERGENCIES

- Extreme hyperglycemia occurs with oliguria, most commonly from volume depletion; therefore it is treated with resuscitation and IV insulin:
  - 500 mL boluses of normal saline IV (regardless of the serum sodium) repeated until heart rate (HR), blood pressure (BP), and urine output are normalized—usually 2–4 L
  - Insulin drip, bolus 5–10 U, and run the drip at 5–10 U/hr based on weight and likelihood of insulin resistance
  - Adjust drip based on (at least) q 1 hour finger stick blood glucose (FSBG) measurements
- Large anion gap (ie, >25 mEq/L) and severe metabolic acidosis (ie, pH < 7.2), with measurable serum ketones, occurs with insulinopenia (relative or absolute):
  - **IV Insulin** is the **mainstay of therapy:**
    - Bolus 5–10 U of insulin IV
    - Run an insulin drip at 5–10 U/hr based on weight and likelihood of insulin resistance
    - Adjust drip based on (at least) q 1-hour FSBG measurements
    - The drip should be continued until the gap closes
      - This often requires the addition of D_5W to prevent hypoglycemia (glucose clamp) when the BG levels are <250 mg/dL
  - No routine role for serial serum ketone assessment
    - Only useful when ketones should have cleared (24–48 hours later) and a gap acidosis persists; lactate normal

- Differential diagnosis (DDx): ongoing ketosis vs renal failure
  - The absence of urine or serum ketones points to uncleared organic acids; associated with renal failure as the cause of the acidosis
- Sodium bicarbonate (Na HCO$_3$) is only administered when the pH and/or the serum HCO$_3$ are **very low** (ie, <7.1, and 10 mmol respectively) or there is a strong suspicion that the acidosis is causing hypotension or arrhythmia
- NaHCO$_3$ administration should be avoided, and insulin therapy delayed, in the setting of ketoacidosis with hypokalemia, to allow for the initiation of potassium repletion
  - In an attempt to avoid a critical drop in potassium as pH rapidly improves and potassium is shifted into cells

- Mild lactic acidosis, typically <5 mmol/L, occurs as hepatic ketogenesis competes with hepatic lactate clearance:
  - May be higher in individuals with concomitant hepatic disease and poor clearance, as in alcoholic or viral hepatitis or cirrhosis
  - The lactate should be trended until it reaches the normal range (typically <24 hours)

- Serum sodium must be corrected to account for the osmotic effect of extreme hyperglycemia and to establish the presence of a water deficit:
  - Na$^+$ of 143 mmol/L with a BG of 900 mg/dL corrects to 152 mmol/L, confirming a large water deficit (>3 L)
  - Na$^+$ of 129 mmol/L with a BG of 900 mg/dL corrects to 137 mmol/L (pseudo hyponatremia); no water deficit
  - Estimate the free water deficit (corrected sodium 150 mmol/L, deficit ~3 L, 160 mmol/L ~6 L, and 170 mmol/L ~9 L) and aim to replace roughly half the deficit in the first 24 hours:
    - Give 250–500 mL of water q 2–4 hours via NG tube (in those unable to drink) over 24 hours
    - Recheck sodium q 4 hours and continue enteral water replacement until patient is awake and able to drink

- Serum potassium level must be interpreted in light of the serum pH, and rapid potassium intracellular shift must be anticipated with pH normalization:
  - Hyperkalemia from acidotic shift and renal failure
    - Will correct as pH and renal function improve
  - Hypokalemia is **very** dangerous (ventricular arrhythmia)
    - A potassium of 3.5 mEq/L on admission with a pH of 7.10 **will fall to <2.5 mEq/L** as the acidosis resolves
    - 20–40 mEq/L should be added to 1 L of saline and infused as rapidly as tolerated with the initiation of insulin therapy for a serum potassium ≤3.5 mEq/L on presentation
      - If the admission potassium is extremely low (<2.0 mEq/L), insulin therapy may be delayed to allow for some degree of potassium repletion before treatment of the acidosis
  - Never give NaHCO$_3$ before potassium chloride (KCL) in an acidotic hypokalemic patient for fear of precipitating ventricular tachycardia and a cardiac arrest

- Hypotension is typically caused by volume depletion (secondary to glycosuria); otherwise it may be related to the triggering event (eg, sepsis, hemorrhage) or to a loss of vascular tone secondary to the acidosis itself, which is uncommon in DKA and unlikely to occur at a pH >7.1
  - Resuscitate with 500 mL boluses of normal saline IV (regardless of the serum sodium) repeated until HR, BP, and urine output are normalized (typically 2–4 L)
    - Long-duration illness causes more volume depletion, increasing resuscitation needs
      - The higher the corrected sodium, the greater the degree of volume depletion (in addition to water)

- Fluid unresponsiveness concerning for an additional process (eg, sepsis, hemorrhage, symptomatic acidosis)
- Decreased mental status (lethargy to obtundation) is caused by hypernatremia and the hypertonicity it causes:
  - Therefore one must demonstrate hypertonicity before attributing obtundation to a diabetic presentation
    - Measured serum osms will include the BUN and ineffective osm (does not draw water out of cells)
    - A measured serum osm >360 mOsm/kg **does not** confirm a hypertonic state if the patient is uremic
      - The calculation for serum osmolality is:
        - Serum osmolality = $(2 \times [Na^+ + K^+]) + (BUN/2.8) + (glucose/18) + (ethanol/4.6)$
      - This calculation is used to screen for an osmolar gap (as seen in ethylene glycol and isopropyl alcohol ingestion) by comparing the result with the measured serum osms
      - This calculation is **not** used to confirm symptomatic hypertonicity, because BUN is an ineffective osm
    - To ensure that obtundation can be attributed to hypernatremia, one should calculate the tonicity
      - Tonicity = $(2 \times [Na^+ + K^+]) + (glucose/18) + (ethanol/4.6)$
        - Tonicity >360 mOsm/kg is required to cause obtundation in individuals with a normal baseline mental status
    - Do not attribute coma to a hyperosmolar state from uremia or hyperglycemia
      - BUN is **not** an effective osm, and BG would have to approach 2000 mg/dL to cause neurologic symptoms (ie, for serum osms to rise above 360 mOsm/kg from glucose alone)
    - Decreased mental status (lethargy to coma) is from **hypernatremia** or is related to the stressful triggering event (eg, infection, CNS event)
- Renal failure is most commonly caused by volume depletion and a decreased RBF, often in the setting of preexisting chronic kidney disease (CKD):
  - May have superimposed ATN component in individuals taking potentially nephrotoxic medications like angiotensin blockers and NSAIDS
  - Leads to extremely elevated glucose levels (600–1600 mg/dL), as oliguria ends glycosuria, allowing blood glucose to spike
    - Extreme hyperglycemia causes dilutional hyponatremia (from the osmotic pull of glucose), which will correct as BG falls

ALCOHOLIC KETOACIDOSIS: CLASSIC PRESENTATION AND PATHOPHYSIOLOGY

- Alcoholic ketoacidosis represents a pathologic transformation of normal starvation ketosis (a regulated safe process)
  - Alcoholics may ingest only ethanol, depleting glycogen stores
  - Hepatic metabolism of ethanol profoundly depletes NAD^+, relative to NADH, inhibiting gluconeogenesis and leading to low levels of insulin
  - Increased catecholamines from volume depletion (water diuresis and vomiting), often complicated by alcohol withdrawal, causes further insulin suppression, resulting in unregulated ketogenesis and ketoacidosis

- A preexisting metabolic alkalosis is common and is caused by volume depletion and vomiting
  - This can be spotted in a chemistry panel by a high-gap, low-chloride, normal HCO_3 pattern (eg, A-g 30, serum HCO_3 24 mmol/L, Cl 80 mEq/L)

Classic alcoholic ketoacidosis presentation illustrating:
1. Large anion gap acidosis, clears with IV dextrose administration (given after or with thiamine and folate)
2. Preexisting metabolic contraction alkalosis (from the water diuresis and vomiting of alcohol abuse) HCO_3 often much higher (40s)
3. Potassium shift with pH where the K^+ of 4.4 is actually ≤ 3.0 (at a normal pH), seen after recovery
4. Critical hypophosphatemia ($PO_4 < 1$) occurs as glucose administration causes ATP generation which utilizes phosphate, stores of which, have been depleted by starvation (refeeding syndrome)

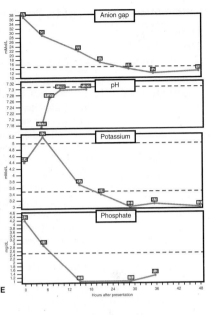

```
ASSESSMENT AND CARE PLAN: 48 yo man with Hx of EtOh abuse
who presents with abdominal pain, vomiting, found to have
acidosis and ketosis.
# Metabolic acidosis with ketosis. ABG 7.17/28.7/86/10.4
with 4+ ketones on dipstick. Large delta-delta
c/w superimposed metabolic alkalosis, likely from vomiting.
Suspect alcoholic ketosis,
- Admit DOU on tele
- Treat ketosis with D5/NS at 200/hour (s/p 100mg thiamine)
```

SODIUM	137	mMol/L	UREA NITROGEN	4 L	mg/dL
POTASSIUM	4.4	mMol/L	CREATININE	0.59	mg/dL
CHLORIDE	92 L	mMol/L	GLUCOSE	132 H	mg/dL
HCO3	8 L	mMol/L	PO4	4.2	mg/dL
			ANION GAP	37 H	mMol/L

The DELTA-DELTA (Δ)

Anion Gap (AG) = $Na^+ - (Cl^- + HCO_3^-)$ = 137−(92+8) = 37
ΔGap = Patients AG − Normal AG = 37−**10** = 27
ΔHCO₃ = Normal HCO₃ − Patients HCO₃ = **24**−8 = 16
Delta-Delta = ΔGap − ΔHCO₃ = 27−16 = **11**
Normal HCO₃ + (Delta-Delta) = **24** + 11 = 35, **THEREFORE**
Serum HCO₃ before the gap acidosis was ~ 35 mMol/L=
Preexisting metabolic alkalosis

Fig. 23.2 Classic presentation of alcoholic ketoacidosis (AKA), highlighting the typical electrolyte and acid–base disturbances encountered. A unique feature of AKA is the preexisting contraction alkalosis, caused by water depletion (ethanol inhibits antidiuretic hormone) and vomiting (gastritis, pancreatitis). This can be detected by the delta–delta calculation, which predicts that the patient's HCO_3 was elevated before the onset of ketoacidosis. As expected, the patient's potassium and phosphate plummet in the first 24 hours. Interestingly the patient's potassium increased after admission (suggesting worsening acidosis). His ABG, obtained at the time of worsening acidosis/increased potassium, showed a metabolic acidosis with a superimposed respiratory acidosis (pH 7.17/Pco_2 29 mm Hg) as evidenced by a Pco_2 29 mm Hg. Although a Pco_2 of 29 mm Hg is low, it is inappropriately high in relation to the pH. A metabolic acidosis producing a pH of <7.25 should trigger a maximal ventilatory response, capable of lowering Pco_2 to the low 20s mm Hg. Because the patient appeared comfortable (ie, no increased work of breathing or obtundation), his worsening hypercarbia was correctly attributed to a shot of hydromorphone he was given for abdominal pain, causing a mild degree of central hypoventilation.

- The "delta–delta" can quantify this by calculating the amount of acid accounted for by the drop in HCO_3 compared with the size of the anion gap
  - This number, added to a normal HCO_3 (ie, 24 mmol/L), predicts the serum HCO_3 before the acidosis occurred (Fig. 23.2)
- **Avoid NaHCO₃ administration**; it is dangerous in this group because the acidosis may clear, rapidly leaving a severe alkalosis in its wake

- Treat with IV dextrose, but make sure to infuse thiamine and folate first/simultaneously (ie, banana bag)
  - Resuscitate with D_5NS, and change to D5 ½NS once volume status is normalized
  - Insulin is **not** required because the pancreas is still functioning (unless also diabetic)

- Watch potassium and phosphate closely; anticipate profound drops secondary to alkalotic shift and the refeeding syndrome respectively
  - A potassium level <2 mmol/L may cause QT prolongation and R-on-T mediated ventricular tachycardia (cardiac arrest)
  - A phosphate level <1 mg/dL is life-threatening, causing diaphragmatic weakness and hypercarbic respiratory failure

Diabetic/Alcoholic Metabolic, Physiologic and Electrolyte Emergencies

Metabolic and Electrolyte Derangement	Physiologic Explanation	Treatment
Extreme hyperglycemia	**Oliguric renal failure** As GFR decreases to zero, **glycosuria stops** and blood glucose **skyrockets** (this is **all** that extreme hyperglycemia implies)	**Restore circulating volume and urine output with 500 mL NS boluses (2–4 L)** Insulin drip bolus 5–10 U, run drip at 5–10 U, q 1 hr FSBG
Large anion-gap Metabolic acidosis with measurable serum ketones	**Unregulated hepatic ketone generation** As a response to unchecked free fatty acid mobilization from adipose tissue secondary to relative or absolute insulinopenia Occurs in type 1 diabetics who administer too little or no insulin, or type II diabetics with, pancreatic exhaustion, and/or overwhelming sympathetic/counterregulatory stimulation (ie, epinephrine, glucagon)	**Insulin drip bolus 5–10 U, run drip at 5–10 U, q 1 hr FSBG** Chemistries q 4 hours (calculating AG) D_5W at 100–200 mL/hr if blood glucose <250 mg/dL and anion gap still present
Mild elevation of lactate	**Hepatic lactate metabolism competes with ketone generation**	No specific therapy, treat ketoacidosis, trend lactate to normal
Hypernatremia	**Hypovolemic hypernatremia from glycosuria** Weeks of an osmotic diuresis (water loss > sodium loss); produces severe dehydration (water deficit may be >10 L), and volume depletion (as Na+ is also lost)	**Restore circulating volume and urine output with 500 mL NS boluses** Then replete water 2–4 L in 24 hrs; enteral route preferred Chemistries q 4 hrs, adjusting water replacement as necessary (based on speed of correction and improvement in mental status)
Hyponatremia	**Pseudohyponatremia** Dilutional, secondary to extreme hyperglycemia and the water it draws into plasma	No specific therapy, treat hyperglycemia
Hyperkalemia	**Acidosis** Causes potassium to shift out of cells	No specific therapy, treat ketoacidosis
Hypokalemia	**Total body potassium store depleted** Seen in the malnourished and alcoholics; more common in AKA overlap syndromes; may be life-threatening as potassium drops further when acidosis is corrected, causing arrhythmia	Treat hypokalemia at presentation with 20–40 mEq of KCL added to 1 L NS infused as rapidly as tolerated Chemistries q 2–4 hours, adjusting KCL replacement May delay insulin therapy until repletion has begun if hypokalemia is severe (ie, K+ <2.0 mEq/L)

Metabolic and Electrolyte Derangement	Physiologic Explanation	Treatment
Hypophosphatemia	**Total body phosphate store depleted** Seen in alcoholics and AKA overlap syndromes; may be life-threatening as phosphate drops further when acidosis is corrected, causing diaphragmatic weakness and hypercarbic respiratory failure	**Use oral phosphate repletion** unless patient suffering weakness and or hypoventilation For symptomatic hypophosphatemia use IV phosphate Use potassium phosphate if hypokalemia present, otherwise sodium phosphate Give 6–12 mmol/L IV phosphate (max 30 mmol/24 hr) Chemistries q 2–4 hours Continue IV phosphate repletion until phosphate >2 mg/dL (max 30 mmol/24 hrs) Then continue oral repletion
Hypotension	**Volume Depletion** From the osmotic diuresis (salt follows water) **Presenting stressor** Sepsis, hemorrhage, myocardial infarction **Symptomatic acidosis** Unusual in DKA, rarely seen until pH <7.1	**Restore circulating volume and urine output with 500 mL NS boluses (2–4 L)** Treat sympathetic stressor (if present) $NaHCO_3$ can be administered to test for symptomatic acidosis (suggested by a rapid, transient improvement in BP)
Renal failure	**Volume depletion** Often in a setting of CKD (from diabetes) and angiotensin blocker use	**Restore circulating volume and urine output with 500 mL NS boluses (2–4 L)** Avoid nephrotoxins (ie, no angiotensin blockers, NSAID, or contrast agent)
Decreased mental status	**CO_2 narcosis** Seen when acidotic patients develop hypercarbic respiratory failure from diaphragmatic fatigue **Increased serum sodium** Seen when osmolality rises >360 mOsm/kg **Presenting stressor** Infection/sepsis, CNS bleed **Drug toxicity** Toxic accumulation of medication or metabolites in the setting of renal failure	**CO_2 narcosis from diaphragmatic fatigue requires intubation** **Enteral water repletion for hypernatremia** Treat presenting (obtunding) stressor if present Search for and hold all possible offending agents (eg, gabapentin, commonly prescribed for diabetic neuropathy)
Abdominal pain, nausea, vomiting	Symptoms caused directly by ketosis	Treat ketoacidosis Antiemetics H_2 blockers Reglan

- Hypokalemia (K^+ <3.5 mEq/L) should be treated first, with 20–40 mEq placed in 1 L of D_5NS infused as rapidly as tolerated
- Hypophosphatemia is common among alcoholics and the malnourished, and oral phosphate repletion should be routine
  - IV phosphate repletion can cause a life-threatening drop in calcium and should be reserved for those individuals with symptomatic hypophosphatemia (ie, PO_4 < 1.0 mg/dL and weakness), which is associated with diaphragmatic fatigue and respiratory arrest
    - In this setting infuse 6–12 mmol of phosphate, rechecking values q 4–6 hours for a maximum infusion of 30 mmol/24 hrs

COMMON QUESTIONS GENERATED BY THIS TEACHING

1. Are liters of IV fluids always the first line of therapy in diabetic emergency presentations?
   No, straightforward DKA often comes with very little volume depletion, and insulin infusion is the most important aspect of the initial care. IV fluids are given for resuscitation and to infuse dextrose as necessary to facilitate IV insulin administration until the anion gap closes (a.k.a. glucose clamp)

2. I thought ketone production and thus circulating ketones were a normal part of fasting. Why are measurable serum ketones always pathologic?
   Ketogenesis is a normal part of fasting, **but** it is well regulated and never causes a significant metabolic acidosis or ketone concentrations high enough to be detected by traditional laboratory analysis.

3. Is the demonstration of serum ketones required for the diagnosis?
   The demonstration of serum ketones (at any dilution) is both the gold standard and classically required for the diagnosis of ketoacidosis. Unfortunately many hospital systems have moved to offsite ketone analysis, where the exact concentration of beta-hydroxybutyrate will be reported days to weeks later (not clinically helpful). When this is the case, ketoacidosis can be inferred in the appropriate clinical setting (diabetes or alcoholism) by demonstrating a large anion gap acidosis (>25 mEq/L) with a near normal lactate (<5 mmol/L) and urine ketones positive. At this point the only reasonable differential is ketoacidosis or an alcohol ingestion. This should be screened for by obtaining a measured serum osm and comparing it to the calculated serum osm. A large osmolar gap should shift concern to ethylene glycol or isopropyl alcohol ingestion.

CHAPTER 24

THE OBTUNDED INPATIENT WITH NORMAL VITAL SIGNS

COMMON MISCONCEPTIONS AND MISTAKES

- All unarousable patients should be immediately intubated because "they are not protecting their airway"
- Failing to realize that only a finite number of processes can cause obtundation with normal vital signs
- Checking for a gag reflex in an unarousable patient
- Placing a nasogastric tube in an unarousable patient

OBTUNDATION WITH NORMAL VITAL SIGNS

- The inability to arouse an individual is a medical emergency
- Obtundation that is **not** obviously attributable to either brainstem (reticular activating system) hypoperfusion (ie, shock) or respiratory failure (hypercarbia or extreme hypoxemia) requires a rapid systematic approach
- The approach to the unarousable patient involves simultaneously looking for rapidly reversible causes (eg, naloxone for opiate overdose) while looking for "good" reasons to immediately intubate (eg, acute hypercarbia)
- In this clinical setting, failure to protect one's airway means that oral and pharyngeal reflexes are suppressed to such a degree that an individual would freely aspirate any material that found its way to the pharynx (ie, emesis)
  - Therefore if an obtunded patient is not vomiting, he or she does not need to be immediately intubated; there is time to rapidly rule out reversible causes
- Never forget to empty the stomach if possible (ie, if the patient already has a nasogastric or gastric tube, place it to suction)
- **Placing a nasogastric tube** in an obtunded patient to empty his or her stomach is **not safe,** given the potential to trigger gagging and emesis
- Do not check for a gag reflex; it is not reliable and may trigger emesis
- In general, patients whose obtundation is **not** from **hypoglycemia, narcotic overdose,** or **postictal state** (ie, quickly reversible conditions) will require intubation and a head CT scan

GOD HELPS OR DOGS HELP

- The typical scenario:
  - You are called to the bedside by nursing, who is visibly concerned because their patient is obtunded

- Temperature, heart rate (HR), blood pressure (BP), and oxygen saturation (O_2 sat) are all normal
- The nurse anxiously reports the patient was fine earlier, adding, "I don't think he's protecting his airway"
- You approach the patient, do a sternal rub, get no response, and begin:
  - Call a rapid response if your institution has a rapid response team
  - Immediately check blood glucose and an arterial blood gas (ABG)
  - Neuroexamination is limited to the eyes and pupils
  - Small (pinpoint) pupils equals opiate effect
  - Disconjugate gaze, fixed deviation, and/or a unilaterally dilated (blown) pupil equals intracranial hemorrhage until proven otherwise (by a stat noncontrast head CT scan)

- **G—Glucose:**
  - Immediately obtain a finger stick blood glucose measurement
  - Severe hypoglycemia is a common, reversible cause of obtundation
    - Blood glucose (BG) <60 mg/dl required (typically <40 mg/dl)
  - Patients should be placed on their side (rescue or recovery position) while waiting for glucose therapy to work
    - Note that oral glucose paste takes several minutes to work

- **0—Overdose:**
  - Inpatient overdose implies oversedation from narcotics, benzodiazepines, antipsychotics, or a GABAergic drug NOS (ie, cyclobenzaprine)
  - *Only* narcotics can be safely and reliably reversed (with naloxone)
    - **Very low** threshold for empiric naloxone use (0.4 mg IV × 1) if there is **any chance** the patient has received an opiate
    - Naloxone response should be dramatic; equivocal response equals no response
  - Benzodiazepine reversal with flumazenil should be reserved for procedure-related oversedation
    - Flumazenil given to a regular benzodiazepine user (most inpatients on benzodiazepines) comes with the risk of seizure
  - The decision to intubate vs observe patients suffering profound sedative medication effects must be individualized (duration of medication, dose, baseline mental status), **but** in general it is safer to intubate
    - Oversedated patients being observed need to be continually screened for hypoventilation with pH/Pco_2 measurements (end-tidal CO_2 is not validated for this use yet but likely has a role)

- **D—Depressed respirations (ie, check ABG for hypercarbia and, to a lesser extent, occult hypoxemia):**
  - Obtain a stat ABG if the patient does not have severe hypoglycemia or naloxone-responsive opiate overdose
    - Obtundation with an acute respiratory acidosis **mandates** intubation

- **H—Hepatic encephalopathy:**
  - In patients with known hepatic encephalopathy, it may be reasonable to attempt treatment with lactulose to prevent intubation
  - However, insertion of an nasogastric (NG) tube in the obtunded patient may cause vomiting; therefore it is safer to intubate if feeding tube access is not available

- **E—Electrolytes (mainly high and low Na^+, but also high Ca^{2+}):**
  - Obtundation from free water imbalance (ie, hyper and hyponatremia) needs to be corrected slowly such that patients should be intubated while the etiology is discovered and correction is made
  - Last chemistry panel may provide clues (Na^+ abnormal)

- Check Na^+ (and possibly Ca^{2+} in the right clinical scenario eg, metastatic squamous cell cancer)
- Hyponatremia: Na^+ <120 mEq/L is typically required to cause obtundation
  - When Na^+ drops quickly, it may cause seizure, with subsequent postictal state
    - Na^+ is most likely to drop quickly when patients with an inability to excrete free H_2O (ie, syndrome of inappropriate antidiuretic hormone secretion [SIADH]) are given hypotonic intravenous fluid (IVF)
- Hypernatremia: Na^+ >150 mEq/L is typically required (but varies, given the baseline mental status)
  - Na^+ rises in inpatients who have excessive free H_2O losses (as in osmotic diuresis, diarrhea, and persistent fevers) and impaired thirst or access to water
    - Because impaired thirst and/or the inability to access water occur in debilitated/demented patients, baseline mental status is often diminished
      - In this situation, intubation is usually **not** required and instead observation while rehydrating is the optimal approach

- **L—Look inside the central nervous system (CNS)** (ie, get a stat noncontrast head computed tomography [CT]; consider lumbar puncture [LP]):
  - Having a nonneurosurgery inpatient develop bacterial meningitis is extremely rare; therefore LP has a very limited role in the general evaluation of the obtunded inpatient
    - In contrast, neurosurgery patients get nosocomial meningitis relatively frequently (often cerebrospinal fluid [CSF] is easy to obtain from preexisting drain)
  - Intracranial catastrophes are relatively common in hospitalized individuals; therefore a head CT without contrast looking for hemorrhage and/or signs of intracranial hypertension needs to be performed stat in all individuals with either:
    - No toxic metabolic reason for obtundation (ie, the GOD HE portion of the algorithm)
    - A neuroexamination demonstrating disconjugate gaze, fixed deviation, and/or unilateral pupil dilatation
  - **Very low threshold** to obtain a noncontrast head CT scan
    - Obtunded patients should be intubated for airway protection before going off the floor for CT scanning

- **P—Postictal state:**
  - Obtundation is common in the **immediate** postictal state and in the absence of emesis, or status epilepticus; intubation should be deferred during observation in the rescue/recovery position
  - The **postictal state** may **precipitate hypoventilation**, especially in people with blunted respiratory drive and/or underlying lung disease, such that one must have a **very low threshold** to obtain an **ABG**
  - The postictal state can be confidently diagnosed in the setting of witnessed seizure and can be reasonably inferred in the right clinical scenarios:
    - Patient with a known seizure disorder who misses medications
    - Patient admitted for alcohol withdrawal
    - Patient undergoing benzodiazepine taper
  - The obtundation portion of the postictal state clears in 5–15 minutes such that protracted obtundation in an individual with a known or suspected seizure should prompt consideration of nonconvulsive status, followed by intubation, stat head CT, and possibly EEG

- **S—Sepsis (early infection in the setting of a poor baseline neurologic function):**
  - Patients with significant baseline cognitive dysfunction may experience obtundation as an initial sign of systemic infection and early sepsis

- In the absence of hypoventilation, one should attempt to avoid intubation because antibiotics and supportive care often lead to significant improvement in just 6–12 hours
- Early intubation (or intubation at all) may not be appropriate given the degree of baseline cognitive impairment in this group
  - Instead, call the family to confirm wishes for aggressive care and consideration of full care and do not attempt resuscitation (DNAR)/do not intubate (DNI) with a plan to change to comfort if respiratory failure ensues

COMMON QUESTIONS GENERATED BY THIS TEACHING

1. **I had a nurse express concern that an obtunded patient might "swallow his tongue", is that possible? what did she mean?**
   Swallowing ones tongue is a colloquial term for upper airway obstruction. Upper airway obstruction occurs commonly in obtunded individuals (often with audible snoring). Head positioning and chin lift should be used to open the airway. Obtundation with refractory upper airway obstruction is a good indication for intubation (with preparation of a difficult airway).

2. **I have seen people bag obtunded patients. Is this a good idea?**
   Positive pressure (either by bag valve mask [BVM] or by bilevel positive airway pressure [BiPAP]) applied to an obtunded individual may lead to excessive gastric air accumulation, leading to disastrous emesis and gastric aspiration. Bagging patients should be primarily reserved for preoxygenation before intubation.

3. **Hey, did you steal this mnemonic from Andrew Lerner? I thought I remember him teaching me something like this.**
   Yes and No. Andrew's *GO TIME* pointed out the necessity (and fun) of a pneumonic in this clinical scenario. I give special credit and thanks to Andrew Learner and his *GO TIME*.

CHAPTER 25

BEDSIDE PRESENTATIONS IN THE ICU

COMMON MISCONCEPTIONS AND MISTAKES

- Giving three complete, separate physical examinations when presenting a single new admission (emegency department [ED] examination, intensive care unit (ICU) admit examination, and the current examination)

- Derailing the presentation by saying things that are very unusual, without specific preface (eg, saying the patient was treated for small-cell lung cancer 10 years ago, instead of just adding "**incredibly**" at the front)

- Reporting a history of the present illness that defies normal human logic, without specifically explaining that follow-up questions were asked and that, yes, this is really the way it occurred (eg, the patient had crushing chest pain, felt like he was going to die, and then returned to bed)

- Not knowing important home medication doses (like prednisone)

- Failing to assess volume status and plan volume goals for every patient, every day (erroneously presuming autoregulation of volume)

- Failing to identify the surrogate decision maker

- Editorializing while giving the labs (ie, "his Cr. is 3.4 up from 1, probably ATN")

- Skipping or glossing over the final overall assessment (instead, launching straight into the plan)

GOAL OF THE BEDSIDE PRESENTATION

- The goal of the bedside presentation is to accurately convey all the necessary facts such that by the end of the presentation, all who are listening have a clear idea of what you think happened to the patient and what you believe needs to be done

- The presentation must never cause the listeners to become confused or distracted, as occurs when the presenter:
  - Violates the anticipated order of the presentation
  - Provides several complete physical examinations ("Wait, was this when you saw him in the ED or this morning?")
  - Says something extremely unusual without special preface (this makes those who are listening concerned that the presenter does not know it is usual)
  - Reads instead of presents—or worse, reads someone else's note

NEW ADMISSION

- History of the present illness (HPI):
  - The goal is for the HPI to elegantly summarize **all** the events from presentation up to that morning at the bedside

- Should contain:
  - Age and demographics
    - 67-year-old white male
  - Relevant comorbidities
    - With a past medical history significant for hypertension (HTN), heart failure with preserved ejection fraction (HFpEF), and chronic obstructive pulmonary disease (COPD) (FEV_1 78% predicted)
  - Relevant recent medical history
    - Recently hospitalized for an non-ST segment elevation myocardial infarction (NSTEMI) (discharged 2 months prior on acetylsalicylic acid [ASA])
  - Presenting scenario
    - ED or floor hospital course before ICU admission
    - A brief summary of the assessment made by the first doctors to see the patient including **pertinent data only** (eg, important vitals, examination findings, test results, ED impression, plan) in a **narrative form**
    - Presented to the ED complaining of a 5-day productive cough and fever. The ED thought he was septic from pneumonia because of a 102 ° F temperature, a white blood cell (WBC) count of 17,000, a lactate of 5 mmol/L, and a new right lower lobe (RLL) opacity seen by chest x-ray (CXR); he was given vanc zosyn and 4 L of IVF before we were called
    - ICU course (narrative form) detailing major events and interventions from arrival right up to the present time (ie, morning rounds)
    - Including important vitals, changes to examination, and new test results in a **narrative form**
    - When we saw him in the ED we noticed his left leg was swollen and had an ultrasound done, which showed a nonocclusive deep vein thrombosis (DVT). His partial thromboplastin time (PTT) was 36 seconds, his platelets (plts) were 180,000 cells/μL, and his hemoglobin and hematocrit (H&H) were at baseline (11 g/dL/33%), so he was given IV heparin after putting in a right internal jugular (IJ) in preparation for pressors. Overnight his blood pressure remained low and his repeat lactate trended up to 7 mmol/L, so we started him on Levophed and then added vasopressin. We also ordered an ECHO for the morning to look for isolated right-sided heart failure because he had DVT and may have had a pulmonary embolism (PE).
- Past medical history (PMHx):
  - Disease/relevant details
    - COPD—report pertinent pulmonary function test (PFT) data (FEV_1/FVC ration [absolute] and FEV_1 %, TLC %, and DLCO %)
    - Heart failure (HF)—report pertinent ECHO data (eg, left ventricular ejection fraction [LVEF], left atrium [LA]-size, pulmonary artery systolic pressure [PAS], right ventricular ejection fraction [RVEF])
- Social history (SHx):
  - Include surrogate decision maker/ durable power of attorney (DPOA) information/ advanced directive status
- Family history (FMHx):
  - Only present relevant information
  - More important in younger patients
- Allergies
- Medications
  - **Outpatient**, **without** dose and interval (unless asked or clearly relevant; based on the medication [eg, prednisone or Lasix])

- **Inpatient** (emphasizing)
  - Pressors/inotropes (dose and trend)
  - Sedation/pain medication (dose and trend)
  - Antibiotics
    - What day, which antibiotics, and for what reason (eg, "Cipro, day 5 out of 10, for *E. coli* UTI")
  - Steroids (dose and indication)
  - Anticoagulation/DVT prophylaxis
- Vitals signs and Fluid Balance (ie I/O)
- Ventilator data—**must have:**
  - For **pressure control mode:**
    - Inspiratory pressure (a.k.a. driving pressure)—**set**
    - Tidal volume (both absolute number in mL and approximate mg/kg value)—**observed (variable)**
      - Example: "tidal volumes **are** 450–510 mL and ~6–7 mg/kg ideal body weight"
    - Rate (set/observed)
    - Minute ventilation (MV): **observed (variable)**
    - Positive end-expiratory pressure (PEEP)
    - Peak airway pressure: **set** (driving pressure + PEEP)
    - Plateau pressure: observed (variable)
    - Fio_2
    - **Low exhaled tidal volume alarm** limit (**critical** in pressure control mode; set as the lowest tidal volume you are willing to accept)
      - This is the alarm that detects a decrease in compliance or an increase in airway resistance in patients placed on a pressure control mode (ie, decreased volumes for the same driving pressure)
  - For volume control mode:
    - Tidal volume (both absolute number in mL and approximate mg/kg value)—**set (fixed)**
      - Example: "tidal volume **is** 450 mL and ~6 mg/kg ideal body weight"
    - Rate (set/observed)
    - MV: **observed (variable)**
    - PEEP
    - Fio_2
    - Peak airway pressure: **observed (variable)**
    - Plateau pressure: observed (variable)
  - Arterial blood gas (ABG) for the previously mentioned settings (pH/Pco_2/Po_2/Fio_2)
- Physical examination (first and **ONLY** complete examination):
  - *Always* look hard **for**, and comment on, the presence or absence of dependent or generalized **edema**
    - The presence of edema has huge clinical significance (by defining volume overload)
- Labs with trends on **abnormal** values (creatinine, Hgb)
  - Do not editorialize
  - Do not trend labs in the normal range (ie, "WBC 9000, up from 6000")
  - **Know** all the microbiology data, including sensitivities, **but only** report new results
- Imaging findings, studies, or other clinical data
- The overall assessment is **very important**
  - The quality of the overall assessment equals your understanding of the case
    - Age and demographics
      - 67-year-old white male

- Relevant comorbidities (clearly related to, or relevant to, the presentation)
  - With a PMHx significant for HFpEF and COPD with a recent NSTEMI
- **"Presented complaining of…"** (clearly related to the presentation)
  - Presented complaining of fever and cough
- **"Found to have…"** relevant abnormal findings in an organized fashion (clearly related to the presentation)
  - Found to have pneumonia, DVT, and shock
- **"Concerning for…"** (differential diagnosis; most likely entities first)
  - Concerning for septic shock with a possible isolated right-sided heart failure component, given venous thromboembolic disease (VTE)
- Trajectory (stable, worse, or better)
  - Stable and improving with a down-trending lactate and Levophed requirement

- Impression and plan **by problem** in descending order of importance (ie, respiratory failure and shock near or at the top)
  - Problem-based organization is superior to systems-based organization for three reasons:
    1. It requires a better understanding of the patient
    2. Patients should be thought of as having a series of problems, interacting in a descending order of importance
    3. It is not possible to make a sensible plan going from head to toe, because you inevitably discuss feeds before getting to the concern for necrotizing fasciitis of the foot

- Systems-based organization argues that in order not to miss anything, one must go head to toe, system by system, in an orderly and systematic fashion
  - Instead, a checklist, like the FAST HUG SSL below, can be used to systematically ensure that nothing is missed

- **Volume status** should **always** be addressed as a problem, with a daily assessment of both:
  - **Total body volume** (ie, a survey for any edema, effusions, and ascites) and
  - **Intravascular volume** assessment (using blood pressure [BP] and urine output, pressor requirement, and possibly central venous pressure [CVP] and/or pulmonary capillary wedge pressure [PCWP] if available)
    - The above volume assessment should lead to **both**:
      - The 24-hour I/O goal:
      - Example: total body volume up and intravascular euvolemic = negative 1-2 L fluid balance over the next 24 hours
      - A simple **algorithm** regarding the initial management of **hypotension, poor urine output, worsening respiratory mechanics**, and/or gas exchange
      - Example 1: **total body volume up** and **intravascular volume up**:
        - Poor urine output = loop diuretic
        - Worsening respiratory mechanics and/or gas exchange = loop diuretic
        - Worsening hypotension = pressors and/or inotropes (ie, no more intravenous fluid (IVF))
      - Example 2: total body euvolemic and intravascular euvolemic:
        - Poor urine output = IVF bolus
        - Hypotension = IVF bolus
        - Worsening respiratory mechanics concerning for a noncardiogenic edema process necessitating an urgent workup

- FAST HUGSSLR (checklist/mnemonic)
  - **F**eeding: discuss
  - **A**nalgesia: ensure analgesia is adequate
  - **S**edation: ensure sedation level is appropriate

- **T**hromboembolic prophylaxis: verify/discuss
- **H**ead-of-bed elevation to >30 degrees: verify
- Peptic **U**lcer prevention: verify/discuss
- **G**lucose control: ensure **no** hypoglycemic episodes and reasonable control (blood glucose [BG] <180 mg/dL)
- **S**kin breakdown: survey for skin breakdown, listing any pressure ulcers, incisions, or wounds
- **S**tool: verify no constipation/no diarrhea
- **L**ines: list every indwelling catheter, ensure no sign of obvious infection, and verify need for continued use
- **R**eadiness to wean: discuss weaning attempts or reasons it is not being attempted (when applicable)

- The mnemonic serves as both a bedside checklist and an excellent way to document (in the daily note) compliance with good practice measures (personalize and add what you like)
  - It allows you to focus on the significant problems, assured that everything else will be covered at the end

DAILY PRESENTATION

- Identifying statement (**only to remind everyone who the patient is**)
  - **Not** a daily recapitulation of all events since hospitalization

- Events of the past 24 hours:
  - Significant events (such as bleeding, need for reintubation, serious arrhythmias, new onset seizures, and hypotension); **not** *simply a rehash of all the routine events of the previous day*

- Vitals signs with net fluid balance (I/O)
  - Range of vital signs (if the range is wide, follow up with "mostly"), but also trends or the most recent findings; for example:
    - "HR was 110–150 bpm, mostly in the 130 s, but was in the 90s in the last hour"

- Ventilator data **must have:**
  - Pressure control mode:
    - Inspiratory pressure (set), tidal volume (TV) (observed), rate (set/observed), MV (observed), PEEP (set), plateau pressure (observed), and Fio_2 (set)
    - **Low exhaled tidal volume alarm limit** (lowest tidal volume you are willing to accept)
  - Volume control mode:
    - TV (observed), rate (set/observed), MV (observed), PEEP (set), peak inspiratory pressure (observed), and Fio_2 (set)
  - ABG on the above settings

- Physical examination (always comment on mental status/level of sedation, pertinent physical findings, and the presence or absence of any edema)

- Labs with trends on abnormal values
  - Have all culture data, including sensitivities, but only report new results

- Imaging or other clinical data

- Overall assessment:
  - **Age**, **PMHx** (clearly related to the presentation), **"Admitted to the ICU with…"** (best guess at what happened), **"Treated with…"** (significant interventions and therapies), **trajectory** (stable, improving, or worsening), **"Active issue remains…"** (eg, list the remaining problems in descending order of importance)

- The overall assessment should be updated daily to reflect trajectory and increased certainty about the disease process
  - Example:
    - Day 1 impression: "fever, infiltrate and decreased BP, concerning for sepsis, likely pneumonia vs UTI"
    - Day 3 impression: "resolving *E. coli* urosepsis"
- Impression and plan by problem in descending order of importance
  - Example:
    - Problem 1: "hypercarbic respiratory failure secondary to sepsis, improving, patient tolerated 6 hours of spontaneous breathing yesterday"
    - Problem 2: "resolving *E. coli* urosepsis, off pressors"
- Volume status should always be addressed as a problem, with a well-thought-out fluid vs. diuretic strategy (as previously outlined)
  - **FAST HUGS SLR** (mnemonic): Feeding, Analgesia, Sedation, Thromboembolic prophylaxis, Head-of-bed elevation, Ulcer prevention, Glucose control, Skin breakdown, Stool, Lines, Readiness to wean

COMMON QUESTIONS GENERATED BY THIS TEACHING

1. I was taught that different people have different styles and some prefer systems-based organization (question implied by tone).
   True, but problem-based organization is objectively superior (your patients deserve the effort)!

2. When your fluid strategy involves fluid bolus (eg, patient dry and hypotensive), how do you "plan" your I/O goal?
   By setting limits—that is, defining the total amount of fluid you will give (in 500 mL boluses) before you reassess the patient's physiology (ie, 2 L).

3. Why FAST HUG SSLR?
   Started as a "give your patient a FAST HUG campaign," it has now morphed into FAST *HUGSSLR* because additional items were added based on ICU performance improvement measures.

CODE STATUS

CHAPTER 26

COMMON MISCONCEPTIONS AND MISTAKES

- Advising your patients to avoid resuscitation based on your assessment of the severity of their baseline cardiopulmonary disease and your "certainty" that resuscitation attempts would fail or that extubation would be impossible

- Accepting a **do not attempt resuscitation (DNAR)/do not intubate (DNI), full care** code status without specific elaboration regarding the desired interventions for sudden ineffective breathing (ie, change to comfort care vs possibly uncomfortable noninvasive ventilation attempts)

- Accepting a **DNAR/DNI** status from a patient without significant chronic disease, daily limitation, or suffering (without vigorously investigating and presuming patient misunderstanding)

- Accepting a split code status request (ie, cardiopulmonary resuscitation (CPR) okay, but DNI) without vigorously investigating and presuming misunderstanding

- Offering advanced care for an exact period of time (eg, 48 hours or 7 days)

- Confusing therapeutic electricity (ie, shocking a symptomatic supraventricular tachycardia [SVT]) with resuscitation

- Asking a patient if he or she "wants to be intubated," failing to mention the alternative (ie, death)

- Believing that once a code status is established, it should **not** be changed

APPROACH TO CODE STATUS

- Patients should **only** be offered one of four possible code statuses:
  1. Full code, full care
  2. Full care, DNAR/DNI
  3. No escalation of care, DNAR/DNI
  4. Comfort as the primary goal, DNAR/DNI

- Establishing the appropriate code status:
  - Full code/full care:
    - The **majority** of individuals seeking medical attention for an acute illness will accept all critical care interventions, assuming:
      - They can be returned to their preillness state of health and functional status
      - They will not have to suffer
    - Therefore the **majority** of patients admitted to the Intensive Care Unit (ICU) should be full code, full care
  - Full care, DNAR/DNI:
    - **Only a minority** of individuals will want to pursue full care **without** resuscitation attempts:

- Typically these are individuals with **a lot of daily suffering** and/or **significant** physical or cognitive **limitation** who are "**ready to die**" comfortably if things go poorly **or** unexpectedly
  - It is **imperative** that full care, **DNI** patients understand that sudden respiratory compromise is typically **uncomfortable** and requires immediate intervention, either:
    - **Noninvasive ventilatory support** (ie, bag valve mask [BMV], oral airway, bilevel positive airway pressure [BiPAP]), which is also **uncomfortable** or
    - **Change to comfort as the primary goal** with immediate administration of narcotics and benzodiazepines, initiating a comfortable death (that often ensues quickly)
  - Patients unhappy to pursue a comfortable (often rapid) death in the setting of sudden respiratory compromise **must** reconsider their code status and are probably more appropriately full code, full care
    - Specifically clarify that intubation does **not** equal ventilator dependence under any circumstances
      - Remind patients that once placed on a ventilator, they (or their surrogate) can decide "enough is enough," choosing compassionate extubation followed by a controlled, comfortable death (at any point)
  - **Full care, DNAR/DNI** patients **should** be offered all possible interventions (unless specifically discussed), assuming they have a pulse:
    - Electrical cardioversion for symptomatic tachyarrhythmias
    - Atropine and/or pacing for symptomatic bradycardia
    - BMV and BiPAP
- No escalation of care, DNAR/DNI:
  - No escalation of care can be considered in a **few circumstances**, where "comfort as the primary goal" is the most appropriate code status, **but**:
    - Loved ones are en route to pay final respects
      - The surrogate must feel and express that the patient would want to wait
      - The patient must not be suffering
    - Deterioration has occurred quickly and the family/surrogate need a little more time to process the information
    - The patient and/or family are "waiting for a miracle"
      - Poor prognosis, further escalation of care futile, but family and/or patient are not ready to change focus to comfort, often because of the sudden unbelievable nature of the catastrophe (eg, drug-induced fulminant hepatic failure in a nontransplant candidate)
  - Comfort as the primary goal, DNAR/DNI:
    - Most appropriate when death is imminent and unavoidable or if the patient is ready to die and wishes no further intervention (may be expressed by the surrogate)
    - Compassionate extubation **must** be a part of changing to comfort as the primary goal
      - Intubation is **not** comfortable
    - Patients should be extubated to room air
      - Postextubation oxygen supplementation **does not** provide comfort and instead may needlessly slow an anticipated death

- Splitting resuscitation attempts makes **no** sense:
  - **CPR okay, but DNI** implies either:
    - Patient misunderstanding regarding intubation (usually equating it with ventilator dependence)
    - The doctor's inappropriate certainty that once intubated the patient will never be extubated
  - **No CPR, but okay to intubate** implies that either:
    - The patient has been threatened by the brutal nature of CPR ("I don't want broken ribs")

- The doctor is inappropriately certain that CPR would be futile
- **No CPR, DNI, chemical code only** implies that:
  - The doctor lacks understanding about the circulatory system (pointless to give medication to a nonperfusing patient in the absence of CPR)

- Do not:
  - **Advise your patients on code status decisions based on your assessment of the severity of their underlying cardiopulmonary disease and your "certainty" that intervention would be futile (eg, $FEV_1 < 1$ L will never get off the ventilator, EF of 10% will never survive CPR)**
    - You will remember all those "certainties" in the coming years as you see other patients defy all your best previous predictions, and you will wonder, "maybe I shouldn't have talked that guy out of intubation, or that gal out of CPR"
  - **Threaten patients with body defiling, rib cracking CPR**
    - Makes no sense (broken ribs are bad, but death is worse) and makes the resuscitation team sound awful
    - Aggressive attempts to avoid CPR should only be made when cardiac arrest is imminent and untreatable (as occurs in refractory acidosis or hypoxemia)
      - The *argument* to the surrogate should be based on the futile nature of CPR in the specific clinical setting (with a clear explanation [ie, "the low oxygen levels are not survivable"])
  - **Offer advanced care for an exact period of time (eg, 48 hours or 7 days)**
    - Life and death decisions must not be arbitrary
      - Very unsatisfying (and untenable) to withdraw care if someone is making significant progress but then "runs out of time!?"
    - Instead, focus on a short (days to a week) or moderate duration (weeks) vs prolonged support
    - This strategy (appropriately) errs on the side of life
  - **Use of the term "withdrawal of care" sounds terrible, and it is not true; instead use "focus on comfort"**
- Code status may appropriately change several times throughout an individual's illness and/or ICU stay based on their clinical course; for example:
  - A patient may be made DNAR because of a refractory hypoxemia and a falling PaO_2 (and the futility that this implies should cardiac arrest occur), only to be changed back to full code if they miraculously improve
  - A patient with a terminal illness who is dying at home on home hospice DNAR/DNI, which practically means no 911 call from home, may wish to be full code when he or she is admitted to the hospital with pulmonary edema, accepting short-term aggressive care with hopes of returning home to die

COMMON QUESTIONS GENERATED BY THIS TEACHING

1. I was taught that patients with severe COPD should be encouraged to be DNAR/DNI because they can "never be extubated" once intubated (question implied by tone). **Everyone** can be extubated. If they cannot be liberated, they can undergo compassionate terminal extubation.

2. What should I do if a full care, DNAR/DNI patient develops acute respiratory failure? This is a common and terrible situation in which patients often endure suffering (needlessly). This situation should be avoided by always planning for it. Unfortunately, if not planned for, the correct answer is to aggressively support the patient with "noninvasive" measures (uncomfortable as this may be) and urgently contact the surrogate to clarify the patient's goals of care. Comfort measures or intubation are always preferable to continued aggressive noninvasive support (this sets the patient up for potential dyspnea and suffering).

CHAPTER 27

ADVANCED CARE PLANNING AND THE FAMILY MEETING

COMMON MISCONCEPTIONS AND MISTAKES

- Parsing out critical care into its individual interventions, asking surrogates what they think their loved one would want (eg, triple-lumen catheter [TLC] placement, nasogastric [NG] tube, continuous veno-venous hemofiltration [CVVHD])

- Mixing advanced care planning with code status discussions (ie, discussions of intubation with discussions of long-term acute care [LTAC])

- Using your **authority** (clutching an advanced directive in your hand) in attempting to get the patient's family and loved ones to limit or withdraw support

ADVANCED CARE PLANNING

- Patients with significant preexisting comorbidities who suffer from a superimposed critical illness should plan for the advanced care they would or would not want to receive

- The physician must first establish a surrogate decision maker in case the patient loses the ability to communicate (ie, intubation)
  - The surrogate is most often a family member **but** may be **any** individual acting in the **patient's best interest** who knows the patient well enough to know how he or she thinks (this vague definition gives the physician enormous discretion in choosing a surrogate)

- Initial advanced care planning discussions with the patient or surrogate should focus on:
  - The patient's preexisting state of health and functional status
  - The postillness limitations that they would **not** be willing to accept (eg, permanent skilled nursing facility residence, hemodialysis, ventilator dependence, severe neurologic or cognitive impairment)
    - It is crucial that the discussion of potential permanent impairment (ie, ventilator dependence) is not misconstrued by the patient to mean that a short-term intervention, like intubation, should not be pursued
    - The physician should provide reassurance that aggressive measures can be stopped at any time should medical certainty predict an unacceptable outcome
      - Specifically, the physician should reassure the patient that the goals of care can be changed to focus on comfort, **including** compassionate extubation (providing a controlled, dignified, and comfortable death)

ESTABLISHING A SURROGATE DECISION MAKER

- When a patient has a catastrophe, the responsible physician should reach out to the patient's loved ones as soon as possible to establish a surrogate decision maker

- If the patient has not designated a surrogate or DPOA, and several family members are available and clearly acting in the best interests of the patient, the priority goes:
  - Spouse → adult child → parent → sibling → adult grandchild → friend

- Relatives may choose to share the responsibility, but an easy-to-reach spokesperson should be insisted on

- The surrogate should be updated daily (in the same way one would update one's patient)

- The surrogate should be continually reminded that his or her responsibility is **not** to make decisions for the patient but rather to "divine" what the patient would choose, say or think based on the surrogates familiarity and knowledge of the patient

THE FAMILY MEETING (HELPING LOVED ONES ACCEPT FUTILITY)

- A family meeting should be held whenever it is requested

- A family meeting **must** be held when there has been a significant clinical deterioration, or significant new "game changing" findings (eg, metastatic cancer), that makes the current care plans futile and thus inappropriate

- Even though the patient may have a single, clearly defined surrogate, decisions regarding the limitation of life-sustaining measures or withdrawal of support are so profound that the physician should attempt to attain a consensus among all involved loved ones **because:**
  - It builds trust
  - It helps ensure a "good death" for the patient and loved ones
  - A first-time conversation with a loved one or a family member **after** you have withdrawn support has a palpable tension ("you killed my love one")

- Consensus can usually be achieved by answering questions and by spontaneously offering explanations and dispelling common misconceptions

- Before the meeting, **always:**
  - Have the most up-to-date patient information (ie, examine the patient right before the meeting)
  - Have a sense of the most appropriate outcome (eg, change to comfort as the primary goal), **but** do not have an agenda

- At the meeting, **always:**
  - Ask about the relationships of those in the meeting to the patient (make no assumptions)
  - Identify yourself as the **responsible physician** (eg, "there are a lot of doctors involved in your loved one's care, but I am ultimately responsible")
  - Ask the family to verbalize their understanding of the current illness, trajectory, and the possible diagnostic and therapeutic interventions they have contemplated or heard discussed
  - **Listen**, picture yourself in their shoes, and make sure that what you are going to tell them will make sense based on their understanding
  - Define the reason for the meeting
    - Significant patient trajectory change as opposed to routine update
  - Do your best to explain the situation in understandable terms
    - Adjust the detail level to the individual family member's needs, but start broad
      - Example: "The cancer has made it impossible to beat the infection, and no more options exist for treating the cancer"

- Attempt to empathize, and do not be afraid to show emotion (within reason); it builds trust, and it usually comes easily after reviewing a patient's recent medical history leading up to the futile point in care
  - Example: "It has obviously been a very difficult few months for your loved one—learning that the cancer has returned after all that painful chemotherapy and then being admitted again after only being home for 2 weeks…"
- Remind the family of the job of the surrogate decision maker
  - To report all previously expressed wishes of the patient
  - And failing any, they are to imagine what their loved one would want
    - **Not** what they would want for themselves or what they would want for their loved one

- The empty chair technique
  - To refocus the discussion, or to bring the meeting to a conclusion, consider "the empty chair" technique
    - Turn and gesture to an empty chair at the table, or in the room, and say, "If your loved one was here right now, sitting in that chair, listening to all we have discussed, what would they say?"

- Discuss your understanding of the patient's wishes and your sense of the most appropriate code status
  - Explain that changing the goals of care to comfort as the primary goal means the discontinuation of all medications and therapies not directly aimed at comfort (eg, pressors and antibiotics), including compassionate extubation

- Then verify that the outcome you have just discussed is what the loved one would have wanted

- Documentation should list all in attendance by name

SPECIAL SITUATIONS

- Changing to comfort is the most appropriate course, but family members are en route
  - Once you verify that "the patient would want to wait," consider no escalation of care (DNAR/DNI) as a reasonable temporary status
  - Assuming no suffering
  - Remind loved ones that we do not have control over life and death and that despite the discussed plans, their loved one may not survive

- Fighting with family (when and why):
  - **Never**
  - Remember, everyone wants the same thing: the best possible outcome for the patient in question; therefore:
    - **Fighting** equals **miscommunication,** and **fighting** is avoided by **communication**
      - **Do not avoid difficult family members;** spend time with them (and **avoid a lawsuit instead**)

COMMON QUESTIONS GENERATED BY THIS TEACHING

1. What if a single family member is irrational and emotional (ie, not acting in the best interests of the patient) and refuses to accept the futility of the situation, rejecting a change to comfort as the primary goal?
   Although he or she ultimately has no power and cannot change the outcome, it is best **not** to demonstrate authority at this point. It is better to give the distressed individual time (within reason), encouraging other family members and loved ones to help him or her accept the reality of the situation. This process helps ensure a "good death" for the family,

which in reality is often all that matters (as is the case when the patient is comatose). It is reasonable to presume that a patient would want **all** his or her family and loved ones to be peaceful at the bedside if possible; thus working toward this end serves the patient. It also prevents complaints, groundless legal letters, or worse.

2. **The family wants to know if they can speak to their loved one after terminal extubation, just for a moment, to say good bye. Can they?**
   By and large, patients undergoing compassionate terminal extubation for respiratory failure would experience extreme dyspnea and suffering if they were allowed to be interactive at terminal extubation. The family usually understands this immediately when it is explained to them.

CHAPTER 28

PULMONARY AND CRITICAL CARE PEARLS

RESPIRATORY MECHANICS AND SOUNDS: (Fig. 28.1)

- Inspiration:
  - Active process in which diaphragmatic contraction generates negative intrathoracic pressure, sucking air into the conducting airways
- Exhalation:
  - Passive process in which intrinsic chest wall and lung compliance generate positive intrathoracic pressure, forcing air out of the thorax
- Extrathoracic stridor:
  - High-pitched, monophonic, **isolated inspiratory** sound implying extrathoracic, upper airway/laryngeal obstruction, as occurs from mucus, swollen tissue, external compression, or tumor
  - Upper airway and laryngeal structures outside of the chest collapse during inspiration and open during expiration
  - Stridor requires urgent evaluation because upper airway obstruction may necessitate an emergency surgical airway
- Wheeze:
  - Harmonic, polyphonic sound indicating **intrathoracic** airway obstruction
  - Airway structures inside the chest collapse during expiration and open during inspiration
    - **Mild airway narrowing** causes an **isolated expiratory wheeze**
    - **Severe airway narrowing** causes an **inspiratory and expiratory wheeze**
  - An isolated inspiratory wheeze equals extrathoracic **stridor** until proven otherwise (examine the neck)
    - It is not possible for an airway structure inside the chest to produce an isolated inspiratory wheeze

SMOKING CESSATION

- Getting a smoker to quit smoking is one of the greatest interventions you can make as a physician
- You must approach smoking cessation with the certainty that every patient will quit
- Your patients must feel your commitment and certainty that they will quit
- Active smokers coming to a pulmonary clinic feel ashamed and want to quit, no matter what they say
- Active smokers with lung disease employ elaborate denial schemes, constantly looking for tacit approval and acceptance from the pulmonologist:
  - "I'll never quit … throw a pack in the grave with me" equals "it's an impossible task doc"
  - "It's too late now … the damage is done" equals "it's not worth it at this point"
  - "I feel great and have no problem exercising" equals "there will be time to quit before trouble"

Extrathoracic upper airway obstruction causes
an isolated inspiratory sound (stridor),
expiration is clear

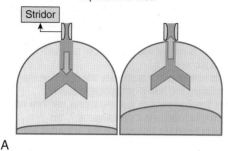

A

Mild to moderate intrathoracic airway
obstruction (e.g. asthma)
expiratory wheeze, inspiration clear

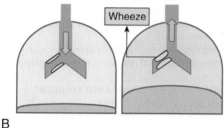

B

Severe intrathoracic airway obstruction
(e.g. asthma) inspiratory and expiratory wheeze,

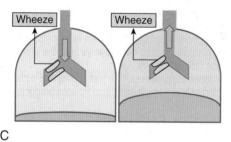

C

Fig. 28.1 **(A)** Schematic diagram depicting the mechanics of stridor, showing how the extrathoracic airway and pharyngeal structures have a tendency to collapse during inspiration and a tendency to open during expiration. **(B)** Demonstrates how mild to moderate airway narrowing will cause a wheeze during expiration only. **(C)** Demonstrates how severe airway obstruction causes an inspiratory and expiratory wheeze. Taken together, it should be clear that an isolated inspiratory wheeze cannot come from inside the thorax.

- "I've cut down to just three cigarettes a day" equals "good enough, eh doc?"
- "It's the only joy I have in my life" equals "have pity on me doc (I am horribly depressed)"
- Tacit approval is given when:
  - You forget to discuss smoking cessation; you might as well light up a cigarette for the patient
    - Counseling works and does not have to take much time

- It should be the first and last thing you discuss with every active smoker, without alienating him or her
  - You accept any of the patient's rationalizations
- Each rationalization must be addressed and exposed for the excuse that it is
  - "I'll never quit" is parried with "everyone quits eventually and wishes they had done it earlier"
  - "It's too late now" is parried with "things can get much worse; imagine getting out of breath taking a shower"
  - "I feel great" is parried with a cautionary tale (based on many true stories) about ventilatory limitation and how it can appear suddenly:
    - "Doc, I was fine 2 weeks ago, got pneumonia, and now can't walk up a flight of steps, and you're telling me it's emphysema?" Yes
  - "I've cut down to just three cigarettes a day" is parried with "fabulous, but now the hard work begins"
- After you make it clear that you are serious about smoking cessation by **not** accepting the patients' initial rationalizations, start by explaining your perspective:
  - Smoking is destroying their lungs and is going to cause cancer, heart attack, or stroke
  - Point out the irrationality of worrying about other disease prevention (ie, daily aspirin, screening colonoscopy) while they are smoking
    - Smoking poses such a grave risk to health that it eclipses the benefits of any primary disease prevention measure
  - Explain that this irrationality in their behavior occurs because it's an addiction:
    - Explain that there is a cluster of neurons in their brain always trying to convince them to smoke
      - "It's a great day ... time to celebrate with a cigarette"
      - "It's a crappy day ... I need a cigarette"
      - "It's such a boring day ... nothing to do but smoke"
    - Ask them if they have ever quit, how they quit, and what made them relapse
      - It is an addiction (with all the shame, lack of self-control, etc), so be empathetic
  - Remind them that the successful ex-smokers quit and relapse an average of 10 times before durable cessation
    - Each failed attempt must be seen as the necessary work required by the difficult process of quitting
      - Each quit-relapse attempt should be seen like a notch in their belt
- Active smokers in a pulmonary clinic must **always** be in the process of quitting
- Common second-line rationalizations:
  - In response to nicotine supplements, "I'm just trading one addiction for another"
    - Nicotine supplements are much safer than tobacco products and not nearly as addictive
      - Almost nobody chews the gum forever
  - "It's not safe for me to smoke and use the supplements, and I *might* cheat"
    - Smoking is not safe
      - Educate patients on nicotine toxicity (potentially incapacitating vertigo, horizontal nystagmus, and nausea)
        - Such that they should not "cheat" while driving or climbing a ladder
        - Nicotine toxicity often produces a conditioned taste aversion to tobacco, which is useful in quitting
- Never let your inpatients go out and smoke:
  - Offer them anything else for their craving while they are an inpatient (from nicotine to lorazepam)
    - If you cannot help them quit in the new context of being an inpatient, you are not trying
  - Nicotine patches in the intensive care unit increase cardiovascular events, such that they should not be used for intubated, sedated patients in attempts to reduce sedation needs

- Helping while they are quitting:
  - Handling the proud report "I've cut down to just three cigarettes a day":
    - Smoking (and addiction in general) is context dependent
      - The last three to five cigarettes a day are the "pillar" cigarettes
        - Those that the smoker falsely believes, they will always long for
        - Typically with their morning coffee, after dinner, during their commute to work, and while on their work break
      - At this stage, cessation efforts must focus on breaking the habit
        - Tell your smokers they can have their three cigarettes a day but **not** at the time they want
    - They must wait at least 2 hours (encourage them to use nicotine supplements [eg, gum] during that time)
  - Encourage them to change their behavior, to avoid contexts that provoke craving (eg, eat, drink, and take breaks in different locations with different, nonsmoking people)
  - Calling a patient on their quit date is a spectacular way to show that you are invested in their quitting (put it on your calendar)
    - Much easier for people to fail themselves than to fail people they respect
  - Remind them that the chemical addiction to cigarettes lasts 2 weeks, and after that point, it is behavioral
    - Creates a concrete, achievable goal that is easier to focus on than lifetime abstinence

BRONCHIECTASIS

- Bronchiectasis is:
  - **Not** related to smoking or chronic obstructive pulmonary disease (COPD)
  - The term used to describe an airway that fails to taper normally, making its lumen abnormally large for its airway generation
    - The vessel traveling alongside the airway gives a good approximation of its anticipated size
  - Caused by either:
    - Fibrosis of the parenchyma surrounding the airway, dilating via traction (ie, traction bronchiectasis), as seen in pulmonary fibrosis, radiation fibrosis, and nontuberculous mycobacteria (NTM) infection
      - Bronchiectasis occurs in the areas of fibrosis
    - Mucus plugging with prolonged airway impaction, as seen in allergic bronchopulmonary aspergillosis (ABPA) or as a sequela of a poorly treated bacterial pneumonia
      - Bronchiectasis occurs focally or multifocally
    - Cystic fibrosis, immune deficiency (eg, IgG), and ciliary dyskinesia (eg, Kartagener syndrome)
      - Bronchiectasis occurs diffusely
  - The most common cause of massive hemoptysis:
    - Areas of bronchiectatic lung are poorly drained, chronically infected, and subject to pathologic angiogenesis, leading to large ecstatic bronchial and intercostal arteries prone to rupture
  - Both a clinical syndrome (chronic daily purulence with intermittent acute infection) and a radiographic finding (which may be insignificant and asymptomatic)
- Bronchiectasis causes disease by impairing the ability of cough to clear secretions (necessary to prevent lung infection)
  - Cough works by collapsing all but the main airways, expelling intraluminal material mechanically and via high expiratory flow rates
  - Bronchiectatic areas fail to collapse and expel material normally, such that secretions pool, promoting chronic airway infection

- Chronic airway infection leads to:
  - Persistent daily purulence (experienced as a chronic productive cough)
  - Acute exacerbations in which patients complain of increased sputum, fever, and hemoptysis
    - Sputum cultures often reveal multiple organisms and/or aerobic gram negative rods
- Outpatient management of bronchiectasis:
  - Reduction of chronic purulence and cough requires daily **airway secretion clearance** via:
    - Position (ie, postural drainage), in which the patient positions himself or herself in such a way that bronchiectatic areas are nondependent, allowing secretions to drain via gravity to more proximal airways where they may be cleared by cough
    - Vibratory kinetic energy, in which the airway is vibrated, dislodging secretions and moving them proximally where they can be cleared by cough
      - Airway vibration may be generated by either:
        - An expiratory flow device with an oscillating resister (eg, flutter valve), in which the patient's slow exhalation generates a vibrating column of air
        - An external thoracic vest or wrap that vibrates the thorax externally
    - Patients should understand that airway clearance devices (working appropriately) do not immediately cause large amounts of phlegm to be expelled, but rather, when performed several times every day, lead to a reduction in chronic purulence over weeks to months (akin to tooth brushing)
      - If this is not explained, individuals may try their flutter valve once, not experience a satisfying episode of phlegm expulsion, and never use it again
    - Nebulized hypertonic saline may be used to further help with secretion clearance
    - Inhaled antibiotics (eg, tobramycin) are often helpful when individuals suffer from persistent/recurrent infection with a resistant organism (eg, pseudomonas)
      - They are typically prescribed on and off for 2–4-week periods (to decrease the chance of resistance)
      - When individuals complain of doing poorly during the off intervals, another antibiotic may be used (eg, ceftazidime)
      - Inhaled antibiotics may still have efficacy (and may be used) even if the organism has demonstrated in vitro resistance, because of the high concentrations achieved in the airway mucosa
      - Inhaled antibiotics may cause severe bronchospasm (necessitating discontinuation)
    - Patients with bronchiectasis invariably develop acute exacerbations with fever, change in sputum (color/volume), and hemoptysis
      - Mild to moderate exacerbations with scant hemoptysis and/or blood-tinged sputum may be treated on an outpatient basis with oral antibiotics
        - Sputum cultures should be obtained in case empiric therapy fails
          - That said, clinical success often occurs despite the presence of resistant organisms cultured (such that antibiotics should not be routinely broadened based on sputum culture results in the face of clinical success)
            - Occasionally the true (sensitive) pathogen is overgrown by the resistant pseudomonas in the culture dish
      - Severe exacerbations and/or those with significant hemoptysis should be treated on an inpatient basis
        - Cultures should be obtained
        - Broad-spectrum antibiotics should be administered intravenously (IV), even though WBC count and temperature are often normal
        - Chest imaging should be performed
          - Individuals with significant hemoptysis should have a chest computed tomography (CT) scan (arterial phase contrast if renal function permits) to localize the bleeding area and plan possible embolization

- Bronchoscopy adds very little to localization and may precipitate respiratory failure (see CH 24)
- Interventional radiology (IR) should be consulted
- ~85% of inpatient exacerbations with hemoptysis respond well to antibiotics with improvement in sputum and hemoptysis over 24–48 hours
  - At this point individuals may be discharged to complete a course of IV antibiotics at home (via peripherally inserted central catheter line) or oral antibiotics if resistance patterns allow
- ~15% of inpatient exacerbations are complicated by massive hemoptysis requiring embolization by interventional radiology
  - IR embolization comes with the risk of spinal cord infarction (see CH 24)

ATYPICAL AND TYPICAL PNEUMONIA (DEFINITIONS AND THINGS TO CONSIDER)

- Atypical and typical pneumonia are terms that carry different meanings in different contexts
- Clinically:
  - Typical pneumonia presentation implies acute onset fever, productive cough, and a new infiltrate
  - Atypical pneumonia presentation implies a more indolent course over weeks to months, involving low-grade temperatures/night sweats, dry cough, and infiltrate(s)
- Radiographically:
  - Typical pneumonia appears as a lobar consolidation or as areas of dense consolidation (with clear air bronchograms)
  - Atypical pneumonia may have many different radiographic appearances, including diffuse or focal ground glass, increased interstitial markings, nodules, and tree and bud opacities
- Organisms and route of infection:
  - Typical pneumonia organisms (eg, *Streptococcus pneumoniae, Haemophilus influenzae, Moraxella catarrhalis,* and *Staphylococcus aureus*) cause the majority of community-acquired pneumonias
    - They tend to have a typical pneumonia presentation and imaging
    - These organisms are present in the naso/oral pharynx in 25% of the population at any time
    - Infection occurs when an individual is carrying an organism in his or her naso/oral pharynx and he or she experiences a microaspiration event in the setting of impaired host immunity (eg, the postviral state)
  - Atypical pneumonia organisms exist in a wider range of species (bacteria and fungi):
    - **Mycoplasma and chlamydia** tend to cause an atypical clinical syndrome with atypical diffuse imaging
      - Infection occurs person to person (likely by droplet)
      - Most infections are very mild, despite radiographic infiltrates (a.k.a. walking pneumonia)
      - Hypoxemia is unusual
      - Self-resolving
    - **Legionella** causes a typical pneumonia presentation with typical imaging (often with rounded, dense consolidations involving the right-middle and right-lower lobes)
      - Initial deterioration after presentation is common, as well as associated gastrointestinal complaints
      - Legionella is contracted by inhalation of contaminated water vapor

- NTM infection may be clinically silent or have atypical pneumonia characteristics
  - Radiographically, NTM causes areas of dense consolidation with traction bronchiectasis and tree and bud nodules ($\pm$ mediastinal adenopathy)
  - NTM infection occurs with inhalation of contaminated water (often during showering)
    - NTM organisms are found in tap water because they are not killed by chlorine
  - Most NTM infections are low grade (involving asymptomatic fleeting nodules) and do not require treatment
  - Indications for treatment include systemic symptoms (weight loss, fevers), progressive parenchymal destruction (increasing areas of traction bronchiectasis), and worsening restriction on pulmonary function tests
- Tuberculous mycobacterial (TB) infection
  - Primary TB has a muted atypical pneumonia presentation with weeks of coughing and typical pneumonia imaging (often with necrosis)
  - Reactivation TB also has an atypical presentation with months of coughing and systemic symptoms (weight loss/night sweats) and imaging showing upper lobe nodular/fibrocavitary infiltrates
- Aspergillus (see CH 10)
- Endemic fungus (inhaled from the environment)
  - Cryptococcus (in the immunocompetent) causes a typical pneumonia presentation with cough, chest pain fever, hemoptysis
    - Imaging shows consolidations that may be mass-like (round and solid)
  - Coccidiomycosis may cause both typical and atypical presentations depending on the individual's ability to handle the organism
    - Radiographically, cocci may cause lobar consolidation, mass-like consolidation, hilar and mediastinal adenopathy, or a cavitary lesion (ultimately persisting as a thin-walled cavity)
- Oral anaerobes (see CH 11)

TROUBLESHOOTING POORLY CONTROLLED OBSTRUCTIVE LUNG DISEASE (ASTHMA AND COPD)

- Asthma
  - When an asthmatic's control worsens, a search for the factors driving airway inflammation should be undertaken, screening for:
    - Environmental allergens (eg, new pet, new living environment, environmental mold exposure, occupational exposures)
    - Allergic rhinitis or sinusitis (eg, nasal congestion, facial pain, headache, tooth pain)
      - Occasionally bacterial sinusitis needs to be treated with prolonged antibiotics before asthma control can be regained
    - Gastroesophageal reflux disease (GERD) (often without symptoms of heartburn)
    - ABPA (see CH 10)
  - Occasionally poor control occurs because the patient has an asthma mimic–like vocal cord dysfunction (VCD)
    - Individuals with VCD will often be intubated on multiple occasions for respiratory distress associated with noisy breathing, only to have normal mechanics on the ventilator immediately after intubation (not compatible with status asthmaticus)
- COPD
  - When COPD patients experience worsening control/multiple exacerbations **before** new medications are added, a search for the factors driving airway inflammation should be undertaken, screening for:
    - Allergic rhinitis (eg, nasal congestion)
    - GERD (often without symptoms of heartburn)

- Chronic Pulmonary Aspergillosis (CPA) or allergic bronchopulmonary aspergillosis (ABPA) (see CH 10)
- NTM infection
- Pseudomonal airway colonization
- When COPD patients experience a subacute worsening of their exercise limitation without symptoms of airway inflammation, they should be screened for superimposed heart failure
  - Heart failure with preserved ejection fraction commonly complicates lung disease (provoked by tachycardia and hypoxemia)
  - They should also be screened for daytime (exertional) and nighttime hypoxemia and obstructive sleep apnea (OSA)
  - CO_2-retaining COPD patients should be offered nocturnal bilevel positive airway pressure to slow the rise of hypercarbia over time
  - Edematous patients or patients with evidence of worsening pulmonary artery pressures deserve a trial of diuresis (see CH 6)

TRACHEOSTOMY

- A tracheostomy tube (trach) accesses the trachea directly through the neck, bypassing the upper airway
- Four standard indications:
  - **Prolonged mechanical ventilation** (continuous or intermittent, eg, only at night)
    - Protects the vocal cords from injury, allowing patients to intermittently talk despite ongoing mechanical ventilation (via a partially deflated cuff in a pressure support mode)
  - **Poor secretion handling** (as seen in neuromuscular weakness or diseases with bulbar involvement)
    - Allows for easy access to the trachea for suctioning
  - **Severe OSA**
    - Tracheostomy collar (TC) at night removes the upper airway obstruction seen in OSA
  - **Loss of upper airway patency** as in malignancy, infection, or trauma
- Most patients require either a #8 or a #6 (based on their size) cuffed or cuffless standard tracheostomy tube
  - **Cuffed tracheostomy tubes** are **only** used for mechanical ventilation:
    - The cuff, or balloon, on the trach inflates to create a soft seal with the tracheal wall
      - This diverts air into the lungs by preventing its escape up through the vocal cords (the path of least resistance)
    - The cuff **does not prevent aspiration** (major misconception)
      - Tracheostomy tubes (and the cuff) **cause** aspiration by mechanically tethering the oral pharynx
        - Impairs the normal pharyngeal rise that occurs with swallowing
      - Occasionally patients are left with a cuffed tracheostomy tube without the need for mechanical ventilation to "prevent" aspiration **(this is always wrong)**
        - Aspiration occurs when material passes below the vocal cords
        - The area above the balloon is not amenable to suctioning such that everything that winds up on top of the balloon, will eventually make its way to the lower airway
  - **Cuffless tracheostomy tubes** bypass the upper airway in patients who do not mechanical ventilation:
    - Often to assist with secretion handling in patients with neuromuscular weakness and poor cough
      - Common after a prolonged episode of critical illness and mechanical ventilation
    - Or to bypass upper airway when swelling, tumor, or infection threaten upper airway patency

- Anticipated course of tracheostomy progress (from consideration, to placement, to decannulation)
  - Should be considered in individuals who will need to be intubated for more than 2–3 weeks
  - Approaching the patient (and/or surrogate) with the pros:
    - Protects against vocal cord trauma and possible permanent disability
    - More comfortable for patients (allowing decreased sedation and pain medication)
    - Allows patients to spend time off of the ventilator, phonating, before complete liberation is achieved
    - Completely reversible (leaving only a small residual scar) when no longer necessary
  - Ensure nobody involved in the decision is erroneously equating tracheostomy with ventilator dependence
  - Percutaneous tracheostomy at the patient's bedside is the preferred approach
    - Surgical tracheostomies may be required for abnormal anatomy, or when tumor or infection are present
  - In the first 5–7 days after placement, the tracheostomy is an **unstable** airway
    - If a "fresh" tracheostomy is dislodged, reinsertion comes with the risk displacing the trachea backward, creating a false plane, where the tracheostomy tube enters the mediastinum
      - Reinsertion of a tracheostomy tube, where the tract is not matured, should be done over a bronchoscope
    - Because of this, tracheostomies remain sutured in place for 5–7 days, until the surgical tract matures
  - After the surgical tract is mature, the tracheostomy is a **stable** airway
    - If a tracheostomy tube is accidently dislodged, it is simply reinserted
      - The tracheostomy hole may significantly narrow and/or close quickly (hours), such that reinsertion should be performed immediately
    - If a patient with a cuffless tracheostomy develops acute respiratory failure, the cuffless trach can be easily (blindly) exchanged for a cuffed trach, allowing for mechanical ventilation
  - In individuals with a tracheostomy, spontaneous breathing trials should move rapidly from pressure support (PS) to TC alone (the preferred mode)
    - The cuff should be deflated during TC trials (allowing the patient to breath around the trach)
    - TC trials should start 1–2 hours three times a day, increasing the duration until it is tolerated all day (or maximum time is achieved)
    - Most patients with critical illness myopathy and deconditioning will be able to be rapidly liberated once they are strong enough to tolerate 12-hour stretches at a time
  - The Passy-Muir valve
    - One-way valve (diaphragm) that fits over the end of the tracheostomy tube that occludes during exhalation, diverting exhaled air around the trach, up past the vocal cords, allowing phonation
    - The valve then opens during inhalation, allowing air to flow through the tracheostomy tube as well as through the oral pharynx
    - It is primarily as a transition device during the few days that the patient is strong enough to talk while on TC trials but not yet ready to have the trach capped
  - Capping the trach (the last step before decannulation) should be attempted in any patient tolerating the Passy-Muir valve for hours at a time (because the cap does not increase the work of breathing much, compared to the valve)
    - Capping provides the benefit of allowing the patient to be free from the humidified oxygen delivery system
    - Patients who are strong enough to cough up secretions, around their capped tracheostomy tube into their oral pharynx (ie, remain capped) for 48–72 hours, continuously deserve consideration for decannulation

- Must ensure respiratory therapy or nursing are not reporting that the cap has been on for 3 days, forgetting to add "except with suctioning," (this is a common misunderstanding)
- When and if to downsize:
  - #8 cuffed (or #6 cuffed) to #6 cuffless (almost always)
    - Patients who are weaned from mechanical ventilation with a #8 cuffed trach should be offered a #6 cuffless trach (as soon as the surgical tract is mature) to facilitate improved swallowing and secretion clearance (ie, coughing secretions around the trach up to the mouth)
  - #6 cuffless to #4 cuffless (rarely)
    - Only done when the patient has swallowing difficulty or fails capping with a #6
      - The smaller the trach, the easier it is to swallow and cough up secretions to the mouth (required to tolerate capping)
      - The disadvantage of the #4 is that it **cannot** be easily exchanged for a cuffed #6 (the tracheostomy hole is too small) If the patient develops recurrent respiratory failure and intubation has to be done from above
- Special tracheostomy tubes
  - Extra-long trachs:
    - Extra-long external portion for large necks at risk of occluding the external trach opening
    - Extra-long internal portion to bypass a tracheal abnormality
      - Focal stenosis from granulation tissue
      - Focal dilation from long-term cuffed trach use
  - Rarely, very abnormal tracheas will require a very specialized tracheostomy tube (eg, Bivona)
    - Allows the balloon and tip to be located precisely in a "sweet spot"

EVALUATION OF THE PRESUMED EXUDATIVE EFFUSION (Fig. 28.2)

- From the standpoint of initial evaluation, a unilateral pleural effusion can be presumed to be exudative, in the same way bilateral pleural effusions can be presumed to transudative
  - Presumed transudates should be treated with a trial of diuresis
  - Presumed exudates should be promptly evaluated further
- A unilateral effusion occurring in a patient with:
  - Signs and symptoms of pneumonia is worrisome for empyema
  - A history of, or significant risk factors for, lung cancer or adenocarcinoma is worrisome for metastatic cancer (or mesothelioma in those exposed to asbestos)
  - Trauma or recent thoracic surgery is worrisome for a hemothorax
  - Rheumatoid arthritis is likely related to his or her disease
  - No obvious acute or chronic diseases associated with an exudative effusion should prompt consideration for:
    - Venous thromboembolic disease (VTE)
      - A unilateral effusion with atelectasis is the most common **abnormal** chest x-ray finding in patients presenting with pulmonary embolism
    - Primary TB pleurisy (a hematogenous spread manifestation of primary TB)
      - TB and granulomatous inflammation line the parietal pleural surface, leading to a large, high-pH, lymphocytic, clear, straw-colored exudate with an ADA >50 U/L
      - Organisms are rarely seen or cultured from the fluid
      - Diagnosis is made by closed pleural biopsy or video-assisted thoracoscopic surgery (VATS)
      - ~25% of individuals with TB pleurisy also have acid-fast bacillus (AFB) in their sputum (despite a paucity of cough or infiltrate seen in a radiograph), such that **respiratory isolation and sputum examination for AFB must be considered** in those with TB risk factors and a unilateral effusion

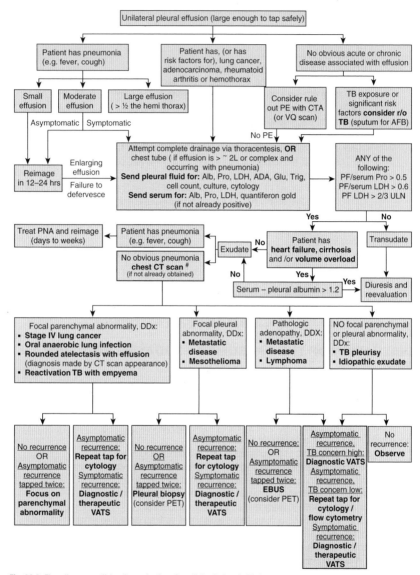

Fig. 28.2 Flow diagram outlining the evaluation of a unilateral pleural effusion.

- The TB pleurisy effusion typically resolves spontaneously; however, failure to make a diagnosis creates a public health problem
  - Individuals with TB pleurisy have a very high reactivation rate (often only a few years after their primary illness)
- Parapneumonic effusions
  - Parapneumonic effusions should be drained if they are:
    - Large (>½ a hemithorax)

- Symptomatic (ie, causing shortness of breath)
- Increasing in size despite therapy
- Possibly responsible for the patient failing to defervesce
- Large parapneumonic effusions (>2 L) or those appearing complex (ie, septated) may be initially drained with a small bore (Seldinger technique–placed) chest tube, ensuring complete drainage and allowing for the instillation of fibrinolytics
- Small to moderate parapneumonic effusions should be initially approached via thoracentesis, aiming for complete drainage
- In general, a unilateral effusion occurring in an individual without pneumonia, should be completely drained
  - Complete drainage may prevent recurrence up to 10% of the time in malignant and idiopathic pleural effusions
  - If the exudate has the fluid characteristics of a complicated parapneumonic effusion, chest tube insertion may be avoided if the space is completely drained (and the fluid does not recur); in other words, complete drainage as the initial approach, almost always, makes more sense than a diagnostic tap
- Complete drainage via a single thoracentesis may not be possible if:
  - The effusion is large (ie, >2 L) because reexpansion symptoms (ie, coughing) invariably necessitate termination of the procedure after removal of 1.5 - 2.0 L
  - The lung is entrapped and unable to reexpand (and instead creates a vacuum) as fluid is removed
    - Trapped lung is detected by thoracentesis via intermittently monitoring pleural pressures during drainage
    - Negative pressure that develops quickly, or a very negative pressure (< −25 cm H2O), suggests trapped lung
      - Further drainage at this point runs the risk of bronchopleural (BP) fistula formation from ex-vacuo injury
    - Trapped lung is often detected by the presence of a hydropneumothorax after drainage (actually a hydro-vacuo thorax) that will ultimately refill with fluid (assuming a BP fistula was not created by generating very negative pressures) (see CH 17)
- If a unilateral effusion is large or complex (septated on CT and/or ultrasound), as seen with complicated parapneumonic effusion, and hemothorax, chest tube insertion (as the initial drainage approach) with hospital admission should be considered
  - This allows for large effusions to be drained completely (ie, 1–2 L every 4–6 hours), as well as facilitating tissue plasminogen activator and DNase administration for complex
- Pleural fluid should be routinely sent for albumin, total protein, lactate dehydrogenase (LDH), adenosine deaminase, glucose, triglycerides, cell count, culture, cytology
- Serum should be sent for albumin, total protein, LDH, QuantiFERON-TB Gold (if not already known to be positive)
- Pleural fluid analysis:
  - If any of the following pleural fluid characteristics are present, the patient may be diagnosed with an exudative effusion:
    - Pleural fluid total protein/serum total protein >0.5
    - Pleural fluid LDH/serum LDH >0.6
    - Pleural fluid LDH > ⅔ upper limit of normal
  - Individuals with volume overload, from heart failure, cirrhosis, or impaired renal function, are at high risk for transudative effusion such that a (serum–pleural fluid) gradient should be calculated
    - A serum–pleural fluid gradient >1.2 g/dL suggests a transudative process such that diuresis (or fluid removal if the patient has end-stage renal disease [ESRD]) should be pursued before reevaluation
  - Other fluid characteristics can help support or refute common etiologies (Table 28.1)

Table 28.1 Exudative Pleural Fluid Characteristics

FLUID CHARACTERISTICS	ASSOCIATED DISEASE STATES
Bloody	Malignant
Cloudy	All entities except TB pleurisy
Straw-colored and clear	TB pleurisy
Milky	Chylothorax
WBC count >10,000	Parapneumonic, pulmonary embolism, pancreatitis, RA
+ Cytology	Malignancy
Adenosine deaminase >50 U/L	TB pleurisy, empyema, RA
Lymphocytic	TB, malignancy
Eosinophilic	Persistent pneumothorax Retained blood (eg, post-CABG)
LDH >1000 IU/L	Malignancy, parapneumonic
Glucose <60 mg/dL	RA, TB empyema, malignancy
Triglycerides >110 mg/dL, or Chylomicrons	Chylothorax

CABG, Coronary artery bypass grafting; *LDH*, lactate dehydrogenase; *RA*, Rheumatoid arthritis; *TB*, tuberculous; *WBC*, white blood cell.

- Evaluation of the confirmed exudate:
  - The most common cause of an exudative pleural effusion is pneumonia, which is treated with antibiotics (± drainage, as previously outlined)
    - A patient with a parapneumonic effusion should be followed clinically and with follow-up chest x-ray imaging (in months) to ensure either complete resolution or development of a stable scar
    - Reimaging can be performed earlier (within weeks) if complete drainage was not achieved to ensure fluid has not reaccumulated
  - Individuals with an exudate who are **not** obviously suffering from pneumonia deserve post drainage chest CT imaging to look for parenchymal, pleural, and/or lymph node abnormalities possibly related to the exudative process
- Postdrainage CT imaging shows a:
  - Focal parenchymal abnormality, DDx:
    - Stage IV lung cancer
      - An asymptotic recurrence of the effusion should prompt a repeat thoracentesis for cytology
      - A symptomatic recurrence of the effusion should prompt consideration for a diagnostic/therapeutic VATS
      - If the fluid does not return and/or repeat thoracentesis for cytology is negative, attention should turn to the primary lesion
        - If the fluid has a white blood cell count >10,000 and/or the lesion may represent a lung abscess (eg, fast growth, air fluid level), consider treatment and reimaging
      - If the fluid is bloody and lymphocytic predominant, and/or the growth characteristics and appearance of the lesion suggest lung cancer, consider biopsy of the primary lesion or any pathologic adenopathy via endobronchial ultrasound

- Oral anaerobic lung infection often presents with effusion and necrotic mass mimicking lung cancer (see CH 11)
  - Growth characteristics, air fluid level, patient risk factors (poor dentition or alcohol/sedative abuse [especially to "aid" sleep]) may increase suspicion
- Rounded atelectasis with effusion
  - Diagnosis made by CT appearance
  - Associated with granulomatous lung infection and asbestos/pneumoconiosis
- Reactivation TB with TB empyema
  - Typically with apical fibrocavitary or nodular disease
  - Diagnosis made by sputum or, less commonly, pleural fluid culture
- Focal pleural abnormality, DDx:
  - Metastatic cancer (especially adenocarcinoma) has a predilection for pleural metastasis and/or thoracic lymphatic involvement such that malignant pleural effusion is a common presenting symptom
    - Effusion may be caused by either the pleural metastases themselves or by microscopic lymphatic obstruction
  - Mesothelioma commonly presents with a pleural effusion (often with chest pain)
    - The effusion may spontaneously resolve
    - Medial pleural thickening and irregular, lumpy pleural thickening are concerning for mesothelioma (See CH 9)
- Pathologic adenopathy, DDx:
  - Metastatic cancer (eg, adenocarcinoma)
  - Lymphoma
    - Flow cytometry should be performed on a sample of the pleural fluid if there is concern for lymphoma (eg, enlarged mediastinal lymph nodes)
- No focal abnormalities or adenopathy DDx TB pleurisy vs. Idiopathic effusion
  - Individuals with risk factors or features suggestive of TB should consider vats for diagnosis, after the initial thoracentesis is diagnostic
  - When a pleural effusion is tapped twice with no etiology discovered, and the CT scan after drainage fails to reveal any abnormalities, the patient can be diagnosed with an idiopathic exudate
  - Idiopathic exudates remain mysterious (or are assumed to be viral) ~25% of the time or ultimately declare themselves in equal parts as malignant (may be years later), related to connective tissue disease, or chronic volume overload (eg, cirrhosis, heart failure, ESRD)
    - TB is much less likely if the patient was initially evaluated appropriately for TB pleurisy
- Role for VATS
  - VATS has a high diagnostic yield for TB and metastatic disease
  - VATS may be nondiagnostic for connective tissue disease, volume overload, or lymphatic obstruction by lymphoma or carcinoma
  - Because of these limitations, patients with a low clinical suspicion for TB pleurisy, in whom the effusion does not symptomatically recur, may be observed expectantly
  - VATS pleurodesis is the most effective way to prevent recurrence of the effusion, and it should be pursued in individuals suffering symptomatic recurrence (pragmatically), regardless of the diagnosis
- Patients with a recurrent exudative effusion who are not candidates for VATS may be offered a tunneled, indwelling thoracic tube (allowing for home drainage), even without a diagnosis (on a compassionate basis)

ROUNDED ATELECTASIS (Fig. 28.3)

- Rounded atelectasis is:
  - An incompletely understood syndrome of pleural inflammation and retractile scarring that gathers up the lung, tethering it to the visceral pleural surface, and thereby creating a rounded consolidation with linear scarring extending to the hilum

ROUNDED ATELECTASIS WITHOUT SIGNIFICANT PLEURAL EFFUSION

- Panel A and B show CT scan images of the right lower lobe in two different individuals with rounded atelectasis.
- Note the round, upside-down mushroom cap shaped appearance to the consolidation, which has air bronchograms, and linear scarring extending to the hilum
- These lesions may grow slowly over time as atelectasis increases
- Rounded atelectasis is a disease of pleural inflammation
- Which leads to retraction, gathering and compression of lung against the visceral pleural surface
- Diagnosis is made based on radiographic appearance
- Rounded atelectasis is associated with granulomatous lung disease and is seen in individuals with asbestos exposure, TB, and endemic fungal infection
- Rounded atelectasis may occur with a pleural effusion, when both the parietal and visceral pleura surfaces become inflamed causing effusion and pleural thickening
- This leads to the 'split pleural sign' where both parietal and visceral pleura are visualized
- Panel C, D and E show Rounded atelectasis with effusion occurring in 3 individuals
- The differential diagnosis is primarily lung cancer (Invasive adenocarcinoma with lepidic growth)

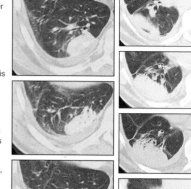
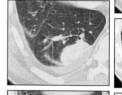
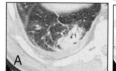
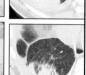

A   B

ROUNDED ATELECTASIS WITH PLEURAL EFFUSION

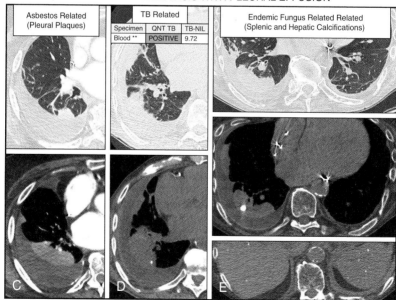

Asbestos Related (Pleural Plaques)	TB Related		Endemic Fungus Related Related (Splenic and Hepatic Calcifications)
	Specimen	QNT TB	TB-NIL
	Blood **	POSITIVE	9.72

C   D   E

Fig. 28.3 A pictorial review of rounded atelectasis and rounded atelectasis with effusion. **(A)** and **(B)** Two different individuals with rounded atelectasis. **(C–E)** Three different individuals with rounded atelectasis and pleural effusion.

- Associated with TB, endemic fungal infection, and asbestos exposure/pneumoconiosis
  - A disease predominately seen in men (80%)
- Rounded atelectasis comes in two varieties, with or without a significant effusion
  - Rounded atelectasis with effusion most commonly occurs at the right base
    - The effusion demonstrates visceral and parietal pleural thickening (split pleura sign)
- Rounded atelectasis without effusion is asymptomatic
- Rounded atelectasis with effusion is often initially symptomatic (dyspnea on exertion) as the effusion accumulates, but symptoms stabilize (and may improve slightly) as the space matures (and VQ relationships adjust)
- Rounded atelectasis is an important entity because the primary differential diagnosis is lepidic predominant invasive adenocarcinoma (a lung cancer that is typically cold on positron emission tomography and has air bronchograms)
- The pleura of rounded atelectasis (especially with effusion) may have FDG avidity, but the atelectatic lung should not
- Rounded atelectasis (with and without effusion) is a diagnosis made primarily based on characteristic CT imaging in the appropriate clinical setting (elderly man with asbestos exposure, TB, or endemic fungal infection) (see Fig. 28.3)
- When tapped, the effusion associated with rounded atelectasis develops negative pressure fast, limiting significant fluid removal and therapeutic benefit
- It is not uncommon to perform a thoracentesis for cytology and ADA, but observation is another reasonable alternative

COMPASSIONATE TERMINAL EXTUBATION

- Withdrawal of life support, specifically terminal extubation, comes with the threat of the highest legal scrutiny, such that most hospitals require additional documentation attesting to the "sound mind" status of the surrogate decision maker and or patient
- Ensure all loved ones agree with the decision (see CH 30)
- It also comes with one of the most important clinical responsibilities, ensuring a comfortable dignified death
- This is achieved when the patient demonstrates the same work of breathing (or improved) after extubation
  - A sudden increased work of breathing after extubation, makes the patient vulnerable to suffering, as medications are increased, but take time to work
- Individuals not on sedation at the time of the decision to withdraw care (eg, anoxic injury):
  - Start a combination of narcotic and benzodiazepine drips, while the patient is on full support
    - For example, Morphine and Ativan, both at 5 mg/hr (at least)
  - After sedation takes effect, the patient should be placed on pressure support (PS) 0/0
  - If this sudden lack of ventilator support produces an increased work of breathing, the patient should be place back on mechanical ventilation and both sedatives should be increased by 2-5 mg/hr, and given time to take effect (20-30 min)
  - Medication increase is followed by PS 0/0 trial, and the cycle is repeated until PS 0/0 is tolerated without causing an increase in respiratory effort
  - At this point the patient can be easily extubated to room air
    - Post-extubation oxygen support provides no significant comfort, in this situation, and may needlessly delay death)
- Individuals on sedation at the time of the decision to withdraw care (eg, ARDS and multiorgan failure):
  - If the patient is on paralytics ENSURE they are stopped, and that time is given for their reversal
    - Document the patient's ability to breath spontaneously before extubation
  - Ensure the patient is on both a narcotic and a benzodiazepine drip

- Place the patient on pressure support (PS) 0/0
- If this sudden lack of ventilator support produces an increased work of breathing, the patient should be place back on mechanical ventilation and both sedatives should be increased by 2-5 mg/hr, and given time to take effect (20-30 min)
- Medication increase is followed by PS 0/0 trial, and the cycle is repeated until PS 0/0 is tolerated without causing an increase in respiratory effort
- At this point the patient can be easily extubated to room air
- Post-extubation oxygen support provides no significant comfort, in this situation, and may needlessly delay death)
- After extubation family are occasionally troubled by upper airway sounds
  - Head positioning can help a lot
  - Family should be reassured that these sounds are similar to snoring, and an indication of the deep level of sedation and comfort there loved one is experiencing

INDEX

Note: Page numbers followed by *f* indicate figures and *t* indicate tables.